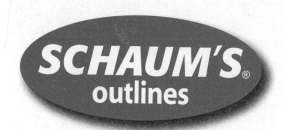

**SCHAUM'S**®
**outlines**

# *Emergency Nursing*

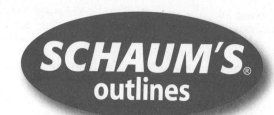

# Emergency Nursing

## James Keogh, RN

Schaum's Outline Series

New York   Chicago   San Francisco   Lisbon   London   Madrid
Mexico City   Milan   New Delhi   San Juan   Seoul
Singapore   Sydney   Toronto

The McGraw·Hill Companies

**James Keogh, RN-BC, AAS, MBA,** is a registered nurse and has written *Schaum's Outline of Pharmacology, Schaum's Outline of Nursing Laboratory and Diagnostic Tests, Schaum's Outline of Medical-Surgical Nursing,* and *Schaum's Outline of Medical Charting* and coauthored *Schaum's Outline of ECG Interpretation.* His books can be found in leading university libraries including Yale University School of Medicine, University of Pennsylvania Biomedical Library, Columbia University, Brown University, University of Medicine and Dentistry of New Jersey, Cambridge University, and Oxford University. He is a former member of the faculty of Columbia University and a member of the faculty of New York University.

1 2 3 4 5 6 7 8 9 10   QDB / QDB   1 9 8 7 6 5 4 3 2

ISBN    978-0-07-178980-6
MHID    0-07-178980-4

e-ISBN  978-0-07-178981-3
e-MHID  0-07-178981-2

Library of Congress Control Number 2012948443

The information contained in this book is intended to provide helpful and informative material on the subject addressed. It is not intended to serve as a replacement for professional medical advice. Any use of the information in this book is at the reader's discretion. The author and the publisher specifically disclaim any and all liability arising directly or indirectly from the use or application of any information contained in this book. A healthcare professional should be consulted regarding your specific situation.

Interior artwork on pages 8, 9, 101, 107, 115, 185, 324 by S4Carlisle Publishing Services

This book is printed on acid-free paper.

*This book is dedicated to Anne, Sandy, Joanne, Amber-Leigh Christine, Shawn, Eric, and Amy, without whose help and support this book couldn't have been written.*

# Contents

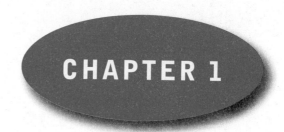

# Triage

## 1.1 Define

- Triage is the systematic process of prioritizing patients based on patient acuity when confronted with limited medical resources. The goal is to allocate medical resources that will result in a positive difference in the patient's outcome.

- Triage was developed by French physicians during World War I to organize treatment of soldiers on the battlefield.

- Triage is a continuous process because the patient's condition can change during interventions to stabilize the patient. In a trauma, a patient's injuries may appear minor at first but may become more serious following the initial triage assessment. Therefore, patients must be continuously evaluated until stabilized.

- There are two models for triage:

  - **Primitive:** the practitioner prioritizes patients based on the practitioner's best guess at the time of assessment. This method is used in the earliest stage of an incident and when there are more patients than can be practically assessed by the practitioner.

  - **Modern:** the practitioner prioritizes patients based on physiological and scientific assessment. This method is used in the later stage of an incident and when the ratio of patients to practitioner is relatively low.

- There are two methods of triage:

  - **Primary:** primary triage requires the practitioner to detect and treat life-threatening conditions.

  - **Secondary:** secondary triage requires the practitioner to detect and treat non-life-threatening conditions.

- The practitioner performs a primary triage assessment when the patient is first presented to him or her. A commonly used primary triage model is Simple Triage and Rapid Treatment (START), which was developed at Hoag Hospital in Newport Beach, California. The results of the primary triage assessment enable the practitioner to assign the patient to one of four treatment categories.

  - **Minor:** these are patients who are likely to live regardless of the care they receive. Sometimes these patients are referred to as the "walking wounded."

  - **Delayed:** these are patients who have a non-life-threatening, serious condition and require medical treatment within a reasonable time frame. Immediate care will not make a positive difference in the outcome.

○ **Immediate:** these are patients who have a life-threatening condition where immediate care can make a positive difference in the outcome.

○ **Deceased:** these are patients who are pulseless and not breathing or who have injuries so severe that they are likely to die regardless of the care they receive.

• Triage raises ethical questions because the practitioner is asked to determine which patient will or will not receive treatment based on the practitioner's assessment. The ratio between patients and practitioners determines the thoroughness of the practitioner's assessment of each patient. In most trauma incidents, there is a favorable patient to practitioner ratio, and therefore ethical implications are not raised. Ethical implications become relevant in disasters where there is a high patient to practitioner ratio. Ethical issues are addressed by the use of systematic assessments that have been developed through evidenced-based practice.

## 1.1.1   Triage Revised Trauma Score (TRTS)

• TRTS is an assessment tool that combines results from the Glasgow Coma Scale, systolic blood pressure, and respiration rate to arrive at a physiological score used to triage a patient quickly. Each assessment value is assigned a TRTS number (Table 1.1). The sum of the TRTS numbers is the patient's TRTS score.

• TRTS score is within the range of 0 to 12.

○ 12 = Delayed: patient is walking wounded.

○ 11 = Urgent: patient can wait a short time for intervention.

○ 10 to 4 = Immediate: patient requires immediate intervention.

○ >4 = Morgue: patient is unlikely to survive even if given intervention.

## 1.1.2   Injury Severity Score (ISS)

• ISS is a system that assigns a triage score based on the severity of injuries to nine body regions. The ISS score ranges from 1 to 75 with a score of 6 or less as not survivable. The score is calculated for the three most severely injured regions.

• The Abbreviated Injury Scale (AIS) is used to identify the nine body regions. These are:

○ head, face, neck, thorax, abdomen, spine, upper extremity, lower extremity, and skin.

• Scores are:

○ 1 = minor

○ 2 = moderate

○ 3 = serious

○ 4 = severe

**TABLE 1.1   TRTS Scoring Table**

| GLASGOW COMA VALUE | TRTS SCORE | SYSTOLIC BLOOD PRESSURE | TRTS SCORE | RESPIRATION RATE | TRTS SCORE |
|---|---|---|---|---|---|
| 3 | 0 | 0 | 0 | 0 | 0 |
| 4 to 5 | 1 | 1 to 49 | 1 | 1 to 5 | 1 |
| 6 to 8 | 2 | 50 to 75 | 2 | 6 to 9 | 2 |
| 9 to 12 | 3 | 76 to 89 | 3 | >29 | 3 |
| 13 to 15 | 4 | >89 | 4 | 10 to 29 | 4 |

- ○ 5 = critical
- ○ 6 = maximal
- Calculating the ISS is performed by using the following formula:
  - ○ Assign a score to each body region.
  - ○ Identify the three lowest scores. These are labeled A, B, and C in the formula.
  - ○ Calculate the ISS score by squaring each score (multiply the score by itself) and then sum the squares.
  - ○ $ISS = A^2 + B^2 + C^2$
  - ○ The lower the score is, the more severe the condition of the patient. If any three body regions are score 6, then the ISS score is 75.

### 1.1.3  Reverse Triage

- Reverse triage is the practice of treating more-stable patients before less-stable patients if those patients are also practitioners whose skills are required by other trauma patients. Reverse triage is used in traumas involving medical and nonmedical patients.
- The goal of reverse triage is to increase medical resources available to assess and treat trauma patients by stabilizing and returning the practitioners to work.

## 1.2  Primary Triage Assessment

- The purpose of primary triage assessment is to systematically assess the condition of the patient to determine the level of care required to stabilize the patient when he or she arrives in the emergency department.
- Primary triage assessment begins by gathering information. Information is gathered by asking questions, observing the patient for signs and symptoms, and making a physical assessment. All occur simultaneously.
- All patients undergo primary triage assessment regardless of whether the patient walks into the waiting room or is brought in by an ambulance. Don't assume that a walk-in patient is not an emergency.
- Acquire information from the patient, first responders, and others who accompanied the patient to the hospital. Learn as much as possible about the situation from those who seem to have firsthand or secondhand information about the situation. Identify
  - ○ What occurred
  - ○ When it occurred
  - ○ How it occurred
  - ○ Why it occurred
  - ○ What led up to the emergency
- Identify interventions provided to the patient by first responders.
  - ○ Extrication
  - ○ Blood pressure
  - ○ Pulse

- Oxygen saturation
- Respirations
- Temperature
- Treatment
- Look for medical alerts on the patient.
  - Medical alert bracelets are found around the neck, wrists, or ankles.
  - Medical alert cards are typically found in the patient's wallet, purse, or pockets.
- Trust but verify given information using critical thinking skills.
  - Ask,
    - Does this information make sense when compared to other information and the clinical assessment of the patient? If it is reported that the young child was found in a swimming pool, then the child's clothes should be damp or wet. If not, then the information is questionable.
    - How did this person arrive at the information told to the practitioner? The information may be secondhand information unless the person actually witnessed the incident.
    - Is the information accurate? Improper procedure may have been used to take vital signs at the scene.
  - Verify the information.
    - Ask the same questions independently of the patient, first responders, and others who accompanied the patient to the hospital, and then compare responses.

## 1.3  Cervical Spine

- The cervical spine supports the skull and enables the head to rotate side to side and forward and back. The cervical spine consists of seven vertebrae (C1, C2, C3, C4, C5, C6, and C7) beginning at the end of the skull and containing cervical nerves.
- The cervical spine contains
  - Ligaments to prevent excessive movement
  - Muscles to provide stability and movement
  - Peripheral nervous system (PNS) that transmits nerve impulses to and from the brain along the spinal cord to parts of the body
  - Cervical nerves control
    - C1: head and neck
    - C2: head and neck
    - C3: diaphragm
    - C4: upper body muscles
    - C5: wrists
    - C6: wrists
    - C7: triceps

### 1.3.1   Assessment

- Assume a cervical spine injury in all major traumas.
- Apply a cervical collar to immobilize and stabilize the cervical spine in a neutral position.
- Do not remove cervical collar until cervical spine injury has been ruled out.

### 1.3.2   Signs and Symptoms

- Difficulty breathing
- Numbness
- Pain
- Sensory changes
- Weakness
- Increased muscle tone (spasticity)
- Paralysis
- Loss of bladder and bowel control
- Constipation

## 1.4   Airway

- The airway consists of the upper respiratory system:
  - Nasal cavities
  - Nose and linked air passages
  - Mouth
  - Larynx
  - Trachea
- The airway can be obstructed by
  - Foreign object
  - Anatomical trauma
  - Inflammation
  - Aspiration

### 1.4.1   Assessment

- Airway is patent if patient is awake, alert, and able to talk.
- The patency of the airway is assessed while immobilizing the cervical spine in a neutral position to decrease the risk of spinal injury.

- Airway may be compromised if patient
  - Is unconscious
  - Has maxillofacial injury
  - Has neck injury
  - Has laryngeal injury
  - Has signs of respiratory distress

### 1.4.2   Signs and Symptoms

- Bluish color (cyanosis) of skin, nail beds, and mucous membranes, indicating inadequate oxygenation
- Agitation, indicating increased carbon dioxide (hypercarbia) in the blood
- Use of accessory muscles, indicating an attempt to increase air flow
- Hoarseness, indicating changes in air flow in the larynx caused by inflammation or injury
- High-pitched wheezing (stridor), indicating turbulent air flow in upper airway
- Crackling noise (crackles, rales, crepitations), indicating fluid in the lungs
- Rapid breathing (tachypnea), indicating increased need for oxygen or increased attempt to remove carbon dioxide
- Snoring, indicating vibration of the soft palate or other object as air flows through the upper airway
- Abnormal breath sounds
- Asymmetrical rise and fall of the chest wall
- Asymmetrical breath sounds
- Restlessness, anxiety, and uneasiness (dysphornia), indicating decreased oxygenation
- Decreased mental capacity (obtundation) related to decreased oxygenation or injury to the brain
- Deviated trachea, indicating asymmetric pleural pressure with the trachea shifting toward the side with high negative pressure caused by injury or disease

### 1.4.3   Intervention

- Perform jaw-thrust maneuver.
- Perform chin-lift maneuver.
- Clear foreign bodies from airway.
- Position patient in lateral, head-down position to prevent aspiration, if patient is at risk for vomiting.

## 1.5   Breathing

- Breathing requires a patent airway and functioning, lower respiratory system.
  - **Bronchi**
  - **Bronchioles:** small thin tubes

- **Alveoli:** air sacs connected to the bronchioles

  - **Capillaries:** a network of tiny blood vessels that covers the alveoli. Capillaries connect to a network of arteries and veins.

  - **Pulmonary artery:** delivers blood containing carbon dioxide to the capillaries of the alveoli

  - **Diaphragm:** main muscle for breathing, located below the lungs and separating the chest cavity from the abdominal cavity

  - **Intercostal muscles:** located between the ribs; assist with breathing

  - **Abdominal muscles:** used to exhale when breathing fast

  - **Accessory muscles (neck and collarbone):** used for breathing when patient is having difficulty breathing

- Respiratory system function

  - Nose and mouth wets and warms the air. Lungs are irritated by cold, dry air in the lungs.

  - Cilia in the nose and airway trap germs and other foreign particles in the air. Particles are swallowed, coughed, or sneezed out of the body.

  - Air then travels through trachea and into two bronchial tubes and then into the lungs.

  - Lungs exchange oxygen and carbon dioxide from blood vessels.

  - Pulmonary artery delivers blood containing carbon dioxide to the capillaries of the alveoli. Gas exchange takes place, replacing carbon dioxide from hemoglobin in red blood cells with oxygen.

  - Pulmonary vein delivers blood containing oxygen from the lungs to the heart.

  - The heart pumps the oxygenated blood throughout the system circulation.

- Respiration

  - Airway carries oxygenated air to the lungs and removes carbon dioxide.

  - Muscle around the lungs expands and contracts to force the lungs to exhale and inhale. These muscles are:

    - Inhalation

      - Diaphragm contracts, moving down to increase space in the chest cavity, enabling lungs to expand. Intercostal muscles pull the rib cage out and up, enlarging the chest cavity.

      - Air sucked through the nose and mouth as the lungs expand travels down the trachea and bronchi, bronchioles, and alveoli where gas exchange occurs.

    - Exhalation

      - The diaphragm and intercostal muscles contract to reduce space in the chest cavity, forcing air out of the lungs.

- Respiratory control

  - The medulla oblongata portion of the brain controls breathing. Sensors in the carotid artery and aorta detect carbon dioxide and oxygen levels in the blood. These sensors signal when respiration should increase or decrease. There are sensors in the airways that detect irritants and trigger the brain to cause coughing or sneezing by tightening smooth muscles around the airway, increasing the air pressure on exhale. Sensors in the alveoli detect fluid buildup and signal the brain to trigger rapid, shallow breathing.

### 1.5.1 Assessment

- Respiratory rate
- Respiratory effort
- Breath sounds
- Movement of chest wall

### 1.5.2 Signs and Symptoms

- Labored respiration
- Abnormal movement of the chest wall
- Abnormal breath sounds

### 1.5.3 Intervention

- Apply bag-valve mask.
- Administer 100% oxygen.
- Suction if necessary.
- Remove obstruction if necessary.
- Insert oropharyngeal airway per institution's training (Figure 1.1).
    - Patient must be unconscious.
    - Oropharyngeal airway may trigger a gag reflex.
    - Jaw muscles relax resulting in obstruction of the airway by the tongue.
    - The oropharyngeal airway prevents the tongue from covering the epiglottis in an unconscious patient.

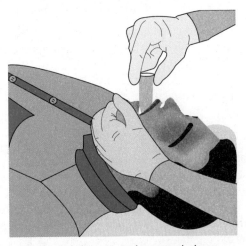

Figure 1.1 Insert oropharyngeal airway.

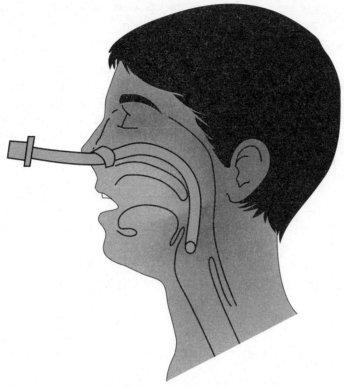

Figure 1.2  Insert nasopharyngeal airway.

- Insert nasopharyngeal airway per institution's training (Figure 1.2).

  ○ Use this airway if the patient's condition prevents the use of the oropharyngeal airway.

  ○ Don't use a nasopharyngeal airway if patient has a severe head or facial injury or if patient has signs of a basilar skull fracture (raccoon eyes, Battle's sign, leakage of blood or cerebrospinal fluid from ears). The nasopharyngeal airway may enter brain tissue.

  ○ The nasopharyngeal airway does not trigger a gag reflex.

- Insert endotracheal tube into the trachea per institution's training (Figure 1.3).

  ○ Patient must be unconscious.

  ○ A cricothyrotomy is performed per institution's training if an airway cannot be inserted.

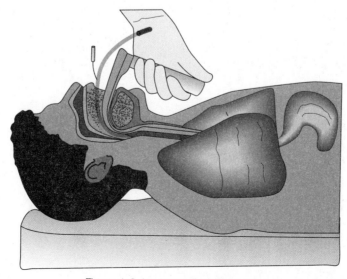

Figure 1.3  Insert endotracheal tube.

- A cricothyrotomy is performed when a patient has severe facial or nasal injuries, midfacial trauma, or cervical spine trauma resulting in airway disruption.

- No manipulation of the cervical spine is necessary.

- A cricothyrotomy is performed as a last, life-saving intervention if other interventions fail.

- A cricothyrotomy has fewer complications than a tracheotomy.

- A cricothyrotomy should not be performed if the patient has acute laryngeal disease, there is an anatomical abnormality at the site, the trachea is transected, or if there is difficulty identifying the cricothyroid membrane.

## 1.6   Circulation

- Patient requires patent circulation to distribute oxygen and nutrients throughout the body and to remove carbon dioxide.

- Patent circulation requires stabilized cardiac function and an intact circulatory system.

- Trauma can result in

  - Decreased or no cardiac output

  - External and internal bleeding

### 1.6.1   Assessment

- It is important to understand the rationale for abnormal values when assessing circulation.

- Presenting condition may be acute or chronic.

- An abnormal value may be considered normal for the patient.

  - A COPD patient may have abnormally low oxygen saturation related to COPD. This abnormal value may not be relevant to the patient's acute presentation.

  - An athlete may have abnormally low blood pressure related to athletic training. This abnormal value may not be relevant to the patient's acute presentation.

- Blood pressure

- Pulse

- Oxygen saturation

- Capillary refill

- Color of skin and mucous membranes

- Cardiac rhythm

### 1.6.2   Signs and Symptoms

- Blood pressure

  - Hypotension: systolic $<90$ and diastolic $<60$

  - Hypertensive crisis: systolic $\geq 180$; diastolic $\geq 120$

- Pulse
  - >100 beats per minute
  - <60 beats per minute
- Oxygen saturation
  - Abnormal: <95% room air or <100% on oxygen
- Capillary refill
  - Abnormal: ≥3 seconds
- Color of skin and mucous membranes
  - Abnormal: cyanotic (bluish)
- Abnormal cardiac rhythm (see Chapter 3)
- Abnormally high heart rate and low blood pressure may indicate bleeding.

### 1.6.3 Intervention

- Open IV access. Use a 12- or 14-gauge cannula to deliver IV fluids and blood quickly.
- Attach a cardiac monitor to the patient.
- Provide advanced life support (see Chapter 3, 3.22.2 Advanced Cardiac Life Support) if necessary.
- Control bleeding.

## 1.7   Disability

The disability component of the primary assessment of the patient focuses on neurological function. The initial component of the primary assessment determines the patency of the cervical spine by immobilizing the cervical spine to ensure that no additional trauma affects the nerves during the triage assessment.

A preliminary assessment of neurological disability is made by determining if the patient is alert and oriented and can react to voices and pain. The simplest way to remember this assessment is by using the mnemonic A Very Practical Use (see 1.7.1 Assessment).

A more involved assessment of neurological disability is performed by using the Glasgow Coma Scale (see 1.7.1 Assessment). The Glasgow Coma Scale provides an objective way to summarize neurological activity in a score. The score is then used to measure the effect of neurological trauma.

### 1.7.1   Assessment

- Mnemonic: **A Very Practical Use**
  - **A** = alert and oriented
  - **V** = reaction to voices
  - **P** = reaction to pain
  - **U** = unresponsive

**TABLE 1.2 Glasgow Coma Scale**

| | 1 | 2 | 3 | 4 | 5 | 6 |
|---|---|---|---|---|---|---|
| Eyes | Does not open eyes | Opens eyes in response to painful stimuli | Opens eyes in response to voice | Opens eyes spontaneously | N/A | N/A |
| Verbal | Makes no sounds | Makes incomprehensible sounds | Utters inappropriate words | Is confused, disoriented | Is oriented, converses normally | N/A |
| Motor | Makes no movements | Exhibits extension to painful stimuli (decerebrate response) | Exhibits abnormal flexion to painful stimuli (decorticate response) | Exhibits flexion/withdrawal to painful stimuli | Localizes painful stimuli | Obeys commands |

- Glasgow Coma Scale
  - The Glasgow Coma Scale (GCS) assesses the conscious state of the patient.
  - GCS was developed at the University of Glasgow's Institute of Neurological Sciences. There are three tests performed to assess the patient using GCS.
    - Eye responses
    - Verbal responses
    - Motor responses
  - Each test results in a score (Table 1.2). The sum of these scores is used to assess the conscious state of the patient.

## 1.7.2  Signs and Symptoms

- The result of the Glasgow Coma Scale enables the practitioner to identify if there are any signs and symptoms of an underlying neurological condition affecting the patient. It is important to remember that a patient's presenting condition in an emergency department can change quickly. The patient's condition should be monitored regularly until the underlying cause is identified, and the patient is stabilized. Expect to reassess the patient throughout his or her stay in the emergency department.
  - A score of 15 indicates that the patient is fully awake and has no current signs or symptoms of a neurological condition.
  - A score of 13 or greater indicates that the patient has minor or no neurological involvement.
  - A score between 9 and 12 is considered moderate neurological involvement.
  - A score of 8 or less is considered severe neurological involvement.
  - A score of 3 indicates deep coma or death.

## 1.7.3  Intervention

- Always assume that the condition is life threatening or is severe until objective test results and assessments prove otherwise. Always err on the side of caution.
- Immobilize the cervical spine if this has not been performed in the field. The cervical spine should be immobilized until an x-ray determines the patency of the cervical spine.

- Support the cervical spine and limbs whenever transferring the patient to avoid misalignment that may result in neurological injury.

- Perform A Very Practical Use assessment (see 1.7.1 Assessment). This can easily be performed when the patient is being moved into the assessment area.

- Perform Glasgow Coma Scale assessment.

## 1.8   Expose and Examine

The last step in the ABCDE assessment is to expose and examine the patient. At this point in the assessment there is a patent airway, the patient is breathing on his or her own or with assistance, circulation is patent, and critical neurological functionality has been assessed.

Exposing and examining the patient is performed to identify any signs or symptoms of injuries not noticed during the initial assessment. This top-down system review of the patient is a more thorough review than previous assessments because critical system deficits have already been identified and stabilized, providing adequate time for systematic patient assessment.

It is important that the patient's clothes be removed and the patient gowned for privacy. Visually examine all areas of the patient's body. Don't assume that the patient is able to report symptoms of the underlying problem because some symptoms such as internal bleeding may at first go unnoticed by the patient.

Remaining chapters in this book explain signs and symptoms to consider when performing a systematic review of the patient.

### 1.8.1   Intervention

- Develop a rapport with the patient before beginning physical assessment.

- Explain to the patient the actions to be performed and any inconvenience that the patient will experience before examining the patient. Be sure to explain that privacy will be ensured during the examination.

- Examination other than that of the abdomen

  ○ **Inspection:** visually examine each area of the body, looking for abnormal signs.

  ○ **Palpation:** touch areas of the body, assessing body parts for location, size, texture, and consistency.

  ○ **Auscultation:** listen to body sounds with a stethoscope.

  ○ **Percussion:** use fingers to tap areas of the body, listening for repercussion sounds.

- Examination of the abdomen

  ○ **Inspection:** visually examine each area of the body, looking for abnormal signs.

  ○ **Auscultation:** listen to body sounds with a stethoscope.

  ○ **Palpation:** touch areas of the body, assessing body parts for location, size, texture, and consistency.

  ○ **Percussion:** use fingers to tap areas of the body, listening for repercussion sounds.

## 1.9   Quick Assessments

An emergency department can be chaotic when an acute patient who has yet to be assessed arrives. The emergency room staff is expected to focus on assessing the patient and ignore distractions commonly seen in an emergency situation.

The way to stay focused is to follow standard procedures that ensure that the right assessment is performed in the right sequence based on the most urgent need and most likely scenario. Earlier in this chapter the ABCDE assessment procedure was explained, which organizes the assessment based on critical systems of the body.

Typically, the patient has a patent airway and is breathing with adequate circulation and relatively patent neurological function. Therefore, the practitioner can use a different assessment procedure that helps narrow the underlying cause of the patient's instability. One of the most commonly used procedures is called SAMPLE. SAMPLE is an acronym that helps the practitioner remember steps to quickly assess the patient.

Also important to a quick assessment is the order in which the practitioner asks the patient questions. The OPQRST acronym is a handy way to remember the sequence of questions. Remember that SAMPLE and OPQRST are assessment tools that help organize the assessment approach in a chaotic situation where the patient knows something isn't right and it is the practitioner's job to identify the problem and fix it.

### 1.9.1 Intervention

- SAMPLE

    ○ **S**igns and **s**ymptoms: ask the patient to describe what hurts and then assess the patient for signs of the underlying cause. Chapters throughout this book present a systematic approach to common causes of conditions that bring patients to the emergency department.

    ○ **A**llergies: ask the patient if he or she has any allergies and the reactions that occur when the allergen is present. Allergic reactions are a common reason why patients seek emergency medical care.

    ○ **M**edication: ask the patient what if any medications he or she takes regularly. The patient's response can help identify the patient's acute or chronic medical conditions. Ask if the patient has taken any new medication. The patient's condition may be a side effect or adverse side effect of the medication.

    ○ **P**ertinent medical history: the patient's condition might be related to the recurrence of a previous medical condition.

    ○ **L**ast oral intake: a sudden onset of instability might be caused by something the patient recently ingested. Identifying what food, fluid, or medication was last taken helps to narrow the cause of the patient's condition.

    ○ **E**vents leading up to the current problem: ask the patient what happened prior to the patient noticing the problem. As the patient describes recent events, he or she may recall exposure to an allergen, eating something that didn't taste right, or exposure to an environmental hazard.

- OPQRST

    ○ **O**nset: when did the problem start?

    ○ **P**rovocation: what makes the problem worse?

    ○ **Q**uality: how does the patient feel?

    ○ **R**adiation: does the pain or discomfort move?

    ○ **S**everity: how bad is the problem?

    ○ **T**ime: how long has this problem persisted?

### 1.10  Emergency Severity Index (ESI)

The emergency severity index is a five-level triage scale that was developed by Dr. Richard Wuerz and Dr. David Eitel and is widely adopted by emergency departments. ESI triage is based on stability first, then resources that are anticipated to be used to care for the patient. A patient is selected for Level 1 or Level 2 based on acuity. Levels 3, 4, and 5 are assigned based on use of resources.

A resource is

- IV fluids
- IV, IM, or nebulized medication
- Labs
- Simple or complex procedures
- ECG
- CT scan
- MRI
- Angiograph
- X-ray
- Ultrasound

A resource is not

- PO medications
- Point-of-care testing
- Slings
- Crutches
- Splints
- Simple wound care
- Tetanus
- Immunization
- Saline or hep-lock
- History and physical

## 1.10.1   Intervention

The patient is triaged based on the following levels:

- **Level 1:** patient requires lifesaving intervention.
- **Level 2:** patient is
  - Confused
  - Lethargic
  - Disoriented
  - In severe pain or distress
  - In a high-risk situation
- **Level 3:** patient requires two or more resources.
- **Level 4:** patient requires one resource.
- **Level 5:** patient doesn't require any resources.

## Solved Problems

**1.1**   What is triage?

Triage is the systematic process of prioritizing patients based on patient acuity when confronted with limited medical resources. The goal is to allocate medical resources that will result in a positive difference in the patient's outcome.

**1.2**   What is the primitive model of triage?

The practitioner prioritizes patients based on the practitioner's best guess at the time of assessment. This method is used in the earliest stage of an incident and when there are more patients than can be practically assessed by the practitioner.

**1.3**   What is the modern model of triage?

The practitioner prioritizes patients based on physiological and scientific assessments. This method is used in the later stage of an incident and when the ratio of patients to practitioner is relatively low.

**1.4**   What is the difference between primary and secondary triage?

Primary triage requires the practitioner to detect and treat life-threatening conditions. Secondary triage requires the practitioner to detect and treat non-life-threatening conditions.

**1.5**   What are the four treatment categories of the START triage model?

- **Minor:** these are patients who are likely to live regardless of the care they receive. Sometimes these patients are referred to as the walking wounded.

- **Delayed:** these are patients who have a non-life-threatening, serious condition and require medical treatment within a reasonable time frame. Immediate care will not make a positive difference in the outcome.

- **Immediate:** these are patients who have a life-threatening condition where immediate care can make a positive difference in the outcome.

- **Deceased:** these are patients who are pulseless and not breathing or who have injuries so severe that they are likely to die regardless of the care they receive.

**1.6**   What is the TRTS assessment tool?

TRTS is an assessment tool that combines results from the Glasgow Coma Scale, systolic blood pressure, and respiration rate to arrive at a physiological score used to triage a patient quickly. Each assessment value is assigned a TRTS number (Table 1.1). The sum of the TRTS numbers is the patient's TRTS score.

**1.7**   What is Injury Severity Score (ISS)?

ISS is a scoring system that assigns a triage score based on the severity of injuries to nine body regions. The ISS score ranges from 1 to 75 with a score of 6 or less being not survivable. The score is calculated for the three most severely injured regions.

**1.8**   How do you calculate an ISS score?

- Assign a score to each body region.

- Identify the three lowest scores. These are labeled A, B, and C in the formula.

- Calculate the ISS score by squaring each score (multiply the score by itself) and then sum the squares.

- ISS = $A^2 + B^2 + C^2$

- The lower the score indicates the more severe the patient's condition. If any three body regions are scored 6, then the ISS score is 75.

**1.9** When would you use reverse triage?

Reverse triage is the practice of treating more stable patients first before less stable patients if those patients are practitioners whose skills are required by other trauma patients. Reverse triage is used in traumas involving medical and nonmedical patients.

**1.10** What is the purpose of primary triage assessment?

The purpose of primary triage assessment is to systematically assess the condition of the patient to determine the level of care required to stabilize the patient when the patient arrives in the emergency department.

**1.11** Where would you look for medical alerts on a patient?

- Medical alert bracelets are found around the neck, wrists, or ankles.

- Medical alert cards are typically found in the patient's wallet, purse, or pockets.

**1.12** How can you verify information received from the patient?

- Ask yourself,

  - Does this information make sense when compared to other information and your clinical assessment of the patient? If you are told that the young child was found in a swimming pool, then the child's clothes should be damp or wet. If not, then the information is questionable.

  - How did this person arrive at the information told to you? The information might be secondhand information unless the person actually witnessed the incident.

  - Is the information accurate? Improper procedure may have been used to take vital signs at the scene.

- Verify the information.

  - Ask the same questions independently of the patient, first responders, and others who accompanied the patient to the hospital, and then compare responses.

**1.13** How does the healthcare provider know if the patient's airway is patent?

Airway is patent if patient is awake, alert, and talking.

**1.14** When would the practitioner suspect the patient's airway is compromised?

- Patient is unconscious.

- Patient has maxillofacial injury.

- Patient has neck injury.

- Patient has laryngeal injury.

- Patient has signs of respiratory distress.

**1.15**  What are signs of cyanosis?

Bluish color of skin, nail beds, and mucous membranes indicate inadequate oxygenation.

**1.16**  What is stridor?

High-pitched wheezing indicates turbulent airflow in upper airway.

**1.17**  What does hoarseness indicate?

Hoarseness indicates changes in airflow in the larynx caused by inflammation or injury.

**1.18**  What does a crackling noise in the patient's lungs indicate?

Crackling noise indicates fluid in the lungs.

**1.19**  What might sudden agitation indicate?

Agitation indicates increased carbon dioxide (hypercarbia) in the blood.

**1.20**  What is the purpose of the Glasgow Coma Scale?

The Glasgow Coma Scale (GCS) assesses the conscious state of the patient.

**1.21**  What does a GCS score of 15 indicate?

A score of 15 indicates that the patient is fully awake and has no current signs or symptoms of a neurological condition.

**1.22**  What procedure is used to assess parts of the body other than the abdomen?

- **Inspection:** visually examine each area of the body, looking for abnormal signs.
- **Palpation:** touch areas of the body, assessing body parts for location, size, texture, and consistency.
- **Auscultation:** listen to body sounds with a stethoscope.
- **Percussion:** use fingers to tap areas of the body, listening for repercussion sounds.

**1.23**  What is the purpose of the OPQRST method of asking the patient questions?

The OPQRST acronym is a handy way to remember sequence of questions.

**1.24**  What is the purpose of the SAMPLE quick assessment method?

SAMPLE helps to focus on areas that are the most common causes of visits to the emergency department.

# CHAPTER 2

# *Multisystem Emergencies*

## 2.1 Define

- A multisystem emergency is a condition that results in the instability of two or more systems.

- A multisystem emergency is caused by trauma such as a motor-vehicle accident, battle wound (i.e., stabbing, gunshot), accident (i.e., fall, work-related injury), or a medical disorder that causes secondary disorders (i.e., cancer, sclerosis of the liver).

- The patient's physiology can be disrupted by an inflammation, infection, or trauma.

- A multisystem emergency can be life threatening if each affected system is not stabilized.

- The focus is on the whole patient rather than the site of the injury after the patient's airway, breathing, circulation, and cervical spine are stabilized.

- A multisystem emergency requires immediate, quick assessment and frequent reassessments. Signs and symptoms of some system instability are delayed minutes, hours, or days following the initial assessment.

### 2.1.1 Goal of Treating Multisystem Emergencies

- Identify the multisystem emergency and stabilize the patient.

- Assess the patient completely before beginning treatment and address all life-threatening emergencies first.

- Don't stop the assessment when the first disorder is found. Assume that all systems are affected. Approach the assessment by ruling out disorders of all systems.

- Diagnose the acute problem(s). There is likely more than one acute problem.

- Stabilize the patient by relieving pain, and prioritize and treat the acute problem(s).

- Refer the patient to follow-up care.

### 2.1.2 Multisystem Assessment

- The multisystem emergency assessment interview
  - The patient may provide little information related to the trauma because the patient may be unaware of what specifically occurred.

- Third parties, such as EMS and police, can provide more accurate information about the trauma.
- The patient's response provides insight into the patient's mental status.
- The healthcare provider asks open-ended questions.
    - Do you remember what happened?
    - What do you remember?
- The healthcare provider looks for clues for underlying cause of the multisystem emergency.
    - What happened prior to this incident?
    - Does the patient have any allergies?
    - Does he or she take any medications?
        - What medications?
            - Prescribed?
            - Over-the-counter?
            - Cultural?
            - Herbal?
        - Why does the patient take these medications?
        - How much medication did the patient take prior to the incident?
    - Has the patient been diagnosed with any medical condition?
        - What medical condition?
            - Is the patient being treated for the medical condition?
                - What is the treatment?
    - Has the patient recently undergone any medical procedure?
        - What medical procedure?
        - When was the medical procedure performed?
- Follow-up questions help probe further into the presenting, multisystem emergency.
    - What hurts?
    - Can you describe the problem?
    - Is the problem spreading, or does the problem remain in one place?
    - Does anything make the problem worse?
    - Does anything make the problem better?
    - Did patient have this problem or a similar problem in the past?
        - Explain.
- Perform a physical assessment as described in Chapter 1 (1.9 Quick Assessments).
    - Inspection
        - Ask the patient to show the site by pointing to the injury or to confirm the site if the injury is visible.
        - Remove the patient's clothes and inspect the patient, beginning with the head. Look for other sites of injury besides those presented by the patient. Be sure to keep the patient warm.

- Percussion
  - Percuss the patient's thorax for infiltrates.
  - Percuss the patient's abdomen for abnormalities.
- Palpation
  - Palpate the surface of the patient's body to assist in identifying injuries.
  - Ask the patient, "Does this hurt?" as site is palpated.
- Auscultation
  - Listen to the patient's lungs for abnormal or adventitious lung sounds and respiration.
  - Listen for bowel sounds in all four quadrants.

### 2.1.2.1  Signs and Symptoms

Multisystem emergency assessment requires the nurse to recognize common signs and symptoms of underlying causes and then prepare for the anticipated treatment that the practitioner is likely to order.

Commonly seen multisystem, emergency signs and symptoms are:

- Internal bleeding
  - Light-headedness
  - Weakness
  - Shortness of breath
  - Decreased blood pressure
  - Increased heart rate
  - Cullen's sign (bruising surrounding the umbilicus due to intra-abdominal bleeding)
  - Turner's sign (bruising of the flanks caused by intra-abdominal bleeding)
  - Vomiting bright red blood or coffee-grounds-like blood (gastrointestinal bleeding)
  - Black and tarry stools or bloody stools (gastrointestinal bleeding)
  - Tense, rigid abdomen (bleeding into the peritoneum)
  - Blood in urine (kidney or bladder bleeding or infection)
  - Difficulty moving joints below the injury and loss of sensation (compartment syndrome–bleeding within the muscle)
- Multiple fractures
- Sepsis
  - Fever
  - Chills
  - Shaking
  - Mottled skin
  - Increased heart rate
  - Increased breathing
  - Decreased blood pressure (in septic shock)

- ○ Agitation
- ○ Confusion
- ○ Dizziness
- ○ Disorientation
- ○ Decreased urination
- ○ Reddish rash
- ○ Joint pain
- Brain injury
  - ○ Asymptomatic
  - ○ Loss of consciousness
  - ○ Prolonged confusion
  - ○ Multiple episodes of vomiting
  - ○ Difficulty concentrating
  - ○ Mood swings
  - ○ Lethargy
  - ○ Aggression
  - ○ Altered sleep habits
  - ○ Seizure
  - ○ Coma

## 2.2   Multisystem Tests

Multisystem emergency tests are designed to assess the effectiveness and capability of the cardiovascular and respiratory systems to function. Emergency-department practitioners order tests to collect objective data to further assess and assist in stabilizing the patient.

The following are commonly ordered environmental tests and procedures by the emergency department's practitioners.

### 2.2.1   Arterial Blood Gas (ABG)

The arterial blood gas is a test where an arterial blood sample is taken and assessed for levels of oxygen ($Pao_2$), carbon dioxide ($Paco_2$), bicarbonate ($HCO_3-$), saturation oxygen ($Sao_2$), and pH levels in the blood. Normal ranges are:

| | |
|---|---|
| $Pao_2$ | 80 to 100 mm Hg |
| $Paco_2$ | 35 to 45 mm Hg |
| $HCO_3-$ | 22 to 26 mEq/L |
| $Sao_2$ | 95% to 100% of hemoglobin |
| pH | 7.35 to 7.45 |

The pH value measures the concentration of hydrogen ions in arterial blood. A value greater than 7.45 indicates alkalosis and a value lower than 7.35 indicates acidosis. The patient's blood must be within normal limits to be considered stabilized. Abnormal values indicate that the patient's body is trying to reestablish the acid-base (alkalosis) balance by having the metabolic system work together with the respiratory system to compensate for the acid-base imbalance.

The imbalance can be caused by a problem with the respiratory system. This is referred to as respiratory acidosis or respiratory alkalosis. The imbalance can also be caused by a problem with the metabolic system. This is referred to as metabolic acidosis or metabolic alkalosis. The results of the arterial blood gas can help identify the underlying cause as shown in Table 2.1.

It is important that any supplemental oxygen administered to the patient shortly before or when the sample is taken is noted on the sample documentation. This enables the lab to adjust the results accordingly.

**TABLE 2.1  Acid-Base Values**

| | pH | Paco$_2$ | HCO$_3$- | SIGNS | CAUSES |
|---|---|---|---|---|---|
| Respiratory acidosis (too much carbon dioxide retained) | <7.35 | >45 mm Hg | >26 mEq/L (metabolic system compensating) | Flushed face Sweating Restlessness Tachycardia Headache | Hypoventilation Asphyxia Decreased central nervous system function Acute/chronic lung disease Sedatives Trauma Neuromuscular disease |
| Respiratory alkalosis (too little carbon dioxide retained) | >7.45 | <35 mm Hg | <22 mEq/L | Anxiety Rapid, deep breathing Light-headedness | Hyperventilation Gram-negative bacteria infection Increased respiratory function related to medication Anxiety Liver failure Sepsis |
| Metabolic acidosis (too little bicarbonate retained) | <7.35 | <35 mm Hg (respiratory system compensating) | <22 mEq/L (metabolic system compensating) | Drowsiness Vomiting Nausea Rapid, deep breathing Fruity breath Headache | Diarrhea Hyperkalemia Renal disease Hepatic disease Medication intoxication Shock Endocrine disorder |
| Metabolic alkalosis (too much bicarbonate retained) | >7.45 | >45 mm Hg (respiratory system compensating) | >26 mEq/L | Ringing in the ear Confusion Slow, shallow breathing Irritability | Severe vomiting Gastric suctioning Steroid administration Diuretic therapy Decreased potassium levels (hypokalemia) |

Since the sample is taken from an artery, the practitioner must apply pressure to the puncture site for 5 minutes and apply a pressure dressing for 30 minutes once the bleeding stops. The site then needs to be monitored regularly to ensure there is no residual bleeding.

## 2.2.2  Electrocardiograph (EKG, ECG)

The electrocardiograph shows a graphic representation of the electrical activity of the heart in a three-dimensional perspective. An electrical signal is generated each time the heart contracts. Small pads containing electrodes are placed on the surface of the skin and detect the electrical signal. Six are placed on the chest, and six electrodes are placed on the arms and legs. Each electrode is connected with wires to an electrocardiograph machine that draws up to 12 different graphical representations of the electrical signal. Figure 2.1 illustrates a normal electrocardiograph showing normal sinus rhythm. *Schaum's Outline of ECG Interpretation* provides details on how to administer an electrocardiograph and how to interpret the results.

- **P wave:** the first deflection is recorded as the P wave and starts when there is electrical activity at the SA node of the heart, indicating atrial contraction (depolarization).

- **PR interval:** the period between the beginning of the P wave and the beginning of the QRS complex is called the PR interval (PRI). This is the time from the start of atrial depolarization to the start of ventricular depolarization.

- **QRS complex:** this represents ventricle contraction (depolarization).

- **T wave:** this represents the wave of repolarization when myocardial cells restore electronegativity enabling restimulation (contraction).

- **ST segment:** the ST segment is the straight line that connects the end of the QRS complex with the beginning of the T wave. This represents the time between ventricular depolarization and ventricular repolarization.

- **QT interval (QTI):** this represents the complete cycle of ventricle contraction and ventricle relaxation.

## 2.2.3  Blood Chemistry

Blood chemistry is a laboratory test of venous blood and an examination of levels of enzymes and other elements in blood to develop a profile of the patient's health. This test is usually performed routinely for emergency department patients because results provide the healthcare provider with objective information about how well the patient's systems are functioning.

Blood chemistry results typically include

- Electrolyte balance (sodium, potassium, bicarbonate, magnesium, calcium, phosphorus)

- Kidney function (BUN, creatinine)

- Liver function (AST/ALT)

- Diabetes (serum glucose)

- Cholesterol level (cholesterol, LDL, HDL, triglycerides)

Enzymes are normally inside the cell. As cells rupture during normal events, enzymes leave the cell and enter the blood stream. The laboratory determines the normal level of a particular enzyme in the blood. A level greater than the normal level indicates more than the normal number of cells were injured, indicating something unusual is happening with the patient.

Enzyme levels might increase gradually and then return to a normal level. This might occur with a myocardial infarction, when blood supply to a part of cardiac tissue is interrupted, leading to the death of some cardiac tissue. Several hours may pass before the abnormal enzyme levels return to normal when no more cardiac tissue is injured.

It is important to look for obvious reasons why enzyme levels or other values are abnormal before assuming that the patient is unstable related to the test results. For example, a patient who exercised before coming to

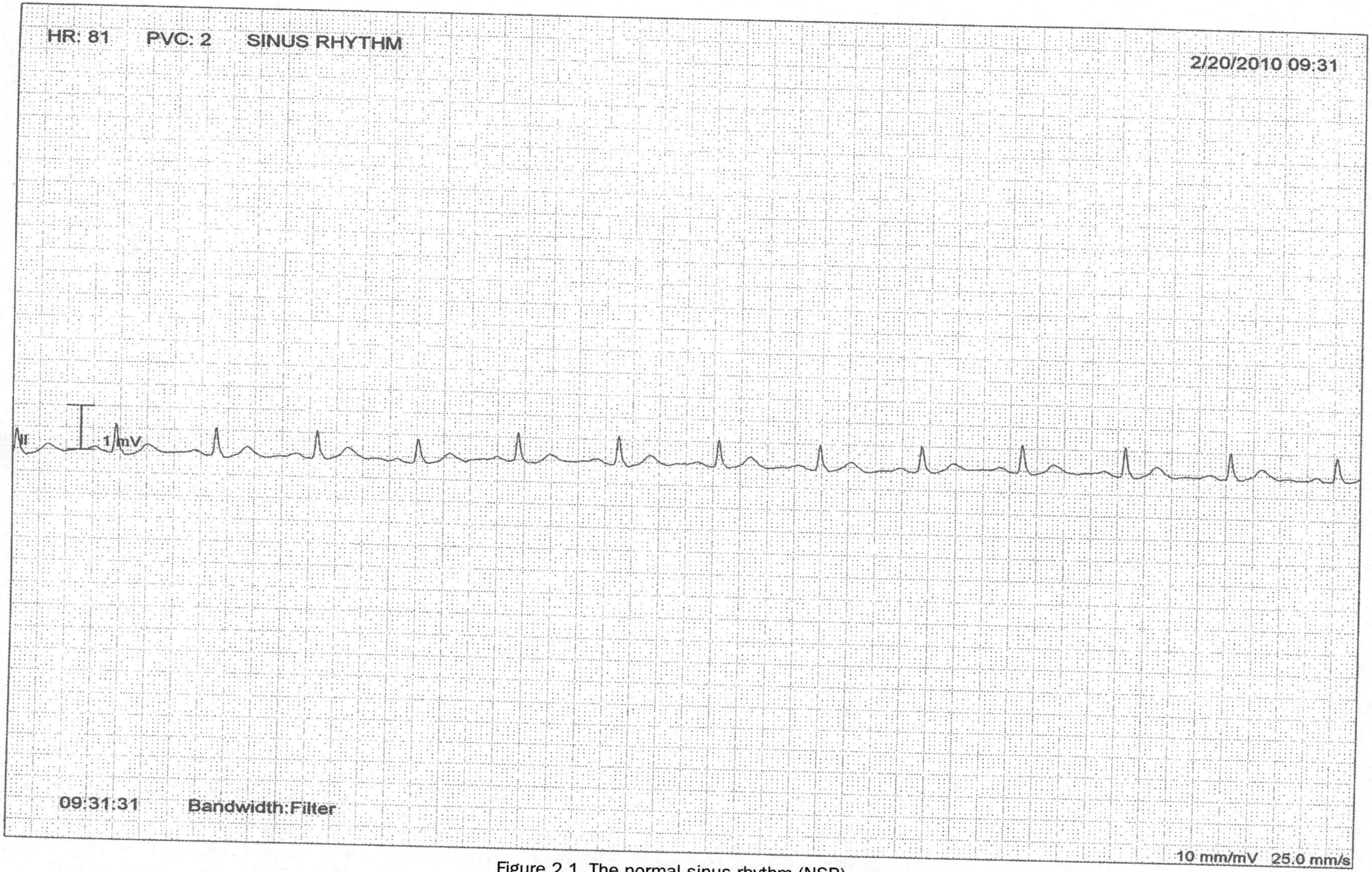

Figure 2.1 The normal sinus rhythm (NSR).

the emergency department will have elevated muscle cell enzymes because exercising injures muscles. Likewise, a patient who ate a normal breakfast before visiting the emergency department will have high blood-glucose levels.

### 2.2.4 Hematologic Studies

Hematologic studies profile the patient's blood and include

- Red blood cell (RBC) count

- White blood cell (WBC) count indicating inflammation

- Erythrocyte sedimentation rate (ESR)

- Bleeding (prothrombin time, INR, partial thromboplastin time, platelet count)

- Hemoblogin and hematocrit (Hgb, Hct)

### 2.2.5 X-Ray

During an x-ray, x-ray particles are beamed through the patient onto a photographic film or to a computer. Dense structures such as bone block x-ray particles, causing those structures to appear white. Less-dense structures such as fluid, foreign bodies, tumors, and infiltrate block some x-ray particles, causing those structures to appear gray. Tissue does not block x-ray particles and appears dark.

The chest x-ray procedure is

- Be sure the patient is not pregnant.

- Remove all jewelry in the area, since jewelry may appear on the x-ray image.

- Assess if the patient has scars in the area. If so, note the location of the scar since the scar may appear on the x-ray image.

- The patient removes clothes. Provide the patient with a gown.

- The x-ray machine is positioned in front of the patient. An x-ray can also be taken while the patient lies down on the x-ray plate.

- Multiple views of the area may be taken.

- The initial result, called a "wet read," provides a relatively superficial assessment of the image. A more thorough reading is taken hours or days later.

### 2.2.6 CT Scan

A CT scan provides a three-dimensional image using x-rays, enabling the healthcare provider to visualize normal and abnormal structures within the body. A CT can be performed with or without a contrast agent. A contrast agent is iodine-based and enhances images of blood vessels and less-dense areas of the system.

The CT scan procedure is

- Assess the patient for allergies to iodine or shellfish if the patient is undergoing a CT scan with contrast. Patients who are allergic to iodine or shellfish have a high likelihood to experience an allergic reaction to the contrast agent.

- Administer diphenhydramine (Benadryl) and prednisone (Deltasone) before the CT scan to reduce the risk of an allergic reaction to the contrast agent, if a contrast agent is ordered.

- Administer the contrast agent through an IV. The patient may feel flushed and have a salty or metallic taste in his or her mouth.

- Explain to the patient that the contrast material typically discolors the urine for upward of 24 hours following the CT scan. The patient should increase fluid intake after the CT scan to flush the contrast agent from his or her body, if a contrast agent is used for the CT scan.

- Assess the patient for claustrophobia, as the patient will be placed in an enclosure during the test.

- Assess the patient's ability to remain still for up to 30 minutes during the CT scan.

- Inform the patient that the CT scanner encircles the patient for up to 30 minutes.

### 2.2.7   Ultrasound

An ultrasound uses sound waves to provide an image that enables the healthcare provider to visualize normal and abnormal structures within the body. Sound waves are transmitted from a handheld device, called a transducer, through the body. Parts of the body absorb some sound waves and reflect other sound waves. The transducer detects reflected sound waves, which are used to depict an image on the screen. Practitioners use the ultrasound as a fast way to assess internal bleeding and structural damage.

The ultrasound procedure is

- The area of the body is exposed.

- A conductive gel is placed on the site.

- A conductive gel is placed on the transducer.

- The transducer is moved up and down the area, resulting in an image of the underlying structure displayed on the screen.

## 2.3   Multisystem Medication

Commonly used medications and supplements in multisystem emergencies are blood products, nonsteroidal anti-inflammatory drugs, corticosteroids, analgesics, and antibiotics. These medications reduce pain and discomfort by reducing pressure on nerves caused by inflammation and by blocking neurological transmission. Antibiotics assist the immune system in combatting bacterial infection.

### 2.3.1   Whole Blood

Whole blood is typically infused in an emergency. Donor blood must match the patient's blood type and Rh factor. However, infuse type O whole blood if patient's blood type is unavailable. Infuse type O Rh negative if the patient is pregnant. Make sure

- Blood is warm.

- Infusion is limited to less than four hours.

### 2.3.2   Packed Red Blood Cells

Packed red blood cells are whole blood where 80% of the plasma has been removed from the blood. Donor's blood must match the patient's blood type and Rh factor. However, infuse type O whole blood if patient's blood type is unavailable. Infuse type O Rh negative if the patient is pregnant. Make sure

- Blood is warm.

- Infusion is limited to less than four hours.

### 2.3.3   Platelets

Platelets are infused when the patient has decreased or ineffective platelets to stop bleeding. Donor blood must match the patient's blood type and Rh factor. However, infuse type O if patient's blood type is unavailable. Infuse type O Rh negative if the patient is pregnant. Make sure

- The same donor platelets are used for each infusion of platelets.
- A microaggregate filter is not used.

### 2.3.4   White Blood Cells

White blood cells are whole blood where 80% of plasma has been removed, and all red blood cells have been removed. White blood cells are used to treat sepsis that does not respond to antibiotics. Donor blood must match the patient's blood type and Rh factor. However, infuse type O if patient's blood type is unavailable. Infuse type O Rh negative if the patient is pregnant. Make sure

- Blood is administered slowly over four hours.
- Vital signs are monitored every 15 minutes.
- Infusion is continued if patient has fever.
- Antipyretic is administered if the patient has fever.
- One unit of white blood cells is infused each day until the patient is no longer septic or for up to six days.

### 2.3.5   Leukocyte-Poor Red Blood Cells (RBC)

Leukocyte-poor RBC is whole blood with 80% of the plasma removed and 70% of the white blood cells removed. Leukocyte-poor RBC is used to return the patient to normal red-blood-cell levels. Donor blood must match the patient's blood type and Rh factor. However, infuse type O if patient's blood type is unavailable. Infuse type O Rh negative if the patient is pregnant.

### 2.3.6   Corticosteroids

Corticosteroids are used to reduce inflammation and cerebral edema. Corticosteroids increase the risk of pancreatitis, heart failure, and thromboembolism.

- Dexamethasone (Dexasone, Decadron)
- Methylprednisolone (Solu-Medrol)

### 2.3.7   Analgesics

Analgesics are used to reduce pain.

- Oxycodone (OxyContin)
- Morphine (Duramorph)

### 2.3.8  Antibiotics

Antibiotics are used to treat bacterial infections, such as sinus infection and conjunctivitis.

- Bacitracin (Baciguent)
- Cefuroxime (Ceftin)
- Cephalexin (Keflex)
- Ceftibuten (Cedax)
- Erythromycin (Ilotycin)
- Gentamycin (Garamycin)
- Neosporin (Bactrim)
- Tobramycin (Tobrex)

### 2.3.9  Nonsteroidal Anti-Inflammatory Drugs (NSAIDs)

Nonsteroidal anti-inflammatory drugs are medications that reduce swelling, pain, and stiffness without exposing the patient to the adverse side effects that occur when using corticosteroid medication.

- Aspirin (ASA)
- Ibuprofen (Motrin, Advil, Nuprin)
- Naproxen (Naprosyn, Aleve)
- Oxaprozin (Daypro)
- Ketoprofen (Orudis)
- Diclofenac sodium (Voltaren)
- Ketorolac (Toradol)
- Celecoxib (Celebrex)

## 2.4  Penetrating Wound

A penetrating wound is one in which a foreign object enters the body. The object can enter the body in a predictable path or an unpredictable path.

- **Predictable path:** a predictable-path, penetrating wound occurs when an object such as a knife penetrates or impales the body. The pattern is relatively predictable within the body because the projectile typically follows a linear trajectory. The amount of damage increases with the depth of the wound, the size of the object, and if the object moved once the object entered the body.

- **Unpredictable path:** an unpredictable-path wound occurs when a bullet or shrapnel enters the body at high velocity, inflicting damage as the object travels in an unpredictable pattern within the body. The amount of damage increases with the velocity of the bullet or object, which is dependent on the size of the bullet and gun and the power of the explosive that caused the blast.

Three categories of penetrating trauma:

- **Pulseless:** there is major vascular damage.
- **Hemodynamically unstable:** patient is bleeding internally.
- **Hemodynamically stable:** patient is not bleeding internally.

### 2.4.1   Signs and Symptoms

- No sign of penetrating wound
  - Round puncture wounds (i.e., ice pick) may appear to self-heal.
  - Small-caliber-bullet entrance wounds may not be obvious especially if the patient does not know where he or she was shot and there is no exit wound.
- Visible entrance and exit wound
- Burn marks and gunshot residue at entrance site
- Bruising
- External bleeding
- Swelling at the site of the injury
- Light-headedness
- Dizziness
- Headache
- Pain
- Signs of internal bleeding

### 2.4.2   Medical Tests

- Ultrasound assesses internal bleeding and structural damage.
- X-ray assesses structural damage.
- CT scan assesses structural damage.

### 2.4.3   Treatment

- Priority is to maintain airway, breathing, and circulation in all cases.
  - Intubation if the patient is unconscious
  - Ventilator support if necessary
  - Administration of analgesics
  - Infusion of blood products
  - Infusion of IV fluids
- Pulseless indicates major vascular damage. Priority is exploratory surgery to identify and repair the vascular damage.

- Hemodynamic instablity indicates priority is to identify the bleeding site and control the bleeding.

- Hemodynamic stablity indicates priority is to identify and repair structure and organ damage.


### 2.4.4  Intervention

- Monitor airway, breathing, and circulation.

- Monitor for shock.

- Focus on replacing fluids to maintain blood pressure before repairing vascular or organ damage.

- Reassess the patient frequently. The patient's condition is dynamically changing. Signs and symptoms of internal bleeding may be delayed.

- Thoroughly assess the patient's body for penetrating wounds. The patient may have multiple wounds. Don't assume there is only one penetrating wound.

- Don't rely on the patient's recollection of the incident. The patient may not recall the number of times he or she was shot or stabbed.

- Penetrating wounds can be located anywhere on the body. Make sure you examine under skin folds.

- The assessment should be deliberate and quick. The practitioner will perform the following; however, steps may be skipped depending on the severity of the patient. For example, the practitioner may immediately order a CT scan or order the patient to undergo exploratory surgery following the physical assessment.

  ○ Perform physical assessment.

  ○ Order ultrasound.

  ○ Order x-ray.

  ○ Order CT scan.

  ○ Order exploratory surgery.

- Instruct the patient

  ○ There will be a lot of people in the room talking, and a number of them will be touching and examining the patient at the same time.

  ○ Who the practitioner-in-charge is.

  ○ What is happening and why each procedure is being performed. Keep the explanations concise and focused on what the patient needs to know to help the patient make informed decisions.

  ○ When to expect that he or she may feel discomfort.

  ○ To inform the staff when he or she feels pain, and reassure the patient that everything will be done to reduce pain and discomfort.


## 2.5  Hypovolemic Shock

Hypovolemic shock is the loss of 20% or more of the total volume of intravascular blood caused by internal or external hemorrhage, dehydration, infection, or obstruction leading to decreased tissue perfusion. As intravascular blood volume decreases, there is a decreased return of blood to the heart, resulting in decreased cardiac preload and causing a decreased cardiac stroke volume. Mean arterial pressure (MAP) also decreases, and as a result oxygen and nutrients do not reach cells throughout the body sufficiently to maintain metabolism, and necrosis may result. A systolic blood pressure of <80 mm Hg indicates reduced cardiac output from a decreased venous supply and can lead to thready pulse and decreased oxygen. Hypovolemic shock can occur as a result of burns, diarrhea, vomiting, or trauma.

Hypovolemic shock is classified as one of four stages.

## Stage 1

- Loss of up to 15% blood volume
- Constricting vascular structures maintain cardiac output.
- Blood pressure maintained
- Normal:
  - Urine output
  - Capillary refill
  - Mental status
  - Respiratory rate
  - Skin pallor

## Stage 2

- Loss of between 15% and 29% blood volume
- Constricting vascular structures do not maintain cardiac output.
- Blood pressure maintained
- Increased:
  - Diastolic pressure
  - Respiratory rate
  - Heart rate (>100 bpm)
  - Restlessness
- Urine output between 21 and 30 ml/hr
- Delayed capillary refill

## Stage 3

- Loss of between 30% and 40% blood volume
- Blood pressure cannot be maintained. Systolic ≤100 mm Hg
- Increased:
  - Heart rate (>120 bpm)
  - Respiratory rate (>30 bpm)
  - Agitation, confusion
- Delayed capillary refill
- Urine output between 20 and 30 ml/hr
- Skin pallor: clammy and cool

**Stage 4**

- Loss of 40% blood volume
- Increased:
  - Heart rate ($>$140 bpm)
  - Respiratory rate
- Decreased:
  - Level of consciousness, coma
  - Systolic blood pressure $\leq$70 mm Hg
- Skin pallor: clammy, cool, moribund
- No urine output
- No capillary refill

## 2.5.1  Signs and Symptoms

- Anxiety
- Agitation
- Confusion
- General weakness
- Loss of consciousness
- Hypotension
- Decreased body temperature
- Respiration: increased and shallow
- Skin: pale, clammy, cold
- Pulse: increased and thready
- Urine output: $<$25 ml/hr
- Pulse pressure: narrow
- Mean arterial pressure (MAP): $<$60 mm Hg
- Central venous pressure (CVP): decreased

## 2.5.2  Medical Tests

- Arterial blood gas
  - Decreased:
    - pH
    - $Pao_2$

- Increased:
  - $Paco_2$
- Complete blood count
  - Decreased:
    - Hematocrit (Hct)
    - Red blood cells (RBC)
    - Platelets
    - Hemoglobin (Hgb)
  - Increased:
    - Serum potassium
    - Serum sodium
    - Blood urea nitrogen (BUN)
    - Creatinine
- Urine
  - Decreased:
    - Sodium
    - Creatinine
- Occult blood: positive
- Ultrasound: shows accumulation of blood
- X-ray: shows accumulation of blood
- Echocardiogram: shows decreased cardiac function
- CT scan: shows accumulation of blood

### 2.5.3   Treatment

- The goal is to
  - Maximize oxygen delivery
  - Control blood loss by replacing blood and fluids
- Add fluids, blood, and plasma expanders to maintain blood pressure.
- Insert two large-bore IV catheters.
- If there is severe hemorrhage, insert an arterial line to provide continuous blood-pressure monitoring.
- Administer
  - Lactated Ringer's solution or normal saline
  - Type O blood, if lactated Ringer's solution or normal saline does not return normal vital signs, or type O Rh-negative blood if patient is pregnant
  - Oxygen
  - Norepinephrine to increase cardiac contractions
  - Dopamine to increase cardiac contractions

## 2.5.4   Intervention

- Monitor airway, breathing, and circulation.

- Monitor vital signs.

- Insert an indwelling urinary catheter.

- Monitor fluid intake and output.

- Place patient in a flat position with feet elevated if no cervical spine injury is suspected.

- Type and crossmatch the patient's blood.

- Monitor cardiac function using an ECG.

- Keep the patient warm to maintain body temperature.

- Instruct the patient

  - He or she is receiving IV fluids and blood to replace the loss of blood.

  - Emergency surgery may be required to identify the source of the bleeding and to stop the bleeding.

  - He or she must remain calm to conserve oxygen consumption.

## 2.6   Cardiogenic Shock

Cardiogenic shock occurs when blood flow is greatly impeded by failure of the heart to produce sufficient cardiac output to perfuse tissues. As the heart rate increases to compensate for the decreased cardiac output, workload on the heart increases, resulting in increased oxygen demand. The patient initially stabilizes until the decrease in oxygen to the heart causes cardiac arrest. Cardiogenic shock is usually irreversible and fatal.
   The most common causes of cardiogenic shock are

- Failure of the heart to pump effectively

- Arrhythmia disease

- Cardiac valve disease

- Acute myocardial infarction

- Myocarditis

- Left ventricular dysfunction

- Cardiomyopathy (end stage)

- Myocardial ischemia

## 2.6.1   Signs and Symptoms

- Anxiety

- Restleness

- Altered mental state

- Distended jugular veins

- Low or no (oligunia) urine output

- Fatigue

- Pulmonary edema

- Pulse: rapid and thready

- Skin: pale, cold, clammy

- Respiration: rapid and shallow

- Decreased senses

- Heart: faint gallop rhythm

## 2.6.2  Medical Tests

- Mean arterial pressure (MAP): <60 mm Hg

- Blood pressure: narrow pulse pressure <80 mm Hg systolic pressure

- Urine output: <20 ml/hr

- Electrocardiography (ECG): shows myocardial infarction, abnormal ventricular function, ischemia

- Echocardiography: shows abnormal ventricular function

- Emergency cardiac catheterization

- Lab tests

  - Arterial blood gas: shows hypoxia, respiratory acidosis, metabolic acidosis

  - Creatininase (CK): shows elevated level

  - Alanine aminotransferase: shows elevated level

  - Lactate dehydrogenase (LD): shows elevated level

  - Aspartate aminotransferase: shows elevated level

## 2.6.3  Treatment

- Percutaneous transluminal coronary angioplasty

- Coronary artery bypass graft

- Intra-aortic balloon pump to assist circulation

- Left ventricular assist device to improve circulation

- Administer

  - Inotropic medication to increase contractility

  - Antiarrhythmic medication for cardiac arrhythmia

  - Normal saline IV

  - Oxygen

  - Sodium bicarbonate, if the patient is acidotic

  - Electrolytes

  - Diuretic

    - Bumetanide (Bumex)

    - Furosemide (Lasix)

### 2.6.4   Intervention

- Monitor vital signs every five minutes until the patient stabilizes.

- Insert an indwelling urinary catheter.

- Monitor intake and output.

- Instruct the patient

  - About each test and procedure

  - About surgery that may be required to address the problem

## 2.7   Anaphylactic Shock

Anaphylactic shock is rapid, vascular swelling leading to respiratory distress and resulting from an immune reaction to an allergen. The allergen can be any substance, including foods or medication, that causes the release of histamine, leukotrienes, and serotonin and may lead to vascular collapse and systemic shock. Anaphylactic shock may occur within seconds or up to 24 hours following exposure to the antigen. Early onset of symptoms indicates severe anaphylactic shock.

### 2.7.1   Signs and Symptoms

- Skin redness (erythema)

- Report of lump in throat

- Wheezing

- Tightness of the chest

- Wheals

- Weakness

- Anxiety

- Sneezing

- Difficulty breathing (dyspnea)

- Itchiness (pruritus)

- Hives (urticarial)

- Sweating

- Stomach cramps

- Nausea

- Incontinence

- Diarrhea

- Restlessness

- Hypotension

### 2.7.2   Medical Tests

- Electrocardiogram (ECG): to rule out cardiogenic shock
- Blood tests:
  - Serum IgE: elevated

### 2.7.3   Treatment

- The goal is to
  - Maintain airway, breathing, and circulation
  - Counteract antigen reaction
  - Maintain vascular volume
- Administer
  - Histamine blockers to decrease histamine reaction
    - Corticosteroids
    - Diphenhydramine (Benadryl)
    - Famotidine (Pepcid)
  - Bronchodilator to reduce vasoconstriction, bronchoconstriction, and bronchospasm
    - Epinephrine (Adrenalin)
    - Aminophylline (Truphylline)
    - Albuterol (Proventil)
  - Vasopressor for blood-pressure stabilization
    - Norepinephrine (Levophed)
    - Dopamine
  - Plasma volume expander
    - Normal saline
    - Lactated Ringer's solution
  - Oxygen

### 2.7.4   Intervention

- Maintain patent airway and provide ventilation support.
- Administer endotracheal intubation if necessary.
- Monitor vital signs, including capillary refill, every five minutes until patient stabilizes.
- Monitor level of consciousness.
- Position patient in semi-Fowler's position or a comfortable position.
- Monitor lung sounds. Decreased wheezing may indicate severe bronchoconstriction or may indicate that the patient is stabilizing.
- Apply cool compresses on itchy sites for relief.

- Instruct the patient
  - ○ Avoid food, medication, and substances that may contain the allergen.
  - ○ Talk with the healthcare provider to determine if allergy skin testing is appropriate.

## Solved Problems

**2.1**   What should be done once the healthcare provider's assessment identifies a disorder in a multisystem emergency?

Don't stop assessment when the first disorder is found. Assume that all systems are affected. Approach the assessment by ruling out disorders of all systems.

**2.2**   What is the initial step once the assessment is completed?

Stabilize the airway, breathing, and cardiovascular system; relieve pain, prioritize symptoms, and treat the acute problems.

**2.3**   What kind of follow-up care is expected in a multisystem emergency?

- Surgery
- Intensive care
- Cardiac care

**2.4**   What should the healthcare provider assume when a patient who has a multisystem emergency arrives in the emergency department?

Assume all systems are affected.

**2.5**   How does the healthcare provider identify disorders in a multisystem emergency?

Approach the assessment by ruling out disorders of all systems.

**2.6**   Is the patient the best source of information regarding a traumatic event?

No. The patient may provide little information related to the trauma because he or she may be unaware of what specifically occurred.

**2.7**   Why are the patient's responses to assessment questions important?

The patient's responses provide insight into the patient's mental status.

**2.8**   Why is it important to remove the patient's clothes before the assessment if the evidence of the trauma is on the patient's hand?

There may be other injuries in addition to the obvious injury. The patient may not realize other injuries exist. Removing the patient's clothes facilitates a complete examination of the patient.

**2.9**   What would the healthcare provider suspect if the patient has bruising surrounding the umbilicus?

There may be intra-abdominal bleeding.

**2.10**    What would the healthcare provider suspect if the patient reports a tense, rigid abdomen?

There may be bleeding into the peritoneum.

**2.11**    How would the emergency department practitioner assess if there is internal organ damage or bleeding in the abdomen while the patient is in the emergency department?

An ultrasound is used to quickly assess internal structures.

**2.12**    What would the practitioner order if he or she suspects organ damage?

A CT scan shows the detailed structure of the organ and other structures in the patient.

**2.13**    What would the healthcare provider suspect if the patient has difficulty moving joints below the injury and is experiencing a loss of sensation?

Compartment syndrome, which is bleeding within the muscle leading to edema, is a possibility.

**2.14**    What would the healthcare provider suspect if the patient is aggressive and agitated while the trauma team is working on the patient?

Aggression and agitation can be signs of a brain injury.

**2.15**    Why might a practitioner order an injection of Benadryl and prednisone before the patient is sent for a CT scan?

The CT scan may require that a contrast material be administered to the patient. In an emergency, the patient may be unable to tell the practitioner that he or she has a shellfish allergy, which means that there is a high probability that the patient will have an allergic reaction to the contrast material. Benadryl and prednisone are used to reduce a possible allergic reaction to the contrast material.

**2.16**    What blood type is infused in an emergency?

Type O blood is infused in an emergency; type O Rh-negative blood if patient is pregnant.

**2.17**    What are packed red blood cells?

Packed red blood cells are a concentrated preparation of whole blood where 80% of the plasma has been removed from the whole blood.

**2.18**    Why might the practitioner order platelets to be infused?

Platelets may be ordered to decrease or stop bleeding.

**2.19**    What might the practitioner order if the patient has sepsis?

Initially the practitioner will order antibiotics. If the patient is not responsive, the practitioner may order white blood cells. White-blood-cell transfusions are whole blood where 80% of the plasma has been removed and all the red blood cells have been removed.

**2.20**    Why might the practitioner order Solu-Medrol?

Solu-Medrol is a corticosteroid and is used to reduce inflammation and cerebral edema.

**2.21**   What are the two general classifications of a penetrating wound?

The two classifications are a predictable path (as with a knife or a projectile wound to the body) and an unpredictable path (as with a gunshot wound).

**2.22**   What are the three categories of penetrating trauma?

- Pulseless: there is major vascular damage.

- Hemodynamically unstable: the patient is bleeding internally.

- Hemodynamically stable: the patient is not bleeding internally.

**2.23**   What is the primary treatment for a pulseless, penetrating wound?

Priority is exploratory surgery to identify and repair the vascular damage.

**2.24**   Why might a practitioner order an exploratory surgery for a patient who is hemodynamically unstable?

The most effective way to identify internal bleeding is through exploratory surgery. Surgeons are often able to identify and stop the bleeding. The emergency department practitioner must weigh the severity of the patient's condition against time delay of testing.

# CHAPTER 3

# *Cardiovascular Emergencies*

## 3.1 Define

- A cardiovascular emergency is a condition that has the potential of disrupting circulation throughout the patient's body, resulting in decreased blood flow to organs and causing malfunction of other systems in the body.

- There is a distinction between a cardiac emergency and respiratory arrest. If the patient has a pulse but is not breathing, then the patient is in respiratory arrest. There is no cardiac emergency, although respiratory arrest can lead to a cardiac emergency if rescue breathing does not occur.

- Hypertension is an emergency if the systolic pressure is ≥160 mm Hg or diastolic pressure is ≥100 mm Hg. The patient experiences headache, drowsiness, confusion, vision disorders, nausea, and vomiting.

- Hypotension is an emergency if the systolic pressure is <90 mm Hg or the diastolic is <60 mm Hg. The patient experiences light-headedness, dizziness, fainting, loss of consciousness, and fatigue.

- A cardiac emergency is a condition that disrupts the function of the heart. The patient is asymptomatic or experiences discomfort, chest pain, back pain, jaw pain, increased urination at night, swelling of ankles and feet, heart pounding, heart skipping a beat, and shortness of breath.

- Thrombosis is a blood clot that reduces blood flow or prevents blood flow to a part of the patient's body. The patient experiences pain in the area, coughing, swelling below the blood clot, and decreased circulation below the blood clot.

- Embolus is a dislodged blood clot that flows freely through the circulatory system until the embolus enters a small blood vessel causing a disruption of blood flow to that area of the body. The patient is asymptomatic until the embolus no longer moves freely, at which point the patient experiences symptoms of thrombosis.

### 3.1.1 Goal of Treating Cardiovascular Emergencies

- The goal of the emergency department staff is to stabilize the patient, not to treat the underlying cause of the problem, unless the underlying cause can be addressed within the scope of the emergency department staff. For example, angina is chest pain due to ischemia resulting in a lack of oxygen supply to cardiac muscle. The emergency department might alleviate angina by administering nitroglycerin; however, the underlying ischemia is likely to be addressed by follow-up care with other physicians.

  ○ It is essential to maintain airway, respiratory functions, and circulation.

  ○ It is important to diagnose the acute problem. For example, the acute problem might be hypertensive crisis, not the underlying cause of the hypertensive crisis.

○ The emergency department will stabilize the patient by relieving pain and treating the acute problem—e.g., administer medication to decrease hypertension immediately.

○ The emergency department will refer the patient to follow-up care to treat the underlying cause of the problem.

### 3.1.2 Cardiovascular Assessment

- Limit the assessment to identifying the problem area and then directing assessment to the problem area.

- Stop the assessment if it is necessary to intervene to stabilize the patient.

- Ask the patient to describe the problem.

- Ask questions that help to quickly identify the problem. Questions should be short and to the point, enabling the patient to answer "yes" or "no." Remember that the patient is typically distressed and anxious because the patient is experiencing an unusual problem that has not been identified.

  ○ Are you in pain? Pain might be a sign of decreased circulation to the heart muscle.

    ▪ Where is the pain?

    ▪ On a scale of 1 to 10, how bad is the pain?

    ▪ Is the pain burning, tight, or squeezing?

    ▪ Does the pain radiate?

    ▪ When did you notice the pain?

    ▪ What were you doing before you noticed the pain?

    ▪ What aggravates the pain?

    ▪ What relieves the pain?

  ○ Are you dizzy? Dizziness is a sign of decreased oxygenation related to decreased circulation.

  ○ Do you urinate frequently at night? Frequent night urination is possibly a sign of right-side heart failure.

  ○ Do you have nausea?

  ○ Are you short of breath? Shortness of breath is a sign of decreased oxygenation related to decreased circulation.

  ○ Do you feel your heart fluttering? Heart fluttering is a sign of irregular heart rhythm.

  ○ Do you feel your heart pounding? Heart pounding might be a sign of hypoxia.

  ○ Do you feel that your heart skips a beat? Skipping a beat is a sign of irregular heart rhythm.

  ○ Do you ever have difficulty awakening? Hypoxia related to decreased circulation is a potential problem.

  ○ Do your ankles or feet swell? Bilateral swelling is a sign of right-side heart failure

- Take vital signs during triage, and monitor vital signs throughout the patient's stay in the emergency department to assess changes in the patient's condition. Remember that anxiety and pain cause changes in vital signs. The emergency-department staffs' therapeutic demeanor can decrease patient anxiety, thereby reducing the anxiety effect on vital signs and enabling the staff to develop baseline vital signs for the patient.

- Inspection

  ○ Look for signs of cyanosis in extremities such as nail beds, tip of the nose, and earlobes. These are signs of deoxygenation of the blood, possibly caused by inadequate circulation.

- Look for clubbing of fingers, which is possibly a sign of chronic deoxygenation of the blood.

- Look at mucous membranes for pallor in dark-skinned patients, a possible sign of inadequate circulation.

- Look at hair distribution on arms and legs. If hair is missing, then decreased arterial circulation to the area is likely.

- Look for swelling of legs, ankles, and feet. Bilateral swelling is a possible sign of right-side heart failure, venous insufficiency, varicosities, or thrombophlebitis.

- Look for flushed skin, which is a possible sign of increased circulation related to fever.

- Look at the chest wall for indentations, called retractions, that can be related to heart failure or congenital heart defect.

- Look for abnormal thoracic cavity, which may inhibit cardiac movement.

- Palpation

  - Squeeze the nail bed to assess capillary refill time. More than three seconds may indicate decreased circulation.

  - Feel the skin temperature. Cold or cool skin temperature may indicate decreased circulation. Hot or warm skin temperature may indicate increased circulation.

  - Feel the precordium of the chest to assess the apical pulse.

    - Fine vibrations might indicate turbulent blood flow related to an aneurysm or heart valve malfunction.

    - Strong, longer pulse might indicate increased cardiac output.

    - Diffused pulse might indicate left ventricular hypertrophy.

  - Feel each of the carotid arteries separately to compare results. Both pulses should be symmetric and equal; otherwise there may be decreased circulation through one of the carotid arteries.

  - Feel pulse sites throughout the body. Compare bilateral pulses.

    - Weak pulse might indicate decreased cardiac output or increased peripheral vascular resistance.

    - Bounding pulse might indicate hypertension and high cardiac output.

- Percussion

  - Percuss the patient's lung fields. A dull sound might indicate pleural effusion possibly caused by biventricular failure in the heart. This allows fluid to build up between the lung and the chest wall.

- Auscultation

  - Listen for fine vibrations throughout the cardiac region of the chest, which might indicate an aneurysm or ventricular hypertrophy.

  - Listen for abnormal heart sounds.

    - S3 heart sound might indicate myocardial infarction, left- or right-side heart failure, intracardiac blood shunting, pulmonary congestion, hyperthyroidism, or anemia.

    - S4 heart sound might indicate aortic stenosis, angina, coronary artery disease, cardiomyopathy, or hypertension.

  - Listen to the patient's lungs for pulmonary congestion. Pulmonary congestion is a sign of left-sided heart failure.

  - Listen to the patient's abdominal region for bruits over the abdominal aorta, indicating abdominal aorta aneurysm.

### 3.1.3 Chest Pain Assessment

- A patient presenting with chest pain must be assessed immediately to rule out a cardiac event. The initial assessment is made by asking the patient three questions:

  ○ What does the pain feel like?

  ○ Where is the pain?

  ○ What makes the pain worse?

- Here is a quick way to assess the answers to these questions in order to identify the potential cause and begin immediate treatment to stabilize the patient. Keep in mind that objective testing such as cardiac enzymes and ECG are necessary to reach a diagnosis.

  ○ Sudden, sharp, continuous pain located below the sternum and radiating to the neck or left arm and worsening when patient lies on back or breathes deeply may indicate pericarditis. The patient should sit up and lean forward to reduce the pain. Anti-inflammatory medication may need to be administered.

  ○ Sudden, stabbing pain over the back worsening on inspiration might indicate pulmonary emboli and may require analgesics.

  ○ Sudden, severe pain located at the side of the chest with difficulty breathing and deviated trachea worsening with normal breathing might indicate pneumothorax and may require analgesic and reinflation of the affected lung.

  ○ Sudden, severe tearing pain located in upper abdomen or behind the sternum might indicate dissecting aortic aneurysm and may require analgesics and immediate surgery.

  ○ Squeezing, aching, burning pain below the sternum radiating to the arms, neck, back, and jaw worsening on exertion, stress, eating, or lying down might be caused by angina pectoris and may require rest and administration of nitroglycerin. The pain may continue if the patient experiences unstable angina pectoris.

  ○ Pressure and aching, burning pain across the chest, possibly radiating to the arms, neck, back, and jaw and worsening on exertion and possibly increasing anxiety may be caused by acute myocardial infarction and may require administration of nitroglycerin and opioid analgesic.

- The pneumonic PQRST is another useful method for pain assessment.

  ○ **P**rovokes

    ▪ What causes the pain?

    ▪ What lessens the pain?

    ▪ What makes the pain worse?

  ○ **Q**uality

    ▪ What does the pain feel like?

    ▪ Is the pain sharp?

    ▪ Is the pain dull?

    ▪ Is the pain stabbing?

    ▪ Is the pain burning?

    ▪ Is the pain crushing?

  ○ **R**adiates

    ▪ Does the pain radiate?

    ▪ Does the pain remain in one place?

    ▪ Where does the pain radiate to?

- ○ Severity
    - ▪ On a scale from 0 to 10, how severe is the pain where 0 is no pain and 10 is the worst pain?
- ○ Time
    - ▪ What time did the pain start?
    - ▪ How long did the pain last?

## 3.2 Cardiac Tests

The physical assessment of a patient who enters the emergency department is performed quickly and methodically. The goal of the physical assessment is to determine if the patient is in a life-threatening situation and to find signs and symptoms that lead to a suspected acute disorder or chronic episode of a disorder that caused the patient to be unstable. Suspicions are confirmed by conducting one or more objective tests and analyzing test results.

When a cardiac emergency is suspected, the healthcare provider will likely order an electrocardiograph, a pulse oximetry, an arterial blood gas, a blood chemistry, and hematologic studies. Additional cardiac tests may be ordered once the patient is stabilized in the emergency department.

### 3.2.1 Electrocardiograph (EKG, ECG)

The electrocardiograph shows a representation of the electrical activity of the heart in a three-dimensional perspective. An electrical signal is generated each time the heart contracts. Small pads containing electrodes are placed on the surface of the skin to detect the electrical signal. Six electrodes are placed on the chest, and six are placed on the arms and legs. Each electrode is connected with wires to an electrocardiograph machine that draws up to 12 different graphical representations of the electrical signal. Figure 2.1 in Chapter 2 illustrates a normal electrocardiograph showing normal sinus rhythm. *Schaum's Outline of ECG Interpretation* provides details on how to administer an electrocardiograph and how to interpret the results.

- **P wave:** the first deflection is recorded as the P wave and starts when there is electrical activity at the SA node of the heart, indicating atrial contraction (depolarization).
- **PR interval:** the period between the beginning of the P wave and the beginning of the QRS complex is called the PR interval (PRI). This is the time the electrical impulse takes to travel to the ventricles after atrial relaxation (repolarization).
- **QRS complex:** the QRS complex represents ventricle contraction (depolarization).
- **T wave:** this represents the wave of repolarization of the ventricles and is measured from the beginning of the QRS complex to the apex of the T wave.
- **ST segment:** the ST segment measures the time from the end of ventricular depolarization to the start of ventricular repolarization.
- **QT interval (QTI):** the QT interval measures the time from the beginning of ventricular depolarization to the end of ventricular repolarization.

### 3.2.2 Pulse Oximetry

Pulse oximetry assesses the arterial oxygen saturation of the patient's blood by passing an infrared beam of light through the patient's nail bed or skin. The amount of infrared light absorbed by the patient's blood provides an estimate of arterial oxygen saturation. This is referred to as an abbreviated arterial oxygen saturation value.

The pulse oximetry value should be between 95% and 100% if the patient is breathing room air and does not have chronic pulmonary disease such as COPD. A patient who has a chronic pulmonary disease may have a lower pulse oximetry value, which may be normal for that patient. A patient who is sedated or sleeping may also have a lower pulse oximetry, which is not alarming because the cause of the low value is known.

A patient who has supplemental oxygen should have a pulse oximetry value between 95% and 100%. A lower value may indicate cardiac or respiratory problems. It may also indicate that a mechanical problem such as a crimped nasal cannula tube prevents the patient from receiving the supplementary oxygen.

A value less than 95% on room air or on supplemental oxygen indicates there is instability in the cardio-respiratory systems. If the underlying cause is not obvious, such as the patient hyperventilating, then the health-care provider is likely to order an arterial blood gas.

### 3.2.3  Arterial Blood Gas (ABG)

The arterial blood gas is a test where an arterial blood sample is taken from the patient and assessed for oxygen, carbon dioxide, bicarbonate, and pH levels. It is important that any supplemental oxygen or ventilation assistance administered to the patient shortly before or when the sample is taken is noted on the sample documentation. This enables the lab to adjust the results accordingly.

Since the sample is taken from an artery, the healthcare provider must apply pressure to the puncture site for 5 minutes and apply a pressure dressing for 30 minutes once the bleeding stops. The site then needs to be monitored for one minute following removal of manual pressure to ensure there is no residual bleeding. Check for hematoma formation and then reassess the pulse.

### 3.2.4  Blood Chemistry

Blood chemistry is a laboratory test of venous blood that examines levels of enzymes and other elements in the blood to develop a profile of the patient's health. This test is usually performed routinely for emergency-department patients because results provide the healthcare provider with objective information about how well the patient's systems are functioning.

Blood chemistry results typically include

- Electrolyte balance (sodium, potassium, bicarbonate, magnesium, calcium, phosphorus)

- Kidney function (BUN, creatinine)

- Liver function (AST/ALT)

- Diabetes (serum glucose)

- Cholesterol level (cholesterol, LDL, HDL, triglycerides)

Enzymes are normally inside the cell. As cells rupture during normal events, enzymes leave the cell and enter the blood stream. The laboratory determines the normal level of a particular enzyme in the blood. A level greater than the normal level indicates more than the normal number of cells were injured, and something unusual is happening with the patient.

Enzyme levels might increase gradually and then return to a normal level. This might occur with a myocardial infarction when blood supply to a part of cardiac tissue is interrupted, leading to the death of some cardiac tissue. Several hours may pass before the enzyme levels are abnormal and then decrease hours later when no more cardiac tissue is injured.

It is important to look for obvious reasons why enzyme levels or other values are abnormal before assuming that the patient is unstable related to the test results. For example, a patient who exercised before coming to the emergency department will have elevated muscle cell enzymes because exercising injures muscles. Likewise, a patient who ate a normal breakfast before visiting the emergency department will have a higher blood glucose level.

### 3.2.5  Hematologic Studies

Hematologic studies profile the patient's blood and include

- Red blood cell count

- White blood cell count, indicating inflammation

- Erythrocyte sedimentation rate (ESR)

- Bleeding (prothrombin time, INR, partial thromboplastin time, platelet count)

- Hemoblogin and hematocrit (Hgb, Hct)

## 3.2.6  Cardiac Enzymes and Markers

When a patient is suspected of having a myocardial infarction, the healthcare provider will order cardiac enzymes and cardiac marker tests to determine if cardiac muscle enzymes appear in the patient's blood.

- Cardiac muscle contains enzymes.

- In a myocardial infarction, cardiac muscle is damaged, causing the release of cardiac enzymes into the bloodstream.

- It can take between 2 and 24 hours for cardiac muscle enzymes to reach a detectable level in blood.

- The cardiac enzymes and cardiac marker tests are used to confirm a previous acute myocardial infarction.

### 3.2.6.1  Brain Natriuretic Peptide (BNP) Test

The heart produces the hormone brain natriuretic peptide (BNP).

- Low levels of BNP are normally found in blood.

- BNP level increases when the heart works harder for long periods such as in heart failure.

- The brain natriuretic peptide test measures the level of BNP in the blood.

- The healthcare provider may order the N-terminal pro-brain natriuretic peptide (NT-proBNP) test that measures the NT-proBNP hormone and provides similar diagnostic results as the BNP test.

### 3.2.6.2  Cardiac Enzyme Studies

The cells of heart muscles and other tissues contain the enzyme creatinine phosphokinase (CK, CPK) and the protein troponin (TnT, TnI).

- Creatinine phosphokinase and troponin enter the blood when heart muscle and other tissues are damaged.

- If levels of creatinine phosphokinase and troponin are abnormal, the healthcare provider orders an electrocardiogram to differentiate between heart muscle damage and other tissue damage.

- Troponin and CPK-MB (creatine phosphokinase myocardial band) are mostly found in cardiac muscle.

- Blood samples are taken every eight hours for two days following a suspected heart attack.

- It takes 3 to 12 hours for troponin levels to rise after a heart attack.

- The healthcare provider may order a myoglobin test with the cardiac enzyme test to help diagnose a heart attack.

- High troponin values may indicate

  ○ Cardiac muscle injury. Troponin level increases for 3 to 12 hours and reaches its highest level 12 to 24 hours after the cardiac muscle injury. Troponin level returns to normal in 10 to 14 days following the cardiac muscle injury.

- High total creatine phosphokinase values may indicate

  ○ Cardiac muscle injury or tissue injury. Total creatine phosphokinase increases for 4 to 12 hours and reaches its highest level 10 to 24 hours after the cardiac muscle injury. Total creatine phosphokinase level returns to normal in three days following the cardiac muscle injury.

- High creatine phosphokinase-MB values may indicate

  ○ Cardiac muscle injury. Creatine phosphokinase-MB increases for 1 to 6 hours and reaches its highest level 18 hours after the cardiac muscle injury. Creatine phosphokinase-MB level returns to normal in three days following the cardiac muscle injury. If levels are high after three days, then additional cardiac muscle is being damaged, and the heart attack is continuing.

### 3.2.7   Renin Assay Test for Hypertension

Blood pressure is regulated by the renin-angiotensin system (RAS).

- Low blood pressure causes the secretion of the renin enzyme by the kidneys, which increases angiotensin I, which constricts blood vessels and results in increased blood pressure.

- Angiotensin II causes vasoconstriction and stimulates the adrenal cortex to replace aldosterone, leading the kidneys to retain water and sodium and resulting in an increased intravascular fluid volume, decreased urine output, and increased blood pressure.

- The renin assay test measures the level of renin in blood.

- The healthcare provider may also order the aldosterone test.

- The renin stimulation test may be ordered if the renin level is low.

- High renin assay test results may indicate

  ○ Malignant high blood pressure

  ○ Kidney disease

  ○ Blocked artery

  ○ Cirrhosis

  ○ Addison's disease

  ○ Hemorrhage

## 3.3   Cardiac Procedures

There are several cardiac procedures that are used to restore blood flow to the heart and reestablish cardiac rhythm.

- **Percutaneous transluminal coronary angioplasty (PTCA):** this is a nonsurgical procedure used to open a blocked coronary artery by inserting a balloon-tipped catheter into the femoral artery and moving the catheter into the blocked coronary artery using a fluoroscope to help guide the catheter into position. Once in position, the balloon is inflated, pushing plaque that causes the blockage against the coronary artery wall and allowing blood to flow again.

- **Coronary artery bypass graft (CABG):** this is a surgical procedure performed when a patient experiences myocardial ischemia. Before this procedure is performed, the patient typically undergoes catheterization to determine the severity of the myocardial ischemia. In severe ischemia, the blockage is bypassed by grafting a segment of the saphenous vein from the leg.

- **Cardiversion:** this is a nonsurgical procedure used to treat atrial fibrillation, atrial flutter, supraventricular tachycardia, and ventricular tachycardia. A low-energy-level shock is administered that is synchronized with the patient's heart cycle, causing interruption of the reentry circuit and enabling control to resume by the SA node.

- **Transcutaneous pacemaker:** this is a nonsurgical procedure that uses an external, electrical generator to send impulses through electrodes placed on the patient's chest to the patient's heart to provide external impulses to the heart in an emergency. The transcutaneous pacemaker remains active until a transvenous pacemaker is implemented.

## 3.4   Cardiac Medication

There are several classifications of medication that are commonly used to stabilize a patient who is experiencing cardiac instability. It is important that the emergency-department nursing staff be familiar with each medication.

### 3.4.1   Adrenergics

Adrenergic medication stimulates contractions similar to the fight or flight response of the sympathetic nervous system. There are two classifications of adrenergic medication: catecholamines and noncatecholamines.

Adrenergic medication can stimulate one or more receptors, depending on the medication. These receptors are:

- Alpha-adrenergic receptors

- Beta-adrenergic receptors

- Dopamine receptors

#### 3.4.1.1   Catecholamines

Catecholamines stimulate the nervous system and increase the depolarization of the SA node, resulting in an increased heart rate and increased blood pressure related to constriction of peripheral blood vessels and causing bronchial dilation. Catecholamines are referred to as inotropes because these medications increase the force of cardiac contractions and cause the heart to work harder and use more oxygen than when at rest. Table 3.1 lists commonly used catecholamines.

**TABLE 3.1  Commonly Used Catecholamines**

| CATECHOLAMINE | USE |
|---|---|
| Dobutamine (Dobutrex) | Increases heart rate and cardiac output |
| Dopamine | Increases cardiac contraction and output. Used in conjunction with cardio shock. |
| Epinephrine | Restores cardiac rhythm in cardiac arrest |
| | Reverses anaphylaxis reaction to an antigen |
| | Relaxes bronchial muscles in bronchospasm |
| Norepinephrine (Levophed) | Increases blood pressure in acute hypotension caused by peripheral vasoconstriction |

#### 3.4.1.2   Noncatecholamines

Noncatecholamines also stimulate the nervous system but focus on a local or systematic effect rather than the general effect of catecholamines. Noncatecholamines can affect selected beta-adrenergic receptors and some stimulate alpha-adrenergic receptors. Table 3.2 contains commonly used noncatecholamines.

**TABLE 3.2 Commonly Used Noncatecholamines**

| NONCATECHOLAMINE | USE |
| --- | --- |
| Albuterol (Proventil) | Relaxes bronchial muscles in bronchospasm |
| Metaproterenol (Alupent) | Relaxes bronchial muscles in bronchospasm |
| Isoetharine | Relaxes bronchial muscles in bronchospasm |
| Methoxamine (Vasoxyl) | Increases blood pressure in hypotension |
| Ephedrine | Increases blood pressure in acute hypotension and orthostatic hypotension |
| Phenylephrine (Neo-Synephrine) | Increases blood pressure in hypotensive emergencies |

## 3.4.2 Adrenergic Blockers

Adrenergic blocker is a class of medication that disrupts the function of the sympathetic nervous system by blocking impulses at the adrenergic receptor site. There are two classifications of adrenergic blockers.

• **Alpha-adrenergic blockers** block the alpha-adrenergic receptor sites. There are two types of alpha-adrenergic receptor sites (alpha$_1$ and alpha$_2$). Alpha-adrenergic blocks affect both types. The result is dilation of blood vessels, relaxation of smooth muscles of blood vessels, decreased blood pressure, and increased blood flow to organs.

Alpha-adrenergic blockers are phentolamine and prazosin (Minipress), used for hypertension, peripheral vascular disorders, and pheochromocytoma (an adrenal gland tumor that causes too much epinephrine and norepinephrine to be released).

• **Beta-adrenergic blockers** block the beta receptor sites. There are two kinds of beta receptor sites (beta$_1$ and beta$_2$). Beta$_1$ receptor sites are in the heart. Beta$_2$ receptor sites are in the bronchi, blood vessels, and uterus.

Beta-adrenergic blockers decrease blood pressure, decrease cardiac contractions by slowing conduction of impulses between the atria and ventricles, and, therefore, decrease oxygen requirements for the heart and decrease cardiac output. Peripheral vascular resistance increases.

Beta-adrenergic blockers are further classified as nonselective and selective. Nonselective beta-adrenergic blockers affect both beta$_1$ and beta$_2$ receptors. Selective beta-adrenergic blockers affect beta$_1$ receptors.

Both nonselective and selective beta-adrenergic blockers are used for

- Angina
- Anxiety
- Migraine headaches
- Hypertension
- Essential tremor
- Pheochromocytoma
- Thyroid crisis (throtoxicosis)
- Myocardial infarction complications

Nonselective beta-adrenergic blockers decrease cardiac stimulation and cause constriction of bronchioles in the lungs, resulting in bronchospasm in patients who have chronic, obstructive lung disorders. Nonselective beta-adrenergic blockers are

- Carvedilo (Coreg)
- Labetalol (Normodyne)
- Penbutotol (Levatol)
- Nadolol (Corgard)
- Pindolol (Visken)
- Propranolol (Inderal)
- Sotalol (Betapace)
- Timolol (Blocadren)

Selective beta-adrenergic blockers are called cardioselective beta-adrenergic blockers because they reduce cardiac stimulation. These are

- Acebutolol (Sectral)
- Atenolol (Tenormin)
- Betaxolol (Kerlone)
- Bisoprolol (Zebeta)
- Esmolol (Brevibloc)
- Metoprolol (Lopressor)

### 3.4.3 Antianginal

Antianginal medication is used to decrease oxygen demand by the heart and/or increase oxygen to the heart and is used to treat angina (angina pectoris). Angina occurs when the heart requires more oxygen than is supplied, resulting in cardiac ischemia that presents as chest pain.

There are three classes of antianginal medications.

#### 3.4.3.1 Nitrates

Nitrates are used for acute angina because nitrates relax smooth muscle around veins causing a decrease in return blood to the ventricles during preload, which is when ventricles are full and before the ventricles contract. Since there is less blood in the ventricles, the ventricles are reduced in size and tension and therefore require less oxygen.

Nitrates cause coronary arteries to dilate, increasing the flow of oxygenated blood to cardiac muscle and decreasing the ischemia, resulting in decreased chest pain.

Nitrates also dilate peripheral arterioles, reducing peripheral vascular resistance resulting in a decrease of the cardiac afterload that occurs when the left ventricle contracts pumping blood throughout the peripheral vascular system.

Commonly prescribed nitrates are

- Isosorbide dinitrate (Isordil)
- Isosorbide mononitrate (Imdur)
- Nitroglycerin (Nitro-Bid)

#### 3.4.3.2 Beta-Adrenergic Blockers

Beta-adrenergic blockers are used to prevent angina in addition to treating hypertension (see 3.4.2 Adrenergic Blockers) by decreasing the heart rate and reducing the force of contractions leading to decreased cardiac oxygen demand.

#### 3.4.3.3 Calcium Channel Blockers

Calcium channel blockers are used to prevent angina when other treatments have failed and the patient continues to experience angina. Calcium is used within muscle cells to contract muscles. Calcium channel blockers dilate coronary and peripheral arteries by preventing calcium ions from entering cardiac muscle and smooth muscle of veins and arteries, resulting in decreased resistance against the heart. The workload of the heart decreases, and, therefore, there is a reduced need for oxygen by the heart. Calcium channel blockers also prevent peripheral arterioles from constricting, reducing the afterload oxygen demand. Calcium channel blockers slow conduction of the impulse from the SA to the AV node, resulting in a decrease in heart rate and a lower need for oxygen by the heart.

Commonly prescribed calcium channel blockers are

- Amlodipine (Norvasc)
- Nifedipine (Procardia)
- Diltiazem (Cardizem)
- Verapamil (Calan)
- Nicardipine (Cardene)

### 3.4.4  Antiarrhythmics

Antiarrhythmic medication is used to resolve disturbances of cardiac rhythm, called arrhythmias, by restoring normal heart rhythm. However, there is a risk that antiarrhythmic medication can also cause arrhythmia.

There are four classes of antiarrhythmic medications.

#### 3.4.4.1  Class I

Class I antiarrhythmic medication has three divisions, each of which is a sodium channel blocker.

Class IA antiarrhythmic medication interferes with impulses from the autonomic nervous system with pacemaker cells in the heart. They also block impulses from the parasympathetic nervous system of the SA and AV nodes, resulting in increased impulse speed between the SA and AV nodes. Normally the impulses from the parasympathetic nervous system slow impulses to the SA and AV nodes. There is a risk that patients with atrial fibrillation may experience a critical increase in ventricular contractions. In such cases, Class IA antiarrhythmic medication will not resolve the patient's arrhythmia. Class IA antiarrhythmic medication is used for atrial fibrillation, atrial flutter, paroxysmal atrial tachycardia, and ventricular tachycardia.

Commonly prescribed Class IA antiarrhythmic medications are

- Disopyramide (Norpace)
- Procainamide (Procanbid)
- Quinidine sulfate
- Quinidine gluconate

Class IB antiarrhythmic medication blocks influx of sodium ions when the heart contracts (depolarizes), resulting in a decrease in the time between contractions (refractory period). Class IB antiarrhythmic medications are used for ventricular tachycardia and ventricular fibrillation.

Commonly prescribed Class IB antiarrhythmic medications are

- Lidocaine (Xylocaine)
- Mexiletine (Mexitil)

Class IC antiarrhythmic medication slows cardiac impulses, resulting in a decreased contraction (depolarization) rate. Class IC antiarrhythmic medications are used for ventricular tachycardia, ventricular fibrillation, and supraventricular arrhythmias.

Commonly prescribed Class IC antiarrhythmic medications are

- Flecainide (Tambocor)
- Moricizine (Ethmozine)
- Propafenone (Rythmol)

#### 3.4.4.2  Class II

Class II antiarrhythmic medication slows the automatic firing of impulses by the SA node, thereby slowing impulses of the AV node, too, by blocking the beta-adrenergic receptors in the heart. As a result, Class II antiarrhythmic medication decreases the strength of cardiac contractions and therefore reduces the oxygen requirement of the heart.

Commonly prescribed Class II antiarrhythmic medications are

- Acebutolol (Sectral)
- Esmolol (Brevibloc)
- Propranolol (Inderal)

#### 3.4.4.3  Class III

Class III antiarrhythmic medication converts a unidirectional block to a bidirectional block, resulting in suppression of the arrhythmia in patients with life-threatening arrhythmias and ventricular arrhythmias.

The commonly prescribed Class III antiarrhythmic medication is

- Amiodarone (Cordarone)

### 3.4.4.4 Class IV

Class IV antiarrhythmic medication blocks calcium during the second phase of the action potential, resulting in slowing conduction and slowing the refractory period of the AV node. This results in resolving supraventricular arrhythmias.
　　Commonly prescribed Class IV antiarrhythmic medications are

- Diltiazem (Cardizem)
- Verapamil (Calan)

### 3.4.4.5 Miscellaneous Antiarrhythmic Medication

One medication does not belong to any of the classes and, therefore, is considered under the miscellaneous category of cardiac antiarrhythmic medication. This is adenosine (Adenocard). This medication decreases the SA node's ability to send impulses, resulting in decreased AV node impulses to the atria and ventricles and leading to decreased heart rate. This is used in paroxysmal supraventricular tachycardia.

## 3.4.5 Anticoagulant Medication

Anticoagulant medication is used to decrease the formation of blood clots by interfering with platelet aggregation. There are three categories of anticoagulant medications. All anticoagulant medication presents a risk for bleeding and, therefore, the effectiveness of these medications must be monitored regularly.

### 3.4.5.1 Heparin

Heparin is used to treat deep-vein thrombosis, embolism prophylaxis, and disseminated intravascular coagulation and to reduce the formation of blood clots following a myocardial infarction (MI). Heparin does not dissolve existing blood clots. Heparin prevents new blood clots from forming by inhibiting the body's ability to create fibrin and thrombin. The side effects of heparin are bleeding and decreased platelet count (thrombocytopenia). Heparin is typically administered by IV. If the patient is maintained on anticoagulant medication, then the patient receives oral anticoagulant in conjunction with heparin. Once oral anticoagulant approaches a therapeutic level, the patient is typically placed on low-molecular-weight heparin (Lovenox, Fragmin), subcutaneous injections until the oral anticoagulant is effective. The partial thromboplastin time (PTT) test is used to measure heparin effectiveness. The International Normalized Ratio (INR) and the prothrombin time (PT) tests are used to measure the effectiveness of oral anticoagulants.
　　Commonly prescribed heparin medications are

- Heparin
- Dalteparin (Fragmin)
- Enoxaparin (Lovenox)

### 3.4.5.2 Oral Anticoagulant Medication

Oral anticoagulant medication is used to treat deep-vein thrombosis, prophylaxis, atrial arrhythmias, and complications from malfunctioning heart valves. Oral anticoagulant medications do not have an immediate effect on preventing the formation of blood clots. Oral anticoagulant medications disrupt the ability of the liver to create vitamin-K-related clotting factor. The effectiveness of oral anticoagulant medications occurs once free-floating clots in the blood dissipate.
　　The commonly prescribed oral anticoagulant medication is

- Warfarin (Coumadin)

### 3.4.5.3 Antiplatelet Medication

Antiplatelet medication reduces platelet aggregation and is used for patients who are at risk for complications from prostatic heart-valve surgery or who have experienced acute coronary syndrome or a myocardial infarction (MI).

Commonly prescribed antiplatelet medications are

- Aspirin (low dose)
- Dipyridamole (Persatine)
- Sulfinpyrazone (Anturane)
- Iclopidine (Ticlid)
- Lopidogrel (Plavix)

### 3.4.6 Thrombolytic Medication

Thrombolytic medications dissolve blood clots by transforming plasminogen to plasmin-dissolving plasma proteins thrombi and fibrinogen. Thrombolytic medications are used to treat blood clots related to acute ischemic stroke, catheter occlusion, pulmonary embolus, acute myocardial infarction, and arterial thrombosis.
Commonly prescribed thrombolytic medications are

- Alteplase (Activase)
- Reteplase (Retavase)
- Streptokinase (Streptase)

### 3.4.7 Antihypertensive Medication

Antihypertensive medication is used to decrease blood pressure when beta-adrenergic blockers (see 3.4.2 Adrenergic Blockers) and diuretics (see 3.4.9 Diuretic Medication) are ineffective. There are three categories of antihypertensive medication. These are sympatholytics, vasodilators, and angiotensin-converting enzyme (ACE) inhibitors.

#### 3.4.7.1 Sympatholytic Medication

Sympatholytic medication is used to decrease impulses from the sympathetic nervous system, resulting in dilation of peripheral blood vessels and decreased cardiac output and leading to decreased blood pressure. Sympatholytic medications are classified by their action.
Commonly prescribed sympatholytic medications are

- Clonidine (Catapress)
- Quanabenz (Wytensin)
- Guanfacine (Tenex)
- Ethyldopa (Aldomet)

Commonly prescribed alpha-blocker sympatholytic medications are

- Doxazosin (Cardura)
- Phentolamine (Minipress)
- Terazosin (Hytrin)

Commonly prescribed mixed alpha- and beta-adrenergic blocker sympatholytic medication is

- Labetalol (Normodyne)

Commonly prescribed norepinephrine-depletor sympatholytic medications are

- Guanadrel (Hylorel)
- Guanethidine (Ismelin)

#### 3.4.7.2 Vasodilator Medication

Vasodilator medication is used to decrease systolic and diastolic blood pressure. There are two classifications of vasodilator medication. These are calcium channel blockers and direct vasodilators. Calcium channel blockers decrease calcium flow into cells, resulting in decreased contraction of smooth muscles around the arterioles. Direct vasodilators increase the diameter of blood vessels, resulting in decreased peripheral resistance and therefore decreased blood pressure. Vasodilators are used to treat moderate and severe hypertension.

Commonly prescribed vasodilator medications are

- Hydralazine (Apresoline)
- Minoxidil (Rogaine)
- Nitroprusside (Nitropress)

### 3.4.7.3   Angiotensin-Converting Enzyme (ACE) Inhibitor Medication

Angiotensin-converting enzyme (ACE) inhibitor medication prevents conversion of angiotensin I to angiotensin II. Angiotensin II is a vasoconstrictor that leads to excretion of aldosterone, which retains water and sodium resulting in increased blood volume. By interrupting conversion of angiotensin I to angiotensin II, blood pressure decreases. ACE inhibitors are used to treat hypertension and heart failure.

Commonly prescribed ACE inhibitors are

- Benazepril (Lotensin)
- Captopril (Capoten)
- Enalapril (Vasotec)
- Fosinopril (Monopril)
- Lisinopril (Zestril)
- Quinapril (Accuprill)
- Ramipril (Altace)

## 3.4.8   Medication to Strengthen Cardiac Contractions

Two medications are used to increase cardiac contractions and to treat heart failure. These are cardiac glycoside medication and phosphodiesterase (PED) inhibitor medication.

### 3.4.8.1   Cardiac Glycoside Medication

Cardiac glycoside medication strengthens cardiac contractions by decreasing the electrical impulse between the SA and AV node, resulting in decreased cardiac rate. Cardiac glycoside medications are used for heart failure and supraventricular arrhythmia.

The commonly prescribed cardiac glycoside medication is

- Digoxin (Lanoxin)

### 3.4.8.2   Phosphodiesterase (PDE) Inhibitor Medication

Phosphodiesterase (PDE) inhibitor medication strengthens cardiac contractions by increasing both the movement of calcium into the cardiac cells and the storage of calcium. In addition, PDE inhibitor medication causes smooth muscles of the peripheral blood vessels to relax, resulting in decreased resistance to cardiac output.

Commonly prescribed PDE inhibitors are

- Inamrinone (Inocor)
- Milrinone (Primacor)

## 3.4.9   Diuretic Medication

Diuretic medication causes water and electrolytes to be excreted by the kidneys, resulting in decreased blood pressure. There are three classifications of diuretics: thiazide diuretics, loop diuretics, and potassium-sparing diuretics.

### 3.4.9.1   Thiazide Diuretic Medication

Thiazide diuretic medication prevents the reabsorption of sodium by the kidneys, resulting in excretion of sodium. As sodium is excreted, water is also excreted, decreasing the volume of plasma and leading to an initial decrease in cardiac output. Cardiac output returns to normal when treatment stabilizes with thiazide diuretic medication. Thiazide diuretic medication also causes excretion of potassium chloride and bicarbonate, leading to an electrolyte imbalance. Thiazide diuretic medication is used to treat edema and hypertension.

Commonly prescribed thiazide diuretic medications are

- Hydroflumethiazide (Diucardin)
- Chlorthalidone (Hygroton)
- Indapamide (Lozol)
- Bendroflumethiazide (Naturetin)
- Hydrochlorothiazide (HydroDIURIL)

### 3.4.9.2 Loop Diuretic Medication

Loop diuretic medication increases the secretion of water, sodium, and chloride in the ascending loop of Henle where urine is concentrated in the kidney. Loop diuretic medication produces the most urine of the diuretic medications and therefore can cause an electrolyte imbalance. Loop diuretic medications are used to treat heart failure, edema, and hypertension.

Commonly prescribed loop diuretic medications are

- Bumetanide (Bumex)
- Furosemide (Lasix)
- Ethacrynic acid (Edecrin)
- Ethacrynate sodium (Edecrin sodium)

### 3.4.9.3 Potassium-Sparing Diuretic Medication

Potassium-sparing diuretic medication increases the secretion of water, chloride, calcium, and sodium but not potassium.

Commonly prescribed potassium-sparing diuretic medications are

- Amiloride (Midamor)
- Spironolactone (Aldactone)
- Triamterene (Dyrenium)

## 3.5 Aortic Aneurysm

Atherosclerosis, degeneration of the middle aortic muscle layer, trauma, infection, or congenital defects can cause the weakening of the aortic wall. Pressure from blood flow causes the wall to bulge. Blood becomes turbulent resulting in increased dilation of the weakened wall. The aneurysm may rupture, causing a drop in circulation, severe hypotension, syncope, and possibly death.

### 3.5.1 Signs and Symptoms

- Asymptomatic
- Restlessness and anxiety
- Increased thready pulse and decreased pulse pressure
- Decreased femoral pulses
- Abdominal pulsation
- Back pain radiating to posterior legs
- Abdominal pain

### 3.5.2 Medical Tests

- Chest x-ray, abdominal ultrasound, CT scan, or MRI, used to display the aortic aneurysm
- Accusation of bruit (swishing sound of turbulent blood) over the iliac or femoral arteries or abdominal aorta

### 3.5.3   Treatment

- Administer

    ○ Morphine sulfate or oxycodone to decrease oxygen demand

    ○ Antihypertensives to reduce blood pressure

    ○ Analgesics to reduce pain associated with tearing of the aortic wall and to relieve the pressure the aortic aneurysm is placing on nerves

- Surgically resection the aortic aneurysm.

### 3.5.4   Intervention

- Limit patient's activity and encourage patient to rest in a quiet place to reduce anxiety.

- Palpate abdomen for pulsating mass or distention. Distention may signify imminent rupture.

- Listen for abdominal bruits.

- Monitor for

    ○ Numbness and tingling

    ○ Decrease in temperature of extremities

    ○ Increased thready pulse

    ○ Change in skin color in extremities

    ○ Pale, clammy skin, indicating decreased circulation

    ○ Restlessness, indicating increased anxiety and decreased oxygenation

    ○ Intake and output and urine quality. Low urine output and high specific gravity of urine indicate hypovolemia.

    ○ Hypovolemic shock

        ▪ Decreased blood pressure due to rupture of the aortic aneurysm

        ▪ Decreased peripheral pulse resulting from decrease in blood pressure

        ▪ Increased heart rate as heart tries to meet increased demand for oxygen

        ▪ Increased respiration to meet increased demand for oxygen

    ○ Decreased pulse pressure resulting from less filling time between cardiac contracts and decreased circulating volume of blood

    ○ Severe back pain due to rupture or dissection

## 3.6   Angina (Angina Pectoris)

Arteriosclerosis of the coronary artery narrows blood flow to cardiac muscles. Chest pain, pressure, heaviness, squeezing, or tightness occurs when the cardiac muscle's demand for oxygen exceeds the supply of oxygen. There are three categories of angina.

- **Stable angina:** chest pain occurs following exercise or stress and is relieved by rest or nitrates.

- **Unstable angina:** chest pain occurs at rest with increasing intensity and duration, is not relieved by rest, and is slow to respond to nitrates.

- **Prinzmetal's or vasospastic angina:** chest pain occurs at night at rest with minimal exertion.

### 3.6.1   Signs and Symptoms

- Chest pain, pressure, heaviness, squeezing, tightness for up to five minutes radiating to the jaw, back, or arms. Occurs at rest, after exercise or stress, and increases oxygen demands on the heart
- Shortness of breath (dyspnea) due to increased respiration related to increased demand for oxygen
- Tachycardia due to increased need to pump oxygenated blood
- Increased anxiety resulting from decreased oxygen to cardiac muscles
- Sweating (diaphoresis) due to anxiety and increased cardiac workload

### 3.6.2   Medical Tests

- Electrocardiogram (ECG) during attack:
  - T wave inverted (first sign of initial ischemia)
  - ST-segment changes (indicates myocardium injury)
  - Abnormal Q waves (indicates myocardial infarction)
- Cardiac panel: troponins, CK-MB, electrolytes
- Routine blood workup: CBC, blood chemistry, PT/PTT/INR, BNP, cholesterol panel
- Holter monitoring for 24 to 48 hours: providing continuous cardiac monitoring
- Stress test: assessing cardiac function under pharmacologic or exercise stress
- Coronary arteriography: assessing arteriosclerosis of the coronary artery
- Cardiac PET (positron emission tomography): assessing arteriosclerosis of the coronary artery
- Chest x-ray: assessing for heart failure
- Echocardiogram or stress-echo: assessing cardiac abnormality caused by ischemia

### 3.6.3   Treatment

- Rest: reduces cardiac demand for oxygen
- Administer
  - 2 to 4 liters 100% oxygen as necessary, using non-rebreather face mask to increase oxygen supply
  - Analgesic (morphine) to decrease cardiac workload and to decrease pain
  - Nitrates (nitroglycerin) to dilate blood vessels, increasing blood flow to cardiac muscles
  - Beta-adrenergic blocker to decrease cardiac workload
  - Inderal (propranolol), Corgard (nadolol), Tenormin (atenolol), Lopressor (metoprolol)
  - Aspirin to reduce formation of platelets
- Procedures
  - Percutaneous, transluminal coronary angioplasty: an inflated balloon within coronary artery compresses blockage against the artery wall.
  - Coronary artery stent: a mesh tube is inserted into the coronary artery and reduces the blockage.
  - Coronary artery bypass graph (CABG): a vein from a leg or an artery from an arm or the chest is graphed to coronary arteries, bypassing the blockage.

- Diet
  - Low-cholesterol
  - Low-sodium
  - Low-fat

### 3.6.4   Intervention

- Place patient in a semi-Fowler's position to avoid stress.
- Monitor vital signs
  - Hold nitrate order if systolic blood pressure is <90 mm Hg (risk of reduced blood to brain).
  - Hold beta-adrenergic blocker if heart rate is less than 60 beats per minute (risk of low cardiac output).
- Monitor patient with a 12-lead electrocardiogram (ECG) during each attack.
- Monitor intake and output to assess renal function.
- Instruct the patient
  - Take one sublingual dose every five minutes for maximum of three doses at first signs of angina.
  - Rest immediately.
  - Call 911 if signs of angina continue for more than 10 minutes.
  - Avoid stress that brings about angina.
  - Adhere to prescribed diet.
  - Do not smoke.

## 3.7   Myocardial Infarction (MI)

Blockage of coronary arteries reduces oxygen supply to cardiac muscle resulting in necrosis of an area of cardiac muscle, also known as an infarction. Blockage is caused by atherosclerosis, which results in a buildup of plaque on the wall of the artery.

### 3.7.1   Signs and Symptoms

- Restlessness, feeling of impending doom, anxiety
- Chest pain radiating to arms, jaw, back, and/or neck that is not relieved by rest or nitroglycerin—unlike angina
- Cool, clammy, pale skin due to decreased circulation
- Diaphoresis (sweating) due to anxiety
- Tachycardia due to pain and low cardiac output
- Nausea or vomiting possibly due to decreased cardiac output
- Variable blood pressure due to decreased cardiac output
- Shortness of breath in the elderly and women
- Asymptomatic (silent heart attack) in diabetics

### 3.7.2  Medical Tests

- Labs
  - Increased WBC, as a result of inflammatory response to infarction
  - Elevated creatine phosphokinase-MB (CK-MB) released by injured tissue. Will follow a predetermined curve reflecting tissue damage and repair
  - Elevated troponin I and troponin T-proteins within one hour of infarction, released by injured tissue
- Urine output: <25 ml/hr due to lack of renal blood flow
- ECG
  - T wave: inversion indicates ischemia.
  - ST segment: elevated or depressed indicates cardiac tissue injury.
- Decreased pulse pressure due to decreased cardiac output

### 3.7.3  Treatment

- Administer
  - 2 to 4 liters 100% oxygen, as necessary, using a non-rebreather face mask to increase oxygen supply
  - Aspirin to reduce formation of platelets
  - Antiarrhythmics to control cardiac arrhythmias
    - Cordarone (amiodarone), lidocaine, Pronestyl (procainamide)
  - Antihypertensive to decrease blood pressure
    - Apresoline (hydralazine)
  - Thrombolytic therapy within 3 to 12 hours of an attack to reduce blockage
    - Activase (alteplase), Streptase (streptokinase), Eminase (Anistreplase), Retavase (reteplase)
  - Heparin to prevent clots following thrombolytic therapy
  - Calcium channel blockers for non-Q-wave infarction to prevent reinfarction
    - Isoptin (Verapamil), Cardizem (diltiazem)
  - Beta-adrenergic blockers to decrease duration of pain
    - Inderal (propranolol), Corgard (nadolol), Lopressor (metroprolol)
  - Analgesics decrease pain and cardiac workload
    - Morphine
  - Nitrates for dilation of blood vessels
    - Nitroglycerin
- Electrical cardioversion in unstable ventricular tachycardia to reestablish sinus rhythm
- Percutaneous revascularization to restore cardiac blood flow

### 3.7.4  Intervention

- Assign bed rest without bathroom privileges.
- Place patient in a semi-Fowler's position and instruct patient to avoid stress.
- Monitor vital signs.

- Monitor cardiac function with a 12-lead ECG.
- Instruct the patient
  - Eat a low-fat, low-cholesterol, low-sodium diet.
  - Reduce stress, reduce weight, and engage in moderate exercise.
  - Stop smoking.
  - Identify myocardial infarction pain and angina pain.
  - Take nitroglycerin and call 911 as necessary.

## 3.8  Cardiac Tamponade

The pericardium fills with fluid, blood, or pus as a result of trauma, postoperative complications, or complications from an MI, cancer, or uremia. Pressure in the pericardium reduces filling of the ventricles and results in decreased cardiac output.

### 3.8.1  Signs and Symptoms

- Muffled cardiac sounds due to fluid
- Sweating (diaphoresis), tachycardia, and difficulty breathing (dyspnea), due to the increased demand for oxygen
- Restlessness due to decreased oxygen to the brain
- Pulsus paradoxus (decrease of 15 mm Hg or more in systolic blood pressure on inspiration) due to pressure change within the chest on inspiration
- Fatigue due to increased workload
- Jugular vein distention due to decreased venous return from the jugular veins

### 3.8.2  Medical Tests

- Chest x-ray: to assess for enlarged heart
- Echocardiograph: ultrasound image of the heart to assess cardiac structure and function
- Electrocardiogram: to exclude cardiac disorders
- Cardiac catheterization

### 3.8.3  Treatment

- Pericardiocentesis: aspirate fluid from the pericardium.
- Administer
  - 2 to 4 liters 100% oxygen as necessary using a non-rebreather face mask to increase oxygen supply
  - Beta-adrenergic blockers decrease duration of pain
    - Inderal (propranolol), Corgard (nadolol), Lopressor (metroprolol)

### 3.8.4  Intervention

- Monitor vital signs.

## 3.9  Cardiogenic Shock

Cardiac tamponade, myocardial ischemia, myocarditis, or cardiomyopathies result in the heart being unable to pump blood and a decreased blood pressure. Blood backs up from the left ventricle into the lungs, causing pulmonary edema. Cardiac rate increases to compensate for the decrease in blood flow. Cardiac muscle oxygenation decreases because the lungs are unable to oxygenate the blood.

### 3.9.1  Signs and Symptoms

- Distended jugular veins caused by fluid overload
- Hypotension due to decreased blood flow
- Clammy skin due to tissue deoxygenation
- Confusion due to poor perfusion in the brain
- Crackles in lungs indicating fluid buildup and pulmonary edema
- Skin pallor (decreased skin temperature) due to decreased circulation
- Cyanosis due to poor perfusion
- Arrhythmias due to irritability of cardiac muscle from decreased oxygenation
- Oliguria (urine output <30 ml/hr) due to decreased kidney perfusion
- Tachycardia due to increased cardiac demand for blood

### 3.9.2  Medical Tests

- Electrocardiogram
  - Q wave: enlarged due to cardiac failure
  - ST waves: elevated due to ischemia
- Echocardiogram: ultrasound image of the heart to assess cardiac structure and function

### 3.9.3  Treatment

- Use Swan-Ganz catheterization to measure pressure in the pulmonary artery.
- Order labs
  - Arterial blood gas to assess the acid/base balance of blood
- Administer
  - Vasodilator to reduce peripheral aterial resistance and decrease cardiac workload
    - Nitropress (nitroprusside), nitroglycerin
    - Adrenergic agent to increase blood pressure and cardiac rate
    - Epinephrine

- ○ Inotropes to strengthen cardiac contractions

  - ▪ Dopamine, dobutamine, Cordarone (amiodarone), Primacor (milrinone)

- ○ Vasopressor to increase blood flow to the heart and brain and decrease blood flow to other organs

  - ▪ Norepinephrine

### 3.9.4  Intervention

- Place patient on bed rest.

- Administer 2 to 4 liters of oxygen to increase oxygen supply.

- Monitor vital signs. Patient is at risk for respiratory distress.

- Measure fluid intake and output to assess for adequate renal perfusion.

- Check weight daily. Notify healthcare provider if weight increases 3 lb (4.4 kg).

- Instruct the patient

  - ○ Notify the healthcare provider of shortness of breath or signs of fluid retention (dependent edema).

  - ○ Eat a low-sodium, low-fat diet.

  - ○ Rest frequently.

## 3.10  Endocarditis

An invasive medical procedure or IV drug use introduces microorganisms into the blood. An infection by a microorganism develops in the inner lining of the heart (endocardium) and heart valves and results in cardiac inflammation leading to ulceration and necrosis of heart valves. Endocarditis is also secondary to degenerative heart disease and rheumatic heart disease.

### 3.10.1  Signs and Symptoms

- Janeway lesions on the soles and palms

- Petechiae on fingernails and palate

- Osler nodes on pads of fingers and feet

- Fatigue related to the infection

- Murmurs related to turbulent blood flow

- Fever related to the infection

### 3.10.2  Medical Tests

- Echocardiograph: to examine functioning of heart valves

- Transesophageal echocardiogram: to examine functioning of heart valves

- Chest x-ray: to examine pulmonary and cardiac abnormalities

- Blood culture and sensitivity test: three times, one hour apart, to identify the microorganism and treatment

### 3.10.3  Treatment

- Administer antibiotics according to results of culture and sensitivity tests
- Schedule valve replacement for damaged valves.

### 3.10.4  Intervention

- Prescribe bed rest to reduce cardiac demand.
- Monitor for renal failure.
  - Decreased urine output
  - Increased BUN
  - Decreased creatinine clearance
- Monitor for embolism.
  - Hematuria
  - Decreased mentation
  - Cough or painful breathing
- Monitor for heart failure.
  - Weight gain and edema
  - Distended neck vein
  - Crackles in lungs
  - Dyspnea
  - Tachycardia
- Instruct the patient
  - Take all prescribed antibiotics even if he or she is feeling well.
  - Tell a healthcare provider, including dentist, to administer prophylactic antibiotics before, during, and after an invasive medical procedure.

## 3.11  Congestive Heart Failure (CHF)

Ventricles are unable to contract at full capacity, causing decreased circulation and a backup of blood. This is caused by a myocardial infarction, hypertension, valve disorder, or endocarditis. Left-side congestive heart failure results in the backup of blood into the lungs. Right-side congestive heart failure results in the backup of blood in systemic circulation, causing edema.

### 3.11.1  Signs and Symptoms

**Early Signs**

- Fatigue
- S4 heart sounds
- Nocturia

- Dyspnea on exertion

- Bilateral rales in lungs

- Hepatojugular reflux

**Advanced Signs**

- Orthopnea

- Cardiomegaly

- Hepatomegaly

- Cough

- Anasarca (edema)

- Cardiac rales

- Frothy or pink sputum due to capillary permeability

## 3.11.2  Medical Tests

- ECG: T-wave sign of ischemia or tachycardia

- Labs

  - Increased B-type natriuretic peptide

  - Decreased Hgb

  - Hct less than three times Hgb

  - Increased BUN, decreased creatinine clearance, decreased urine output

- Chest x-ray

  - Enlarged left ventricle (left-side heart failure)

  - Pulmonary congestion

  - Pleural effusion (right-side heart failure)

  - Cardiomegaly (right-side heart failure)

## 3.11.3  Treatment

- Administer

  - Diuretics: to decrease fluid volume

    - Lasix (furosemide), Bumex (bumetanide), Zaroxolyn (metolazone), Aldacton (spironolactone)

  - ACE inhibitors: to decrease pressure in the left ventricle

    - Prinivil (lisinopril), Capoten (captopril), Vasotec (enalapril)

  - Beta-adrenergic blockers: to decrease cardiac contractions

    - Inderal (propranolol), Corgard (nadolol), Lopressor (metroprolol)

  - Inotropic agent: to increase cardiac contractions

    - Dopamine, dobutamine, Cordarone (amiodarone), Primacor (milrinone), digitalis (digoxin)

○ Vasodilator: to reduce peripheral arterial resistance and decrease cardiac workload

   ▪ Nitropress (nitroprusside), nitroglycerin

○ Anticoagulant: to decrease blood coagulation

   ▪ Heparin, Coumadin (warfarin)

### 3.11.4 Intervention

- Indicate rest and place patient in high Fowler's position.

- Administer high-flow oxygen with legs dependent (dangling) and positive end-expiratory pressure (PEEP), by ventilator if necessary.

- Monitor vitals.

- Weigh daily. Notify healthcare provider if weight increases 3 lb (4.4 kg).

- Measure fluid intake and output.

- Prescribe low-sodium diet.

- Administer 2 to 4 liters of oxygen to increase oxygen supply.

- Instruct the patient to elevate legs to reduce dependent edema.

## 3.12 Hypertension and Hypertensive Crisis

Hypertension occurs when blood-vessel pressure increases secondary to an underlying condition or idiopathic cause. Hypertensive crisis occurs when hypertension occurs rapidly, leading to organ damage. A hypertensive crisis is categorized by how significant the end-organ damage is and the estimation of how quickly the blood pressure must be lowered. Causes can be pheochromocytoma, Cushing's syndrome, abnormal renal function, intracerebral hemorrhage, myocardial ischemia, eclampsia, monamine oxidase inhibitor interaction, and abrupt withdrawal of antihyhpertensive medication.

**Classifications of Hypertension**

- Normal: <120 mm Hg systolic/<80 mm Hg diastolic

- Prehypertension: 120–139 mm Hg systolic/80–89 mm Hg diastolic

- Stage 1 hypertension: 140–159 mm Hg systolic/90–99 mm Hg diastolic

- Stage 2 hypertension: ≥160 mm Hg systolic/≥100 mm Hg diastolic

- Diabetic hypertension: 130 mm Hg systolic/80 mm Hg diastolic or higher

- Hypertensive crisis: <180 mm Hg systolic/<120 mm Hg diastolic

### 3.12.1 Signs and Symptoms

- Hypertension

   ○ Asymptomatic

   ○ Dizziness

   ○ Headache

- Hypertensive crisis
  - Dizziness
  - Confusion/disorientation
  - Irritability
  - Nausea/vomiting
  - Shortness of breath on exertion
  - Blurred vision or double vision
  - Seizure
  - Decreased level of consciousness

## 3.12.2 Medical Tests

- Hypertension: blood pressure >140/90 mm Hg on at least three different occasions lying, sitting, and standing, bilaterally
- Hypertensive crisis: diastolic pressure <120 mm Hg one occasion

## 3.12.3 Treatment

- Hypertension
  - First: change lifestyle.
    - Decrease caloric intake.
    - Monitor vital signs.
    - Decrease caffeine intake.
    - Decrease alcohol intake.
    - Follow low-sodium diet.
    - Increase exercise.
    - Stop smoking.
  - Second: administer medication.
    - Diuretics to decrease circulation
      - Lasix (furosemide), Bumex (bumetanide), Zaroxolyn (metolazone), Aldacton (spironolactone)
    - Beta-adrenergic blocker to decrease cardiac output
      - Inderal (propranolol), Corgard (nadolol), Lopresspr (metroprolol)
    - Calcium channel blockers to increase peripheral vasodilation
      - Isoptin (verapamil), Cardizem/Dilacor/Tiazac (diltiazem), Cardene (nicardipine)
    - ACE inhibitors to delay renal disease
      - Prinivil (lisinopril), Capoten (captopril), Vasotec (enalapril)
  - Third: increase medication dosages.
  - Fourth: combine medication.

- Hypertensive crisis

  ○ Reduce blood pressure slowly over days. Reduce blood pressure no more than 25% of the MAP within the first two hours.

  ○ Administer

    ▪ Sodium nitroprusside (Nitropress), nitroglycerin (Nitro-Bid), hydralazine (Apresoline [for preeclampsia])

### 3.12.4  Intervention

- Hypertension

  ○ Measure fluid intake and output.

  ○ Advocate stress-free environment.

  ○ Introduce low-sodium diet.

  ○ Instruct the patient

    ▪ Change lifestyle to avoid need for prescribed medication.

    ▪ Reduce weight.

    ▪ Be aware of possible side effects of medications.

- Hypertensive crisis

  ○ Monitor ECG continuously.

  ○ Monitor blood pressure constantly while administering medication and then every 15 minutes.

  ○ Determine MAP.

  ○ Check pulse oximetry.

  ○ Administer oxygen.

  ○ Monitor fluid output—normal is 1 ml/kg per hour; critical is <0.5 ml/kg per hour.

  ○ Provide quiet, low-lit environment.

  ○ Monitor for symptoms of thiocyanate toxicity if patient is administered Nitropress:

    ▪ Delirium

    ▪ Blurred vision

    ▪ Nausea

    ▪ Fatigue

    ▪ Tinnitus

## 3.13  Hypovolemic Shock

This is the result of a decrease in circulation of blood, plasma, or other body fluids leading to decreased intravascular volume from hemorrhage, dehydration, or fluid moving from blood vessels into tissues resulting in inadequate organ perfusion.

### 3.13.1   Signs and Symptoms

- Tachycardia due to cardiac compensation for reduced blood volume
- Agitation and restlessness due to decreased brain perfusion
- Hypotension due to decreased blood volume
- Decreased skin temperature due to decreased circulation and resulting in peripheral vasoconstriction
- Decreased blood pressure
- Increased heart rate
- Urine output less than 25 ml/hr due to decreased kidney perfusion

### 3.13.2   Medical Tests

- Labs
- Decreased Hgb (anemia)
- Increased BUN
- Decreased creatinine clearance
- Decreased Hct
- Arterial blood gas: decreased pH, increased $Paco_2$, decreased $Pao_2$

### 3.13.3   Treatment

- Administer
  - Catecholamines to increase blood pressure
    - Dopamine, epinephrine, and norepinephrine
  - Inotropic agent to increase blood pressure
    - Dobutamine
      - IV using largest catheter (18 gauge)
      - Crystalloid solutions to expand intravascular and extravascular fluid volume
    - 0.9% normal saline, lactated Ringer's solution (contains electrolytes)
      - Fresh-frozen plasma for clotting
      - Blood replacement (type O negative universal donor)

### 3.13.4   Intervention

- Monitor vital signs every 15 minutes.
- Administer 2 to 4 liters 100% oxygen as necessary using non-rebreather face mask. Increase oxygen if less than 80 mm Hg systolic.
- Measure urine output hourly using indwelling urinary catheter. Increase fluid intake if urine output is less than 30 ml/hr.
- Monitor lungs for crackles and dyspnea due to fluid overflow.
- Instruct the patient on how to avoid hypovolemic shock.

## 3.14 Myocarditis

Infection from chronic alcohol abuse, disease, and drug use causes cardiac muscle to become inflamed. Inflammation can degenerate cardiac muscle, leading to congestive heart failure.

### 3.14.1 Signs and Symptoms

- Dyspnea related to congestive heart failure
- Chest pain due to infection and inflammation
- Fever due to infection and inflammation
- S3 gallop related to congestive heart failure
- Tachycardia due to increased cardiac workload

### 3.14.2 Medical Tests

- Labs indicate increased CK-MB and increased troponins related to cardiac cell injury.
- Chest x-ray shows cardiomegaly.
- Echocardiogram shows cardiomegaly.
- ECG shows abnormal ST segment related to inflammation.
- Endomyocardial biopsy is used to identify microorganism.

### 3.14.3 Treatment

- Treat underlying cause.
- Administer
  - Antiarrhymics to stabilize arrhythmia
    - Quinidine, Pronestyl (procainamide)

### 3.14.4 Intervention

- Indicate bed rest without bathroom privileges.
- Monitor vital signs.
- Instruct the patient
  - Gradually return to normal activities.
  - Avoid competitive activities.

## 3.15 Pericarditis

Pericarditis is the result of an infection by a microorganism, autoimmune disease, acute myocardial infarction, or a reaction from medication causing inflammation of the pericardium. Acute pericarditis is typically caused by a viral infection. Chronic pericarditis is typically caused by disease or medication reaction.

### 3.15.1   Signs and Symptoms

- Acute:
  - Anxiety due to pain and respiratory changes
  - Sharp pain over the pericardium radiating to the neck, shoulders, back, and arm relieved by learning forward or sitting up and related to common nerve
  - Pain in the teeth or muscles related to common nerve
  - Arrhythmias related to irritated heart
  - Dyspnea related to inflammation
  - Tachypnea related to increased oxygen demand
  - Pericardial friction rub due to inflammation
  - General malaise
  - Fever and chills
- Chronic:
  - Hepatomegaly related to decrease in cardiac output and fluid overflow
  - Ascites related to decrease in cardiac output and liver fluid overflow
  - Increased fluid retention related to decrease in cardiac output
  - Pericardial friction rub related to inflammation

### 3.15.2   Medical Tests

- Chest x-ray shows fluid in pericardium.
- Electrocardiogram shows ST segment elevation.
- Echocardiograph shows fluid in pericardium.
- Labs:
  - Increased AST and LST due to injury of liver cells
  - Increased CK due to injury of heart cells
  - Increased WBC due to inflammation
  - Increased SED rate due to inflammation
  - Increased LDH due to tissue damage

### 3.15.3   Treatment

- Pericardiocentesis to remove fluid from pericardium
- Pericardial biopsy to identify infecting microorganism
- Administer
  - Corticosteroids to decrease inflammation
    - Medrol (methylprednisolone)
  - Nonsteroidal anti-inflammatory drug (NSAID)
    - Aspirin, Indocin (indomethacin)

### 3.15.4    Intervention

- Prescribe bed rest without bathroom privileges.

- Prescibe coughing and deep-breathing exercises to decrease discomfort.

- Place patient in high Fowler's position to ease breathing.

- Instruct the patient

  ○ Reduce ongoing fatigue by scheduling rest periods.

  ○ Slowly resume normal activities.

  ○ Ease his or her anxiety by understanding that there will be a recovery.

## 3.16    Pulmonary Edema

This is the result of decreased pumping action of the left side of the heart causing fluid to build up in the lungs. This is caused by congestive heart disease or is the result of acute myocardial infarction.

### 3.16.1    Signs and Symptoms

- Restlessness due to decreased oxygenation of brain

- Capillary permeability resulting in frothy, pink sputum

- Tachypnea due to increased demand for oxygen

- Cool, clammy skin due to decreased circulation

- Crackles in lungs due to increased fluid in lungs

- Distended jugular vein due to fluid overload

- Cyanosis due to decreased oxygenated blood

- Dyspnea when sitting upright due to increased fluid in lungs

- Hypertension

- Tachycardia

- Anxiety

### 3.16.2    Medical Tests

- Chest x-ray shows cardiomegaly.

- Echocardiogram assesses cardiac ejection fraction.

- Oxygen saturation assesses if oxygen saturation is <90%.

### 3.16.3    Treatment

- Treat underlying cause.

- Administer

  ○ Analgesics to decrease cardiac workload and pain

    ▪ Morphine

- Vasodilator to dilate blood vessels and decrease cardiac workload
  - Nitropress (nitroprusside), nitroglycerin, Dilatrate (isosorbide dinitrate)
- Inotropes to improve cardiac contractions
  - Dopamine, dobutamine, Cordarone (amiodarone), Primacor (milrinone), digitalis (digoxin)
- Bronchodilators to decrease bronchospasms
  - Albuterol
- Diuretics to decrease fluid
  - Lasix (furosemide), Bumex (bumetanide), Zaroxolyn (metolazone), Aldacton (spironolactone)

### 3.16.4 Intervention

- Monitor vital signs and capillary refill.
- Administer 2 to 4 liters 100% oxygen as necessary using non-rebreather face mask or high-flow oxygen.
- Place patient in full Fowler's position.
- Prescribe bed rest.
- Place patient on low-sodium diet to prevent fluid retention.
- Decrease patient's fluid intake due to existing fluid overload.
- Measure intake and output of fluids to assess renal perfusion.
- Weigh daily and notify healthcare provider if weight increases by 3 lb (4.4 kg).
- Instruct the patient
  - Elevate head when sleeping by placing blocks under the headside of the bed frame or by using three pillows.
  - Notify the healthcare provider of shortness of breath or fatigue.

## 3.17 Thrombophlebitis

A thrombus (blood clot) in a vein causes inflammation of a vein usually in the lower extremities. This may be caused by trauma, poor circulation, coagulation disorder, or medication.

### 3.17.1 Signs and Symptoms

- Asymptomatic
- Cramps caused by decreased blood flow
- Positive Homan's sign
- Tenderness and warmth in affected area caused by inflammation
- Edema due to decreased blood flow

- Clot moved to lungs
  - Dyspnea due to clot in lungs
  - Tachypnea due to clot in lungs
  - Crackles in lungs due to fluid buildup

### 3.17.2 Medical Tests

- Photoplethysmography to assess blood flow in affected area.
- Ultrasound to detect blood flow in affected area.

### 3.17.3 Treatment

- Administer
  - Nonsteroidal anti-inflammatory drug (NSAID) to decrease inflammation
    - Aspirin, Indocin (indomethacin)
  - Anticoagulant to decrease coagulation
    - Heparin, Coumadin (warfarin), Fragmin (dalteparin), Lovenox (enoxaparin)

### 3.17.4 Intervention

- Elevate affected area.
- Limit activity (bed rest with bathroom privileges; superficial thrombosis).
- Apply warm, moist compresses on affected area to increase blood flow.
- Monitor therapeutic level of anticoagulant.
- Monitor for tachypnea and dyspnea that may indicate emboli in lungs.
- Instruct the patient
  - Refrain from crossing legs as this causes decreased circulation.
  - Do not use oral contraceptives due to increased risk of clotting.
  - Wear support hose.
  - Move frequently once clot has resolved to prevent future clot formation.
  - Contact healthcare provider if experiencing shortness of breath or signs of bleeding.

## 3.18 Atrial Fibrillation

The atria stops beating and quivers, resulting in ineffective contractions. This is caused by abnormal cardiac impulses. It is not life-threatening; however, the patient is at risk for stroke and blood clots.

### 3.18.1  Signs and Symptoms

- Asymptomatic
- Dyspnea due to decreased oxygenation related to decreased circulation
- Faint feeling and light-headedness due to decreased circulation
- Irregular pulse due to arrhythmia
- Palpitations due to arrhythmia

### 3.18.2  Medical Tests

- Echocardiogram: shows structural abnormalities
- Thyroid function tests to rule out hyperthyroidism
- Electrocardiogram
  - QRS complexes: irregular
  - PR interval: barely visible
  - P wave: absent

### 3.18.3  Treatment

- Patient unstable: synchronized cardioversion to reestablish normal sinus rhythm
- Patient stable: internal pacemaker
- Administer
  - Antiarrhymics to stabilize arrhythmia
    - Cordarone (amiodarone); digitalis (digoxin); Cardizem, Dilacor, Tiazac (diltiazem), Isoptin (verapamil)
  - After 72 hours administer:
    - Anticoagulant to decrease coagulation and reduce risk of thromboembolism
      - Heparin, Coumadin (warfarin), Fragmin (dalteparin), Lovenox (enoxaparin)

### 3.18.4  Intervention

- Limit activity to decrease cardiac workload.
- Indicate bed rest to decrease cardiac workload.
- Allow bathroom privileges.
- Monitor for hypoperfusion (cool extremities, increased heart rate, decreased pulse pressure, altered mentation).
- Instruct the patient
  - Contact the healthcare provider if dizziness develops.
  - Do not use nicotine, caffeine, or alcohol, as these can trigger arrhythmia.

## 3.19  Asystole

This is a result of cardiac standstill resulting in no circulation. Asystole can be caused by arrhythmia, cardiac tamponade, pulmonary embolism, sudden cardiac death, acute myocardial infarction, or hypovolemia (Figure 3.1).

### 3.19.1  Signs and Symptoms

- No blood pressure
- No pulse
- Apnea
- Cyanosis

### 3.19.2  Medical Tests

- Electrocardiogram: no wave

### 3.19.3  Treatment

- Cardiopulmonary resuscitation within two minutes
- Advanced cardiac life support within eight minutes
- Transcutaneous pacing
- Endotracheal intubation
- Administer
  - Buffering agent to correct acidosis
    - Sodium bicarbonate
  - Antiarrhythmics to control arrhythmia
    - Atropine, epinephrine, vasopressin, and amiodarone

### 3.19.4  Intervention

- Cardiopulmonary resuscitation

## 3.20  Ventricular Fibrillation

Erratic impulses cause ventricles to quiver, resulting in disruption of circulation. This is caused by electrolyte disturbances, drug toxicities, ventricular tachycardia, electric shock, or myocardial infarction (Figure 3.2).

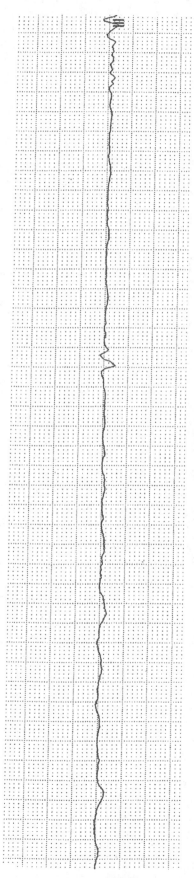

Figure 3.1 Asystole.

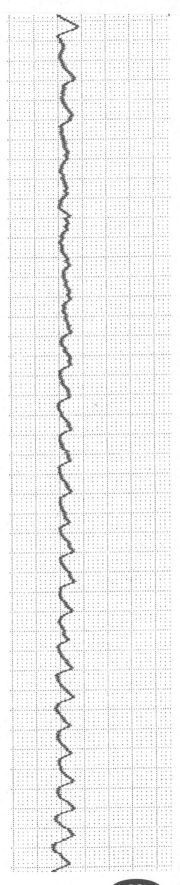

Figure 3.2 Ventricular fibrillation.

### 3.20.1   Signs and Symptoms

- Apnea
- No blood pressure
- No pulse

### 3.20.2   Medical Tests

- Electrocardiogram
  - P wave: not noticeable
  - Ventricular rhythm: chaotic
  - QRS complex: irregular and wide

### 3.20.3   Treatment

- Cardiopulmonary resuscitation
- Endotracheal intubation
- Advanced cardiac life support
- Defibrillation
- Administration of
  - Buffering agent to correct acidosis
    - Sodium bicarbonate
  - Antiarrhythmics to control arrhythmia
    - Vasopressin, epinephrine, lidocaine, and amiodarone

### 3.20.4   Intervention

- Cardiopulmonary resuscitation
- Defibrillation

## 3.21   Ventricular Tachycardia

Erratic impulses cause ventricles to contract more than 160 beats per minute, resulting in inadequate filling of the ventricles and decreased cardiac output. This is caused by mitral valve prolapse, coronary artery disease, and acute myocardial infarction. It can suddenly start and stop (Figure 3.3).

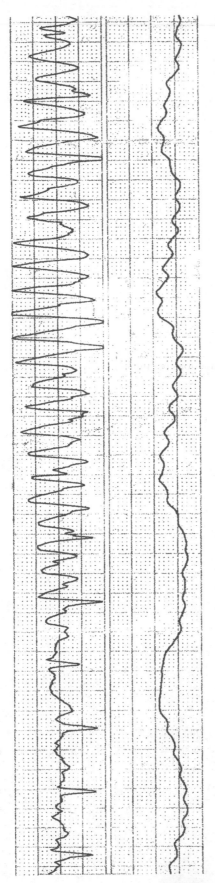

Figure 3.3 Ventricular tachycardia.

### 3.21.1   Signs and Symptoms

- Hypotension due to decreased circulation
- Decreased pulse due to insufficient heart rate
- Decreased breathing
- Dizziness due to decreased oxygenation of blood
- State of unconsciousness
- Apnea

### 3.21.2   Medical Tests

- Electrocardiogram
  - P wave: not noticeable
  - Rhythm: chaotic, >160 bpm
  - QRS complex: abnormal
- Ventricular tachycardia may suddenly start and stop depending on the irritability of the heart.
- Ventricle contracts greater than 160 contractions per minute.

### 3.21.3   Treatment

Treatment consists of establishing a regular rate and rhythm.

- Cardiopulmonary resuscitation
- Endotracheal intubation
- Advanced cardiac life support
- Synchronized cardioversion
- Administer
  - Buffering agent to correct acidosis
    - Sodium bicarbonate
  - Antiarrhythmics to control arrhythmia
    - Vasopressin, epinephrine, lidocaine, procainamide

### 3.21.4   Intervention

- Cardiopulmonary resuscitation
- Synchronized cardioversion

## 3.22   Cardiac Arrest

Cardiac arrest is a condition where the heart is unable to properly circulate blood, resulting in malfunction of cardiac muscle. Ineffective circulation of atrial blood leads to decreased oxygenation of tissues and organs throughout the body, resulting in necrosis, which is dead tissue.

**TABLE 3.3  Common Causes of Cardiac Arrest**

| Acidosis | Hypovolemia | Hypoxia | Hypo/hyperkalemia |
|---|---|---|---|
| Hypoglycemia | Hypothermia | Toxins | Cardiac tamponade |
| Tension pneumothorax | Thrombosis | Trauma | |

Cardiac muscle malfunction can be caused by many underlying conditions that include myocardial infarction, overdose of medication, trauma, respiratory arrest, and improper impulses leading to ventricular fibrillation (ventricles quiver) or ventricular tachycardia (ventricles beat very fast).

Treatment for cardiac arrest depends on staff certification. There are two types of certifications. These are basic life support (BLS) and advanced cardiac life support (ACLS). Basic life support focuses on cardiopulmonary resuscitation and the use of the automated external defibrillator (AED). Advanced life support focuses on recognizing ECG patterns and administering medication and/or manually defibrillating the patient.

The treatment of cardiac arrest differs if the cardiac rhythm is shockable or not shockable. An AED or manual defibrillator is used to send an electrical impulse through the patient's chest to the heart. The impulse stops the heart suddenly, causing the natural pacemaker cells of the heart to reestablish a normal rhythm. However, if the natural pacemaker is not functioning, then the heart is not shocked. The ECG depicts the cardiac wave form that determines if the natural pacemaker cells are functioning. The AED analyzes the wave to determine if this is a shockable wave or not. Advanced cardiac life support staff reviews the ECG to determine if the wave is shockable (see 3.22.2 Advanced Cardiac Life Support).

As CPR and advanced cardiac life support are performed, look for common causes of cardiac arrest (Table 3.3). Treating the underlying cause may return the patient to normal cardiac function.

## 3.22.1  Basic Life Support

Basic life support requires the following algorithm to be performed when presented with a patient who has had a sudden loss of consciousness and respirations are absent. This algorithm is provided by the American Heart Association. Consult with the American Heart Association for updates on this algorithm.

Be sure to push hard and fast, 100 compressions per minute, allowing full chest recoil. One cycle is 30 compressions to two breaths if there is no advanced airway. There should be five cycles every two minutes. Rotate with another person every five cycles.

- **Step 1:** try arousing the patient by calling the patient by name and rubbing the upper portion of the sternum.
- **Step 2:** call 911 or send someone to activate the emergency response system.
- **Step 3:** get an AED or send someone to get an AED.
- **Step 4:** if no response, check for a pulse, lightly feeling the carotid artery for a minimum of five seconds and a maximum of ten seconds.
- **Step 5:** bare the patient's chest and position hands for CPR.
- **Step 6:** deliver first cycle of compressions: 100 compressions per minute at a depth of at least two inches. Allow complete recoil between compressions. Rotate doing compressions every two minutes. Limit interruptions for less than ten seconds.
- **Step 7:** open the airway. Tilt the head back if there is no sign of trauma. If there is a sign of trauma then use a jaw thrust to open the airway.
- **Step 8:** administer two breaths per 30 compressions. Make sure the chest rises.
- **Step 9:** attach AED leads to patient and follow AED's voice instructions.

## 3.22.2  Advanced Cardiac Life Support

Advanced cardiac life support (ACLS) is used when the patient experiences cardiac arrest and requires external electric stimulation and/or medication to reestablish cardiac function. Advanced cardiac life support is performed by staff that are ACLS certified and who are permitted to perform advanced cardiac life support within their scope of practice.

Advanced cardiac life support requires the algorithm in Table 3.4 be performed when presented with a patient who has had a sudden loss of consciousness and who does not have a pulse. This algorithm is provided by the American Heart Association. Consult with the American Heart Association for updates on this algorithm.

**TABLE 3.4  Advanced Cardiac Life Support Algorithm**

**STEP 1**

Continue CPR.

Administer oxygen.

Attach cardiac monitor.

**STEP 2**

Is there a shockable rhythm?

| **STEP 9 NOT SHOCKABLE** | **STEP 3 SHOCKABLE** |
|---|---|
| Asystole/PEA | Ventricular fibrillation |
| | Ventricular tachycardia |
| **STEP 10** | **STEP 4** |
| Give five cycles of CPR over two minutes. | Set manual biphasic defibrillator to device- specific setting. If unknown, set to 200 joules. |
| Open IV/IO access. | Set monophasic defibrillator to 360 joules. |
| During CPR: | Call "clear." |
| • Give epinephrine 1 mg IV/VO. | Give one shock. |
| • Wait three to five minutes. | Give five cycles of CPR. |
| • Give epinephrine 1 mg IV/VO. | |
| • Wait three to five minutes. | |
| • Give epinephrine 1 mg IV/VO. | |
| Or, | |
| • Give vasopressin 40 units IV/IO (can replace first or second dose of epinephrine). | |
| If asystole or slow PEA rate: | |
| • Give atropine 1 mg IV/IO. | |
| • Wait three to five minutes. | |
| • Give atropine 1 mg IV/IO. | |
| • Wait three to five minutes. | |
| • Give atropine 1 mg IV/IO. | |
| • Give five cycles of CPR. | |

*(Continued)*

**TABLE 3.4 Advanced Cardiac Life Support Algorithm (*Continued*)**

| STEP 11 | | STEP 5 | |
|---|---|---|---|
| Is there a shockable rhythm? | | Is there a shockable rhythm? | |
| **STEP 12 NOT SHOCKABLE** | **STEP 13 SHOCKABLE** | **NOT SHOCKABLE** | **STEP 6 SHOCKABLE** |
| If asystole, go to Step 10. | Go to Step 4. | Go to Step 12. | Call "clear." |
| If electrical activity, check pulse. | | | Give one shock. |
| • If no pulse, go to Step 10. | | | Give five cycles of CPR over two minutes. |
| • If pulse, begin post-resuscitation treatment. | | | During CPR IV/IO give first dose of epinephrine 1 mg. |
| | | | Wait three to five minutes and give second dose of epinephrine 1 mg. |
| | | | Or, |
| | | | Give one dose of vaspopressin 40 units IV/IO. |

**STEP 7**

Is there a shockable rhythm?

**STEP 8 SHOCKABLE**

Call "clear."

Give one shock.

Give five cycles of CPR over two minutes.

Give during CPR IV/IO Amidarone 300 mg IV/IO

If, no conversion:

• Give Amidarone 150 mg IV/IO.

Go to Step 5.

## 3.23 Bradycardia Treatment

Bradycardia is a condition where the heart beats slowly, reducing circulation and resulting in decreased oxygenation of tissues and organs. The American Heart Association recommends the following interventions when treating bradycardia (See Figure 3.4 and Table 3.5).

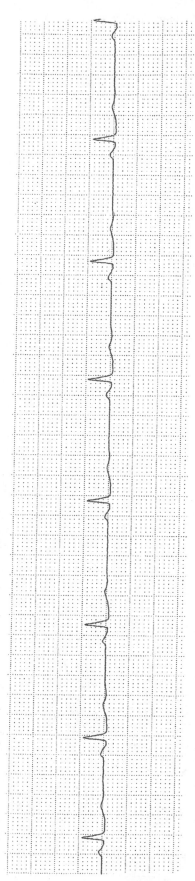

Figure 3.4 Sinus bradycardia.

**TABLE 3.5 Advanced Cardiac Life Support Algorithm for Bradycardia**

| STEP 1 |
| --- |

Maintain a patent airway.

Assist with breathing.

Administer oxygen.

Monitor ECG 12 lead.

Monitor vital signs.

Monitor oximetry.

Establish perfusion.

Monitor signs of perfusion (shock):

- Altered mental state
- Chest pain
- Hypotension

| STEP 2 | STEP 3 |
| --- | --- |
| Adequate Perfusion | If poor perfusion caused by bradycardia, then go to Step 4.<br><br>If poor perfusion not caused by bradycardia, then monitor and observe. |

| STEP 4 | STEP 5 |
| --- | --- |
| Continue monitoring. | Give atropine 0.5 mg.<br><br>If ineffective, repeat. No more than 3 mg.<br><br>Give epinephrine 2 to 10 mcg per minute, or give dopamine 2 to 10 mcg/kg per minute. |

| STEP 6 | STEP 7 |
| --- | --- |
| Treat underlying cause. | If Type II second-degree heart block or third-degree heart block, administer transcutaneous pacing.<br><br>Otherwise, administer transvenous pacing. |

| | STEP 8 |
| --- | --- |
| | Treat underlying cause. |

## 3.24 Fibrinolytic Therapy

Fibrinolytic therapy is used to remove all or a portion of an existing blood clot, resulting in normal blood flow 50% of the time using tPA, reteplase, tenecteplase, or streptokinase. Table 3.6 contains the fibrinolytic checklist used to determine if the patient is a candidate for fibrinolytic therapy.

**TABLE 3.6  Fibrinolytic Checklist**

| ADMINISTER FIBRNOLYTIC THERAPY | DON'T ADMINISTER FIBRNOLYTIC THERAPY | |
|---|---|---|
| Ischemic chest pain | Patient presents more than 12 hours after onset of symptoms. | INR >1.7 <br> PT >15 <br> Platelet count >100,000 <br> Systolic BP >185 |
| Persistent ST segment elevation more than 1 mm in two or more contiguous chest or limb leads | Arterial puncture at a non-compressible site within past 7 days | Warfarin in use by patient |
| Onset of symptoms within 12 hours of presentation and positive ECG waves | Active internal bleeding | Patient received heparin within the past 48 hours. |
| Onset of symptoms within 12 hours and positive posterior MI (ST segment depression in early precordial leads) | Witnessed seizure at time of stroke | Acute trauma |
| 18 years or older | Intracranial hemorrhage assessed with non-contrast head CT | Subarachnoid hemorrhage |
| Ischemic stroke with measurable neurologic deficit | History of intracranial hemorrhage | Arteriovenous malformation |
| <3 hours since patient seemed normal | | |

## 3.25  Acute Stroke

A stroke is referred to as a cerebrovascular accident (CVA) that occurs when there is disturbance in the blood supply to the brain resulting in neurological disturbance. The disturbance can be caused by a blockage that leads to an ischemia, a hemorrhage, or an unknown cause. Decreased blood flow can result in tissue damage in the affected area of the brain. Depending on the area affected, the patient can experience:

- Weakness in the face, arm, or leg, typically on one side of the body
- Confusion
- Difficulty speaking
- Difficulty understanding
- Vision problems
- Dizziness
- Coordination problems
- Severe headache from unknown cause

A patient can experience a transient ischemic attack (TIA), commonly called a ministroke. A TIA is a brief disturbance of the blood supply. Symptoms resolve once blood supply returns. There is no tissue necrosis (infarction). A patient can also experience a silent stroke where there are no outward symptoms of a stroke. A silent stroke causes lesions on the brain that are identified using an MRI.

TABLE 3.7  Cincinnati Pre-Hospital Stroke Scale

THREE SIGNS INDICATE AN ACUTE STROKE

| SIGN | TEST | POSITIVE RESULT |
|---|---|---|
| Facial droop | Patient shows teeth. | One side of the patient's face doesn't move as well as other side of the face. |
| Arm drift | Patient extends both arms, palms up, for 10 seconds. | One arm moves down. |
| Abnormal speech | Patient says, "You can't teach an old dog new tricks." | The patient is unable to speak or words are slurred. |

TABLE 3.8  Los Angeles Pre-Hospital Stroke Scale

| CATEGORY | SIGN |
|---|---|
| Age | >45 years of age |
| History | No history of epilepsy or seizures |
| Duration | Symptoms started within the past 24 hours. |
| Ambulatory | Patient is not bedridden or in wheelchair. |
| Blood glucose | Between 60 and 400 |
| Face | Droop |
| Grip | Weak or no grip |
| Arm | Drifts down |

All signs present indicates an acute stroke.

An acute stroke occurs when the patient suddenly shows signs of a stroke. It is critical that the patient receive treatment immediately in order to minimize the effect of the stroke and to reduce tissue necrosis. There are two pre-hospital stroke assessments. These are the Cincinnati Pre-Hospital Stroke Scale (CPSS) (see Table 3.7) and the Los Angeles Pre-Hospital Stroke Scale (LAPSS) (see Table 3.8).

Table 3.9 is the algorithm recommended by the American Heart Association to treat an acute stroke.

## 3.26  Acute Coronary Syndrome

An acute coronary syndrome is reported by the patient as chest discomfort and described as uncomfortable pressure that may extend to the jaw, neck, between the shoulder blades, shoulders, and arms. The patient may experience shortness of breath, nausea, sweating, and light-headedness that may result in fainting. The acute coronary syndrome may or may not result in chest pain.

Based on these signs and symptoms, the American Heart Association recommends treatment using the algorithm in Table 3.10.

### TABLE 3.9  Treating an Acute Stroke

**START**

Make sure airway, breathing, and circulation are patent.

Assess vital signs.

Administer oxygen.

Open IV access.

Gather blood samples.

Assess blood glucose levels.

Review patient's history.

Determine when symptoms first presented.

Administer an ECG.

**PERFORM CT SCAN OF THE BRAIN**

| NO HEMORRHAGE | | HEMORRHAGE |
|---|---|---|
| Assess if patient is a candidate for fibrinolytic therapy (see 3.24 Fibrinolytic Therapy). | | Consult neurologist/neurosurgeon. |

| YES | NO |
|---|---|
| Administer tPA or appropriate fibrinolytic. | Administer low-dose aspirin. |
| Do not administer anticoagulants or antiplatelet treatment for 24 hours. | Transfer to stroke unit for follow-up care. |

### TABLE 3.10  Advanced Cardiac Life Support Algorithm for Acute Coronary Syndrome

**START**

Monitor airway, breathing, and circulation.

Monitor vital signs.

Administer oxygen 4 liters per minute to maintain oxygen saturation level >90%.

If the patient shows no evidence of recent GI bleed, and

- If the patient does not have nausea, vomiting, or peptic ulcer, then administer aspirin 160 to 325 mg orally and ask the patient to chew the aspirin tablet to increase absorption time.

- If the patient has nausea, vomiting, or peptic ulcer, then administer aspirin 160 to 325 mg rectally.

If the patient is not experiencing hypotension, bradycardia, or tachycardia and has not taken Viagra or Levitra within 24 hours or Cialis within 48 hours and if the patient is hemodynamically stable, then administer nitroglycerin sublingual three doses each, three minutes apart.

If the patient is unresponsive to nitroglycerin, then administer morphine to reduce the left ventricular preload and cardiac oxygen requirements.

*(Continued)*

**TABLE 3.10  Advanced Cardiac Life Support Algorithm for Acute Coronary Syndrome (*Continued*)**

Administer a 12-lead ECG.

Open IV access.

Administer IV fluids if patient is hypotensive.

Perform fibrinolytic checklist (see 3.24 Fibrinolytic Therapy)

Draw blood sample for cardiac marker levels, electrolyte, and coagulation studies.

Administer a chest x-ray within 30 minutes of the patient's arrival.

**REVIEW ECG**

ST Elevation MI (STEMI)

or

Left Bundle Branch Block (LBBB)

**ADMINISTER**

Beta-adrenergic receptor blockers

Plavix

Heparin

If more than 12 hours from onset, then admit patient to the cardiac care unit.

If 12 hours or less from onset, then administer

- Fibrinolytic therapy (within 30 minutes)
- Percutaneous coronary intervention (PCI) to restore blood to the heart (within 90 minutes)
- ACE inhibitors
- HMB CoA reductase inhibitor

**UNSTABLE ANGINA NON-ST ELEVATION MI (UA/NSTEMI)**

**ADMINISTER**

Nitroglycerin

Beta-adrenergic receptor blockers

Glycoprotein IIb/IIIa inhibitor

Plavix

Admit patient to the cardiac care unit.

**NORMAL ST OR T WAVES**

If troponin positive, then administer

- Nitroglycerin
- Beta-adrenergic receptor blockers
- Glycoprotein IIb/IIIa inhibitor
- Plavix

If symptoms of ischemia or infarction persist, then

- Continue monitoring ECG
- Admit patient to the cardiac care unit

If troponin negative and no symptoms of ischemia or infarction, then discharge patient with appropriate follow-up care.

## 3.27  Cardiac Contusion

A cardiac contusion is a blunt trauma injury to the chest that results in bruising of the myocardium, typically the right ventricle.

### 3.27.1  Signs and Symptoms

- Precordial chest pain, due to bruising
- Bruising around the sternum, due to blunt trauma
- Shortness of breath, due to cardiac irritability
- Cardiac arrhythmias, due to cardiac irritability
- Bradycardia, due to cardiac irritability
- Tachycardia, due to cardiac irritability
- Murmurs, due to cardiac irritability
- Hemodynamic instability, due to cardiac irritability

### 3.27.2  Medical Tests

- Echocardiograph: to assess ejection fraction and ventricular viability
- Cardiac enzyme level: to assess CK-MB levels and injury to cardiac muscle
- Cardiac troponin I levels: to assess injury to cardiac muscle
- Electrocardiograph: to assess cardiac rhythm

### 3.27.3  Treatment

- Administer
  - IV fluids to provide hemodynamic stability (systolic blood pressure >90 mm Hg)
  - Digoxin for signs of cardiac failure
  - Lidocaine for ventricular arrhythmias
  - Inotropic medication to increase cardiac output
  - Oxygen

### 3.27.4  Intervention

- Monitor electrocardiograph.
- Assess vital signs each hour until patient is stable, monitoring for decreased peripheral tissue perfusion.
- Assess respiration, monitoring for signs of congestion.
- Assess urine output (1 ml/kg per hour).
- Raise head of bed 30 degrees.

## Solved Problems

**3.1**    What is a cardiovascular emergency?

A cardiovascular emergency is a condition that has the potential of disrupting circulation throughout the patient's body resulting in decreased blood flow to organs and causing malfunction of other systems in the body.

**3.2**    What is the distinction between a cardiac emergency and respiratory arrest?

If the patient has a blood pressure but is not breathing, then the patient is in respiratory arrest. There is no cardiac emergency, although respiratory arrest can lead to a cardiac emergency if rescue breathing is not administered.

**3.3**    What are the signs of thrombosis?

The patient experiences pain in the area, coughing, swelling below the blood clot, and decreased circulation below the blood clot.

**3.4**    What are the goals of treating a cardiovascular emergency?

- The goal of the emergency department staff is to stabilize the patient—not to treat the underlying cause of the problem.

- Maintain airway, respiratory functions, and circulation.

- Diagnose the acute problem. For example, the acute problem might be hypertensive crisis, not the underlying cause of the hypertensive crisis.

- Stabilize the patient by relieving pain and treating the acute problem. For example, administer medication to decrease hypertension immediately.

- Refer the patient to follow-up care to treat the underlying cause of the problem.

**3.5**    What should the healthcare provider do if the patient becomes unstable during the assessment?

The healthcare provider should stop the assessment and stabilize the patient.

**3.6**    How should the healthcare provider phrase questions during the patient assessment?

Questions should be short and to the point, enabling the patient to answer "yes" or "no."

**3.7**    What questions would the healthcare provider ask to assess pain?

- Where is the pain?

- On a scale of 1 to 10, how bad is the pain?

- Is the pain burning, tight, or squeezing?

- Does the pain radiate?

- When did the pain become noticeable?

- What were you doing before you noticed the pain?

- What aggravates the pain?

- What relieves the pain?

**3.8**   What are common signs of decreased oxygenation?

Dizziness, shortness of breath, irritability, and low level of consciousness are signs of decreased oxygenation.

**3.9**   What are signs of right-side heart failure?

Bilateral swelling of ankles and feet or frequently urinating at night are signs of right-side heart failure.

**3.10**   What might be a cause of heart pounding?

Hypoxia may be a cause.

**3.11**   Why would difficulty awakening indicate a cardiovascular problem?

Difficulty awakening can be caused by hypoxia related to decreased circulation and caused by a cardiovascular problem.

**3.12**   What might cause clubbing of fingers?

Chronic deoxygenation of blood may cause clubbing of fingers.

**3.13**   What might cause decreased distribution of hair on arms and legs?

Decreasde arterial circulation to the area may be the cause.

**3.14**   What might it mean if the capillary refill time is greater than three seconds?

Decreased peripheral circulation may be the cause.

**3.15**   Why should the healthcare provider compare carotid arteries?

Both pulses should be symmetric and equal; otherwise there may be decreased circulation through one of the carotid arteries.

**3.16**   What might an increased peripheral pulse indicate?

Increased peripheral vascular resistance may be indicated.

**3.17**   What might the healthcare provider suspect if he or she hears S3 heart sounds?

S3 heart sounds might indicate myocardial infarction, left- or right-side heart failure, intracardiac blood shunting, pulmonary congestion, hyperthyroidism, or anemia.

**3.18**   What is a sign of left-side heart failure?

Pulmonary congestion is a sign of left-side heart failure.

**3.19**   What might it mean if bruits can be heard over the patient's abdominal region?

Bruits heard over the abdominal region may indicate an abdominal aorta aneurysm.

**3.20** What might the healthcare provider suspect if the patient reports sudden, sharp, continuous pain below the sternum that worsens when lying on his back or when he breathes deeply, but the pain reduces when the patient sits up and leans forward?

Pericarditis may be indicated.

**3.21** What would the healthcare provider suspect if the patient reports sudden, stabbing pain over the back that worsens on inspiration?

Pulmonary emboli may be indicated.

**3.22** A patient complains of having a heart attack. The patient reports sudden, severe pain on the left side of the chest with difficulty breathing. The healthcare provider notices a deviated trachea. What would she or he suspect is the problem?

Pneumothorax may be indicated.

**3.23** What would the healthcare provider suspect if the patient reports a sudden, severe tearing pain behind the sternum?

Dissecting aortic aneurysm may be indicated.

**3.24** What is the importance of the CPK-MB level?

CPK-MB is an enzyme found only in cardiac muscle and indicates that cardiac muscle tissue has been damaged.

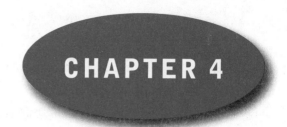

# CHAPTER 4

# *Respiratory Emergencies*

## 4.1  Define

- A respiratory emergency is a condition that alters gas exchange.

- Gas exchange can be disrupted by an obstruction, inflammation, or trauma to the respiratory system.

- A respiratory emergency can be life threatening.

- A respiratory arrest is a respiratory emergency where no gas is exchanged because the patient is not breathing.

- There is a distinction between a respiratory arrest and a cardiac emergency. If the patient has a blood pressure but is not breathing, then the patient is in respiratory arrest. There is no cardiac emergency, although respiratory arrest can lead to a cardiac emergency if rescue breathing is not administered.

- A respiratory emergency requires immediate intervention.

### 4.1.1  Goal of Treating Respiratory Emergencies

- The goal of the emergency-department staff is to identify the respiratory emergency and stabilize the patient's respiration, not to treat the underlying cause of the respiratory emergency, unless the staff is able to do so. For example, a patient experiencing an asthma attack will be referred to a primary-care provider for ongoing treatment. However, the emergency-department staff may prescribe medication self-administered through an inhaler for ongoing treatment and refer the patient to a primary-care healthcare provider.

- Maintain airway and respiratory functions.

- Diagnose the acute problem. For example, the acute problem might be an asthmatic attack, not the underlying cause of the asthmatic attack.

- Stabilize the patient by relieving pain and treating the acute problem. For example, administer bronchodilators and anti-inflammatory medication to relax smooth muscles around the bronchi and reduce inflammation of the bronchi for a patient experiencing an asthmatic attack.

- Refer the patient to follow-up care to treat the underlying cause of the problem.

### 4.1.2 Respiratory Assessment

- Assess airway, breathing, and circulation immediately. Begin cardiopulmonary resuscitation (see 3.22.1 Basic Life Support) if these are not patent.

- Assess for pending respiratory crisis.

  - Does the patient experience problems breathing?

  - Is the patient confused or agitated? Decreased oxygenation causes confusion and agitation.

  - Is the patient sweating (diaphoretic)? This is a sign of increased stress.

  - Is the patient cyanotic? This is a sign of decreased circulatory oxygenation.

  - Is the patient pale? This is a sign of decreased circulation.

  - Are the patient's shoulders elevated? This is a sign that the patient is using accessory muscles to supplement the diaphragm to breathe.

- Limit the assessment to identifying the problem area and then direct the assessment to that problem area.

- Stop the assessment if it is necessary to intervene to stabilize the patient.

- Ask the patient to describe the problem.

- Ask questions that help to quickly identify the problem. Questions should be short and to the point, enabling the patient to answer "yes" or "no." Remember that the patient is typically distressed and is anxious because the patient is experiencing an unusual problem that has not been identified.

  - Are you in pain? Pain might be a sign of pleural inflammation or soreness related to using chest muscles for coughing.

    - Where is the pain?

    - On a scale of 1 to 10, how bad is the pain?

    - Is the pain burning, tight, or squeezing?

    - Does the pain radiate?

    - When did the pain first become noticeable?

    - What were you doing before you noticed the pain?

    - What aggravates the pain?

    - What relieves the pain?

  - Do you have a cough? A cough is a reflex action where short bursts of air are expelled by the lungs to clear the breathing passages.

    - How long have you experienced the cough?

    - Has the cough changed?

    - Is the cough productive?

      - What color is the sputum?

      - Is the sputum liquid or thick?

      - Does the sputum contain blood?

      - How much sputum is produced (i.e., teaspoon)?

    - What time of day do you cough?

    - What aggravates the cough?

    - What relieves the cough?

- Do you have shortness of breath (dyspnea)? This is related to ineffective gas exchange typically associated with an underlying respiratory or cardiac condition and is measured using one of two dyspnea grading scales.

    - On a scale of 1 to 10 where 1 is no shortness of breath and 10 is the worst shortness of breath that you experienced, how would you rate your current shortness of breath?

    - On a scale of 0 to 4, how would you rate your current shortness of breath?

        □ 0 = no shortness of breath

        □ 1 = shortness of breath when walking up a small hill or walking fast on a level surface

        □ 2 = shortness of breath causing you to walk slower than others of the same age or to stop when walking to catch your breath

        □ 3 = shortness of breath causing you to stop every 100 yards to catch a breath

        □ 4 = shortness of breath when changing clothes preventing you from leaving your home

- Do you have shortness of breath when lying down (orthopnea)?

    - How many pillows do you use when sleeping? (Record the answer as two-pillow orthopnea, if the patient uses two pillows.)

- What aggravates the shortness of breath?

- What relieves the shortness of breath?

- Are you drowsy or irritable during the day? This is a sign of temporary stoppage of breathing during sleep (sleep apnea).

    - Do you sleep throughout the night?

    - Are you told that you snore?

- Do you have allergies?

    - What allergies?

    - Have you recently been exposed to the allergen?

    - How do you react when exposed to the allergen?

- Do you smoke?

    - How much do you smoke a day?

    - How long have you smoked?

- Are you exposed to secondary smoke?

    - How long have you been around secondary smoke?

- Do you have any respiratory disease?

- Are you currently or were you previously treated for respiratory disease?

- Were you exposed to environmental conditions that may have caused current respiratory condition?

- Are you immunocompromised?

- Inspection

    - Count the respirations. Normal respiration is between 10 and 20 respirations per minute.

    - Look for breathing patterns. A regular breathing pattern is even and unlabored. Signs are normal. Common abnormal breathing patterns are:

        - **Biot's respiration:** alternating deep, rapid breathing is followed by sudden apnea, indicating a problem with the central nervous system.

- **Cheyne–Strokes respiration:** a cycle of shallow to deep breathing is followed by up to 20 seconds of apnea. This pattern is normal during sleep for some patients. This pattern may indicate kidney or cardiac failure or problems with the central nervous system if the patient is awake.

  - Look for signs of cyanosis in extremities such as nail beds, tip of the nose, and ear lobes, which are indicators of deoxygenating of the blood possibly caused by inadequate gas exchange.

  - Look for clubbing of fingers, a possible sign of chronic deoxygenating of the blood.

  - Look for flaring of the nostrils, a sign of respiratory distress.

  - Look for pursing of lips, a sign that the patient is trying to control shortness of breath and improve ventilation because the airway is opened longer and decreases the effort to breathe.

  - Look for asymmetrical chest movement on inspiration and expiration. There should be little chest movement. Asymmetrical chest movement may indicate uncoordinated respiration and the use of accessory muscles to breathe.

  - Look for a displaced trachea, which may indicate a collapsed lung.

  - Look for signs of agitation, indicators of decreased oxygenation.

  - Look for elevated shoulders, a sign that the patient is using accessory muscles to assist in respiration.

  - Look for abnormal thoracic cavity, which may inhibit cardiac movement.

  - Look at the angle between the ribs and the sternum above the xiphoid process (costal angle). The angle should be less than 90 degrees. An angle 90 degrees or greater may indicate chronic expansion of the lungs related to chronic obstructive pulmonary disease (COPD).

- Palpation

  - Place the palms of hands lightly on the patient's bare back in the thoracic region—one hand over each lung.

  - Don't touch the patient with fingers.

  - Ask the patient to fold his arms across his chest to reposition scapulae away from the thoracic region.

  - Ask the patient to say "99" aloud several times.

  - Healthcare provider should feel vibrations (tactile fremitus).

    - No or little vibration is a sign of bronchial obstruction or fluid in pleural cavity (pleural effusion).

    - Intense vibration is a sign of tissue consolidation.

    - Less vibration is a sign of pleural effusion, emphysema, or pneumothorax.

  - Repeat the assessment on the front of the patient's chest.

    - Place hands on the front of the patient's chest.

    - Position thumbs in the second intercostal space.

    - Ask the patient to breathe normally.

    - Healthcare provider's thumbs should separate equally and simultaneously.

    - Thumbs separating asymmetrically indicate pleural effusion, pneumonia, pneumothorax, or atelectasis.

    - Decreased expansion at the diaphragm indicates emphysema, ascites, respiratory depression, paralysis of the diaphragm, obesity, or atelectasis.

  - Repeat the assessment on the patient's back with thumbs placed at the tenth rib.

- Percussion
  - Percuss the patient's lung fields by placing one finger on the patient and tapping the finger with a finger from the other hand, causing the patient's lung fields to vibrate.
  - On the front of the chest, begin at the upper right, then move left, down, and to the right. Continue this pattern until the end of the rib cage is reached.
  - On the back, move along the shoulder lines then move upper right, across to the right, down, and across to the left until the end of the rib cage is reached.
    - Hyperresonance indicates air in the lungs common in asthma, emphysema, and pneumothorax.
    - Hyporesonance (dull) indicates decreased air in the lungs common in atelectasis, pleural effusion, or tumor.
- Auscultation
  - Listen to air moving through the bronchi with a stethoscope.
  - Over the trachea
    - Normal: harsh, discontinuous sounds on inhalation and exhalation
  - On the front of the chest along the clavicle, begin at the upper right, then move left, down, and to the right. Continue this pattern until the end of the rib cage is reached (Figure 4.1).
  - On the back, move along the shoulder lines, then move upper right, across to the right, down and across to the left, until the end of the rib cage is reached.
  - Normal breath sounds
    - **Bronchial** (next to the trachea): high-pitched, loud, discontinuous, and loudest on exhalation
    - **Bronchovesicular** (between scapulae and upper sternum): medium-pitched, continuous on inhalation and exhalation
    - **Vesicular** (remaining lung area): low-pitched, soft, prolonged on inhalation, and short on exhalation
  - Abnormal breath sounds
    - **Crackles**: non-musical, intermittent sounds on inspiration, resembling a crackling sound related to air moving through secretions
    - **Fine crackles:** a sound like hair rubbing together
    - **Coarse crackles:** a sound like gurgling

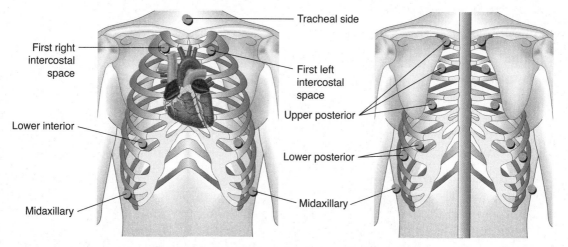

Figure 4.1 Auscultation sites to hear lung sounds.

- **Wheezes:** high-pitched sound on exhalation or inspiration related to blocked airflow

- **Rhonchi:** low-pitched sound, such as snoring on exhalation that alters when the patient coughs

- **Stridor:** high-pitched, loud sound during inspiration

- **Pleural friction rub:** painful, low-pitched grating sound on expiration and inspiration

○ Misplaced breath sounds are normal breath sounds heard in a different area of the lung. For example, normal bronchial sounds in the vesicular area indicate that the vesicular area contains fluid and no air is moving through the vesicular area.

○ Voice sounds are chest vibrations produced when the patient speaks. Listen to voice sounds with a stethoscope. Abnormal voice sounds are:

- **Egophony:** ask the patient to say "E"

  □ Normal: muffled

  □ If the lung area is dense (consolidated): sounds like the patient is saying "A"

- **Bronchophony:** ask the patient to say "99"

  □ Normal: muffled

  □ If the lung area is dense: loud

- **Whispered pectoriloquy:** ask the patient to whisper "1, 2, 3"

  □ Normal: unable to distinguish the numbers

  □ If the lung area is dense: numbers are loud and distinct

### 4.1.2.1  Signs and Symptoms

Respiratory assessment in an emergency situation requires the nurse to recognize common signs and symptoms of underlying causes and then prepare for the anticipated treatment that the practitioner is likely to order. Commonly seen signs and symptoms:

- Stridor (high-pitched wheezing) on inspiration and seesawing or abdominal breathing:

  ○ Upper airway obstruction

  ○ Croup (children)

    - Nebulized epinephrine

    - Corticosteroids

    - Anaphylaxis

    - IM epinephrine—self-administered auto-injection

    - Albuterol

    - Antihistamine

    - Corticosteroids

  ○ Aspiration of foreign body

    - Position the patient for comfort

    - Call the practitioner

- Stridor (high-pitched wheezing) on expiration:
    - Lower airway obstruction
        - Asthma (see 4.6 Asthma)
        - Bronchitis (see 4.9 Bronchitis)
- Rapid respiration rate and grunting
    - Lung tissue disease
        - Pneumonia (see 4.13 Pneumonia)
        - Pulmonary edema (see 4.5 Acute Respiratory Distress Syndrome)
            - Automatic mechanical ventilation
            - Diuretic medication
- Disordered control over breathing
    - Increased intracranial pressure
    - Medication overdose
    - Poisoning
    - Neuromuscular disorder

### 4.1.2.2    Pediatric Respiratory Assessment

At times infants and children are unable to voice symptoms of respiratory disorders; however, there are signs that indicate a respiratory problem. Here are some common signs of respiratory problems in infants and children.

- Decreased oxygen level
    - Irritable
    - Agitated
    - Decreased response
    - Listless
    - Cyanotic
- Difficulty catching breath or working to breathe
    - Nasal flaring indicating respiratory distress
    - Increased respiration indicating inadequate perfusion
    - Sepsis shock (wide pulse pressure)
- Respiratory pauses
    - Disordered control of breathing
- Pale skin
    - Hypoxemia
    - Hypercarbia
    - Increased vascular resistance

- Change in voice or difficulty breathing on inspiration
  - Upper airway obstruction
    - Inability to speak more than one word at a time or prolonged forced exhalation
  - Lower airway obstruction
- Grunting or strange breathing
  - Lung tissue disorder
  - Respiratory failure
- Snoring on inspiration
  - Tongue occlusion
  - Floppy pharynx
- Crackles at the base of the lungs
  - Cardiac shock

## 4.2   Respiratory Tests

Respiratory tests are designed to assess the effectiveness of gas exchange and the capability of the respiratory system to function. Some respiratory tests are also used to assess the structural patency of the respiratory system. Emergency-department healthcare providers order respiratory tests, and those results are used to assess and assist the healthcare team in stabilizing the patient. Once stabilized, the patient is transferred or referred for follow-up care designed to treat the underlying cause of the current episode, which may require additional respiratory tests. The following are tests commonly ordered by the emergency department's healthcare providers.

### 4.2.1   Pulse Oximetry

Pulse oximetry measures the saturation of oxygen in arterial blood by using infrared light passed through a finger, toe, earlobe, or the bridge of the nose. A sensor within the pulse oximeter assesses the color absorbed by arterial blood. The tests assess the saturation of oxygen without the need for arterial blood gas (ABG) test. Don't perform the test if the patient is suspected of having carbon-monoxide poisoning. Carbon monoxide adheres to hemoglobin and is recorded as oxygen by the pulse oximeter device. In cases of suspected carbon-monoxide poisoning, use arterial blood gas to assess oxygen saturation.

- Assess the patient's pulse prior to administering pulse oximetry.
- Perform test intermittently or continuously.
- Rotate the pulse oximetry site every four hours if used continuously.
- Be aware that some pulse oximetry devices have an audible alarm that sounds when arterial blood saturation levels fall to an abnormal range.
- Always record if the patient was on room air or oxygen when the test was performed. If the patient was on oxygen, then note the dose and the delivery method (i.e., nasal cannula).
- Compare pulse displayed on the device with the pulse that healthcare provider manually assessed prior to the test. If there is a material difference, then reposition the pulse oximeter and take another reading.
- Pulse oximetry results are within 2% of saturation results reported from an arterial blood gas test.

- The oxygen saturation level of arterial blood is displayed as a percentage of oxygen to hemoglobin. 100% means that 100% of hemoglobin in the arterial blood contains oxygen.

- Normal:
    - 95% to 100%

- Abnormal:
    - Below 95% may indicate abnormal gas exchange
    - Patients with COPD or other lung disorders may have consistently abnormal saturation that is consider normal for that patient. Saturations lower than the patient's abnormal "normal" saturation level may indicate that the lung disorder has worsened.

- If the oxygen saturation level is abnormal, then assess the patient for factors that may interfere with the test.
    - Fingernail polish
    - Acrylic finger nails
    - Excessive ambient light
    - Hypotension
    - High bilirubin levels in the blood
    - Patient movement during the test
    - Administration of vasoconstrictors

## 4.2.2   Arterial Blood Gas (ABG)

The arterial blood gas is a test where an arterial blood sample is taken from the patient and assessed for oxygen ($Pao_2$), carbon dioxide ($Paco_2$), bicarbonate ($HCO_3-$), saturation oxygen ($Sao_2$), and pH levels in the blood. Normal ranges are:

| | |
|---|---|
| $Pao_2$ | 80 to 100 mm Hg |
| $Paco_2$ | 35 to 45 mm Hg |
| $HCO_3-$ | 22 to 26 mEq/L |
| $Sao_2$ | 95% to 100% of hemoglobin |
| pH | 7.35 to 7.45 |

The pH value measures the concentration of hydrogen ions in arterial blood. A value greater than 7.45 indicates acidosis, and a value lower than 7.35 indicate alkalosis. The patient's blood must be within normal limits to be considered stabilized. Abnormal values indicate that the patient's body is trying to reestablish the acid-base (alkalosis) balance by having the metabolic system work together with the respiratory system to compensate for the acid-base imbalance.

The imbalance can be caused by a problem with the respiratory system. This is referred to as respiratory acidosis or respiratory alkalosis. The imbalance can also be caused by a problem with the metabolic system. This is referred to as metabolic acidosis or metabolic alkalosis. The results of the arterial blood gas can help identify the underlying cause as shown in Table 4.1.

It is important that any supplemental oxygen administered to the patient shortly before or when the sample is taken is noted on the sample documentation. This enables the lab to adjust the results accordingly.

Since the sample is taken from an artery, it is necessary to apply pressure to the puncture site for 5 minutes and apply a pressure dressing for 30 minutes once the bleeding stops. The site then needs to be monitored regularly to ensure there is no residual bleeding or the formation of a hematoma.

**TABLE 4.1 Acid-Base Values**

| | pH | Paco$_2$ | HCO$_3$- | SIGNS | CAUSES |
|---|---|---|---|---|---|
| Respiratory acidosis (too much carbon dioxide retained) | <7.35 | >45 mm Hg | >26 mEq/L (metabolic system compensating) | Flushed face Sweating Restlessness Tachycardia Headache | Hypoventilation Asphyxia Decreased central nervous system function Acute/chronic lung disease Sedatives Trauma Neuromuscular disease |
| Respiratory alkalosis (too little carbon dioxide retained) | >7.45 | <35 mm Hg | <22 mEq/L | Anxiety Rapid, deep breathing Light-headedness | Hyperventilation Gram-negative bacteria infection Increased respiratory function related to medication Anxiety Liver failure Sepsis |
| Metabolic acidosis (too little bicarbonate retained) | <7.35 | <35 mm Hg (respiratory system compensating) | <22 mEq/L (metabolic system compensating) | Drowsiness Vomiting Nausea Rapid, deep breathing Fruity breath Headache | Diarrhea Hyperkalemia Renal disease Hepatic disease Medication Intoxication Shock Endocrine disorder |
| Metabolic alkalosis (too much bicarbonate retained) | >7.45 | >45 mm Hg (respiratory system compensating) | >26 mEq/L | Ringing in the ear Confusion Slow, shallow breathing Irritability | Vomiting Gastric suctioning Steroid administration Diuretic therapy Decreased potassium levels (hypokalemia) |

### 4.2.3 End-Tidal Carbon Dioxide Monitor

End-tidal carbon dioxide monitoring (Figure 4.2) uses infrared light to measure carbon dioxide concentration in gas expired from the patient's breath. The end-tidal carbon dioxide monitor is connected to the patient's airway or endotracheal tube. The measurement is typically displayed as a wave form on a monitor along with other vital signs and can signal the first sign that the patient is having difficulty breathing.

- Normal end-tidal carbon dioxide value is between 35 to 45 mm Hg and is usually 2 to 5 mm Hg lower than the corresponding arterial blood gas value.

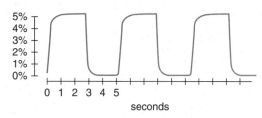

Figure 4.2  Normal wave form from end-tidal carbon dioxide monitoring.

- >10% end-tidal carbon dioxide value indicates an increase in carbon dioxide possibly caused by respiratory depression or partial airway obstruction.

- <10% end-tidal carbon dioxide value indicates decreased carbon dioxide, possibly caused by dislodged ventilator or endotracheal tube or complete airway obstruction.

### 4.2.4   Bronchoscopy

Bronchoscopy is a procedure that enables the healthcare provider to view the patient's larynx, trachea, and bronchi through the use of a bronchoscope. The bronchoscope is a flexible tube that uses fiber optics to display images of the respiratory structure. The healthcare provider uses the bronchoscope to remove airway obstructions, including mucus, tumors, and foreign bodies. The bronchoscope is also used to obtain specimens for further testing.

**Bronchoscopy Procedure**

- Administer atropine to decrease secretions.

- Administer midazolam (Versed) or other sedative and antianxiety medication to help relax the patient.

- Administer a topical anesthetic to the nasopharynx, vocal cords, and trachea to suppress the gagging reflex.

- Administer oxygen.

- Monitor vital signs.

- Insert the bronchoscope through the mouth or nose.

- Suction as necessary.

- Remove the obstruction or sample.

- After the bronchoscope is removed, raise the head of the bed 30 degrees or place the patient on his or her side.

- The patient must refrain from taking anything by mouth until the gag response returns.

- Test for the return of the gag response.

- Monitor the patient's vital signs until the gag response returns.

### 4.2.5   Sputum Analysis

Sputum is mucus produced when the patient coughs and can contain microorganisms if the patient is experiencing a respiratory infection. Sputum can also contain abnormal lung cells. Sputum analysis is the procedure to identify cells or microorganisms in the sputum. The color of the sputum may provide a clue as to the underlying infection.

- Bloody may indicate tuberculosis.

- Rusty may indicate pneumonia.

- Yellow-green may indicate a bacterial infection.

- Frothy pink may indicate pulmonary edema.

- Foamy white may indicate edema or a respiratory obstruction.

- White or opaque (milky) may indicate an infection other than bacterial, such as a viral infection.

**Sputum Collection Procedure**

- The patient takes three deep breaths and forces a deep cough to produce the sputum.

- Sputum is collected in a sterile container; otherwise the contaminants in the container may affect the results of the study.

- Saliva is bubbly (froth) and has a thinner consistency than sputum and should not be collected.

### 4.2.6   Chest X-Ray

During a chest x-ray, x-ray particles are beamed through the patient's chest onto a photographic film or to a computer. Dense structures such as bone block x-ray particles, causing those structures to appear white. Less-dense structures such as fluid, foreign bodies, tumors, and infiltrate block some x-ray particles, causing those structures to appear gray. Lung tissue does not block x-ray particles and appears dark.

Two common reasons healthcare providers use a chest x-ray to assess the lungs are

- To determine if there is fluid, foreign bodies, tumors, scarring, or infiltrate in the lungs

- To compare the current chest x-ray to previous chest x-rays to assess changes that may indicate if the disorder has improved or has worsened

**Chest X-Ray Procedure**

- Be sure that the patient is not pregnant.

- Remove all jewelry in the thoracic area, since jewelry may appear on the x-ray image.

- Assess if the patient has scars in the thoracic area. If so, note the location of the scars since the scars may appear on the x-ray image.

- Instruct the patient to remove clothes above the waist. Provide the patient with a gown.

- Instruct the patient to stand or sit in front of the x-ray machine. An x-ray can also be taken while the patient lies down on the x-ray plate.

- Ask the patient to hold his or her breath while the x-ray is taken.

- Multiple views of the patient's thoracic area may be taken.

- The initial result, called a "wet read," provides a relatively superficial assessment of the image. A more thorough reading is taken hours or days later.

### 4.2.7   Thoracic CT Scan

A thoracic CT scan provides a three-dimensional image of the lung using x-rays, enabling the healthcare provider to visualize normal and abnormal structures within the respiratory system. A CT can be performed with or without a contrast agent. A contrast agent is iodine-based and enhances images of blood vessels and less-dense areas of the respiratory system.

**Thoracic CT Scan Procedure**

- Assess if the patient is allergic to iodine or shellfish if the patient is undergoing a CT scan with contrast. Patients who are allergic to iodine or shellfish have a high likelihood to experience an allergic reaction to the contrast agent.

- Administer diphenhydramine (Benadryl) and prednisone (Deltasone) before the CT scan to reduce the risk of an allergic reaction to the contrast agent if the contrast agent is ordered.

- Administer the contrast agent through an IV. The patient may feel flushed and have a salty or metallic taste in his or her mouth.

- Explain to the patient that the contrast material typically discolors the urine for upward of 24 hours following the CT scan. The patient should increase fluid intake after the CT scan to flush the contrast agent from the patient's body, if the contrast agent is used for the CT scan.

- Assess if the patient is claustrophobic. The patient will be placed in an enclosure during the test.

- Assess if the patient can remain still for 30 minutes during the CT scan. The CT scanner encircles the patient for up to 30 minutes.

### 4.2.8   Thoracic MRI Scan

A thoracic magnetic resonance imaging (MRI) provides a three-dimensional view of the respiratory system using radio waves, a strong magnet, and a computer. An MRI is particularly used to assess fluid-filled soft tissue and to identify tumors from other structures within the thoracic area.

**Thoracic MRI Procedure**

- Remove all metal from the patient. No metal must enter the room containing the MRI scanner. The MRI scanner's magnet is always activated.

- Assess if the patient is claustrophobic. If so, then ask the healthcare provider if an open MRI scanner should be used for the test or if the patient should be sedated before the scan begins.

- Instruct the patient that the thoracic MRI scan takes about 30 minutes.

- Instruct the patient that the thoracic MRI scan is noninvasive. The patient will not feel any discomfort.

### 4.2.9   Ventilation Perfusion Scan

A ventilation perfusion scan assesses the respiratory system's ventilation capacity and perfusion capacity and is used as a less risky alternative to the pulmonary angiograph when evaluating pulmonary function. This test is done to determine if there is abnormal blood flow or a blood clot in the lungs. However, this test is not performed if the patient is on a mechanical ventilator since it is difficult to perform the ventilation element of the test with a ventilator. The pulmonary angiography is performed in lieu of the ventilation perfusion scan if the patient is on a mechanical ventilator.

The elements of the ventilation perfusion scan are

- **Ventilation:** this element determines the ability of air to reach all parts of the lungs.

- **Perfusion:** this element determines how well blood circulates within the lungs.

**Ventilation Perfusion Scan Procedure**

- Assess if the patient is allergic to contrast medium (i.e., iodine, shellfish).

- Keep emergency resuscitation equipment and medication (diphenhydramine [Benadryl] and prednisone [Deltasone]) on hand.

- Place a mask over the patient's nose and mouth for the ventilation portion. The patient breathes gas that contains contrast material, and air and the lungs are scanned.

- Instruct the patient to lie on a moveable table as contrast material is infused by IV while the lungs are scanned.

- Following the test instruct the patient to remain on bed rest, during which vital signs are monitored.

- Signs of adverse reaction to contrast material are:

  - Tachypnea

  - Restlessness

  - Urticaria

  - Respiratory distress

  - Nausea and vomiting

  - Tachycardia

## 4.2.10    Pulmonary Angiograph

Pulmonary angiograph (pulmonary arteriography) is an x-ray imaging test that uses radioactive contrast dye to assess pulmonary circulation and identify abnormal blood flow in the lungs. A pulmonary angiograph has a higher risk than the ventilation perfusion scan because a catheter is inserted through the heart chambers into the pulmonary artery. This procedure may cause ventricular arrhythmias. However, the pulmonary angiograph produces more reliable results than the ventilation perfusion scan.

**Pulmonary Angiograph Procedure**

- Assess if the patient is allergic to contrast medium (i.e., iodine, shellfish).

- Keep emergency resuscitation equipment and medication (diphenhydramine [Benadryl] and prednisone [Deltasone]) on hand.

- Assess that renal functions are normal (creatinine and BUN).

- Assess that bleeding time is normal (PT, PTT, INR, platelet count).

- Assess if the patient is able to lie still during the test.

- Let the patient know that he or she may feel flushed when the contrast material is infused.

- Insert the catheter into the femoral artery.

- Monitor vital signs during and following the test.

- Apply a pressure dressing on the insertion site following the test.

- Compare the insertion site to the opposite leg to assess temperature, sensation, and color. Both legs should have the same assessment; if not, notify the healthcare provider.

- Instruct the patient to increase fluid intake orally or administer through an IV infusion to flush the contrast material from the patient's body.

- Assess the renal function (creatinine and BUN) following the procedure to ensure that the contrast material has not caused renal malfunction.

- Monitor for signs of adverse reaction to contrast material.

  - Tachypnea

  - Restlessness

  - Urticaria

  - Respiratory distress

  - Nausea and vomiting

  - Tachycardia

## 4.3 Respiratory Medication

There are four categories of medication commonly used in respiratory emergencies. These are bronchodilators, anti-inflammatory medications, sedatives, and neuromuscular blocking medications. Bronchodilators relax smooth muscles around the bronchi when the patient experiences bronchospasms. Anti-inflammatory medication is used to reduce the inflammation response around the bronchi. Both of these cause the bronchi to remain open, enabling the flow of air and gas exchange to occur. A sedative is used to reduce anxiety and provide sedation for respiratory medical procedures. A neuromuscular blocking medication is used to inhibit spontaneous breathing when the patient is on a mechanical ventilator.

### 4.3.1 Bronchodilators

There are two types of bronchodilators:

- Beta$_2$-adrenergic agonists

  - Albuterol (Proventil): this is a short-acting bronchodilator commonly used for acute asthma and bronchospasm. Caution: this medication may cause bronchospasm (paradoxical bronchospasm). If this occurs, stop the medication immediately and inform the healthcare provider. The patient may also experience tachycardia and hyperactivity.

  - Epinephrine (Bronaid Mist): this is a fast-working bronchodilator commonly used for bronchospasm, anaphylaxis, acute asthma, and hypersensitivity reaction. Caution: this medication should not be used for patients who have coronary insufficiency, cerebral arteriosclerosis, or angle-closure glaucoma.

  - Pirbuterol (Maxair): this is a fast-working bronchodilator commonly used for asthma and bronchospasm. Caution: this medication may cause bronchospasm (paradoxical bronchospasm). If this occurs, stop the medication immediately and inform the healthcare provider.

- Anticholinergic medication

  - Ipratropium (Atrovent): this is a longer-acting bronchodilator commonly used for emphysema and chronic bronchitis. The action of this medication is delayed. This is not to be used for acute respiratory distress. Caution: this medication should not be used for patients who have bladder neck obstruction, prostatic hypertrophy, or angle-closure glaucoma.

## 4.3.2  Anti-Inflammatory Medication

Anti-inflammatory medication suppresses the immune response to the underlying cause that resulted in the swelling of bronchial tissues. The most commonly used anti-inflammatory medication is corticosteroids. Corticosteroids are categorized by the method that the medication is administered to the patient.

- **Inhalation corticosteroids:** these are long-acting, anti-inflammatory medications used for maintenance treatment of asthma. Caution: these are not used for an acute asthma attack. If the patient experiences hoarseness, bronchospasm, oral candidiasis, or dry mouth, then use a spacer. Make sure that the patient rinses his or her mouth after use to prevent oral candidiasis.
  - Commonly used inhalation corticosteroids are:
    - Fluticasone (Flovent)
    - Salmeterol (Advair)
    - Triamcinolone (Azmacort)
    - Beclomethasone (QVAR)
- **Systemic corticosteroids:** these are fast-acting, anti-inflammatory medications used for acute respiratory distress, COPD, and acute respiratory failure. These medications are administered by IV and then are tapered to oral administration. Monitor patients who have renal disease, hypertension, or gastrointestinal ulcers or patients who have recently experienced myocardial infarction for side effects when administering these medications. Adverse side effects include edema, thromboembolism, circulatory collapse, and arrhythmias.
  - Commonly used systemic administered corticosteroids are:
    - Methylprednisolone (Solu-Medrol)
    - Prednisone (Deltasone)
    - Dexamethasone (Decadron)

## 4.3.3  Sedatives

Sedatives (benzodiazepines) are used to reduce anxiety for patients who undergo respiratory tests and for patients who are placed on mechanical ventilators. Patients who are on a mechanical ventilator receive neuromuscular blocking medication that stops spontaneous breathing, enabling the mechanical ventilator to breathe for the patient. However, the patient's level of consciousness remains unchanged, and he or she is fully aware that natural breathing is paralyzed, which is distressful. Sedatives are administered to reduce the patient's anxiety.

Commonly used sedatives are

- Lorazepam (Ativan): used for anxiety. There is a risk of acute withdrawal symptoms if the patient suddenly stops taking the medication. This is not for use if patient has acute angle-closure glaucoma.
- Propofol (Diprivan): used for sedation in patients who are on a mechanical ventilator. Propofol should not be used with other medications. Monitor vital signs and have emergency respiratory resuscitation equipment available.
- Midazolam (Versed): used for conscious sedation and sedation for intubation and mechanical ventilation. Do not use if patient has acute angle-closure glaucoma. Monitor vital signs and have emergency respiratory resuscitation equipment available.

## 4.3.4 Neuromuscular Blocking Medication

Neuromuscular blocking medication is used to prevent a patient from spontaneously breathing in order for a mechanical ventilator to assist the patient's breathing. Although the patient's natural breathing response is blocked, the patient's level of consciousness remains unchanged. The patient is aware that spontaneous breathing is arrested.

There are two classifications of neuromuscular blocking medication:

- **Depolarizing:** medication causes the plasma membrane of the skeletal muscle fiber to depolarize. Commonly used depolarizing medications are:

  ○ Sccinylcholine (Anectine): used for endotracheal intubation and induction of skeletal muscle paralysis for mechanical ventilation. Do not use for patients who have acute angle-closure glaucoma, penetrating eye injuries, or malignant hyperthermia.

- **Non-depolarizing:** medication blocks the acetylcholine receptors, preventing acetylcholine from depolarizing skeletal muscle fiber. Commonly used non-depolarizing medications are:

  ○ Tubocuraine (Curare): used to induce skeletal muscle relaxation for mechanical ventilation, which reduces dislocations and fractures, and for intubation. Monitor renal function and electrolyte level to establish a baseline before administering the medication.

  ○ Atracurium (Atramed): monitor for bradycardia.

  ○ Pancuronium (Pavulon): a large dose may cause tachycardia. Do not mix with barbituates using the same syringe.

  ○ Cisatracurium (Nimbex): do not use with propofol or ketorolac. Monitor electrolyte and acid-base levels.

  ○ Vecuronium (Norcuron): do not administer intramuscularly, only by IV. Monitor renal and liver functions and electrolyte level to establish a baseline before administering the medication.

## 4.4 Respiratory Procedures

There are several commonly performed respiratory procedures used in emergency situations to ensure that the patient has an open, unobstructed airway and is adequately exchanging gases so that the patient's blood oxygen–carbon dioxide levels are within acceptable range.

### 4.4.1 Oxygen Therapy

Oxygen therapy delivers oxygen to the patient through a nasal cannula, a mask, or a mechanical ventilator to return the patient's blood to an acceptable blood oxygen–carbon dioxide level, thereby reducing the cardiac-respiratory workload related to hypoxemia.

Oxygen is considered a medication and therefore requires a medical order before it can be administered to the patient. Typically in the emergency department oxygen is prescribed by as-needed (PRN) orders or as a standing order. Both types of orders specify the patient's condition under which the order can be carried out and the dose and route to administer to the patient. The nurse has assessed the patient and administers oxygen accordingly if the specified patient condition exists.

- **High-flow system:** a high-flow system delivers a precise mixture of oxygen and air through either a Venturi mask or a ventilator.

- **Low-flow system:** a low-flow system delivers a variable mixture of oxygen and air through a non-Venturi mask or nasal cannula.

Oxygen dose is measured as either liters per minute or a percentage of oxygen concentration delivered to the patient.

- **Nasal cannula:** 2 to 6 liters per minute, 24% to 40% oxygen concentration

- **Simple face mask:** 6 to 12 liters per minute, 28% to 50% oxygen concentration

- **Venturi mask:** 40% oxygen concentration

- **Partial rebreathing mask** (has a reservoir bag): 5 to 15 liters per minute, 40% to 70% oxygen concentration

- **Non-rebreather mask:** 10 liters per minute, 60% to 80% oxygen concentration

When administering oxygen therapy it is important to remember:

- Oxygen therapy can dry mucous membranes. Use an oxygen humidifier if the dose is greater than 3 liters per minute except if the Venturi mask is used to deliver the oxygen. The Venturi mask contains valves that might clog if the oxygen is humidified.

- Do not use more than 2 liters per minute with patients who are diagnosed with COPD. The level of carbon dioxide in their blood causes the desire to breath. Decreasing the level of carbon dioxide through oxygen therapy can decrease the respiratory drive in COPD patients. However, a normal amount of oxygen is given if the patient is in respiratory arrest or is intubated, since the patient is unable to breathe.

- Monitor the patient's level of consciousness and vital signs. Decreased levels of consciousness and increased cardiac and respiratory rates may indicate hypoxemia.

### 4.4.2   Aerosol Therapy

Aerosol therapy is a form of inhalation therapy that delivers liquid medication directly to the patient's airway, enabling the mucosal membrane of the respiratory system to absorb the medication. There are two devices used for aerosol therapy. These are metered-dose inhalers and nebulizers. Listen to the patient's breath sounds prior to administering the medication and then again after the medication is administered to determine if the medication is effective.
Commonly used medications for aerosol therapy are:

- **Bronchodilators:** these relax smooth muscles around the bronchi when the patient experiences bronchospasms.

- **Corticosteroids:** these decrease inflammation around the bronchi, causing a decrease in swelling and resulting in more open bronchi.

- **Mucolystics:** these medications make mucus less viscous by dissolving thickened mucus secretions, enabling the patient to easily cough up the mucus.

### 4.4.3   Continuous Positive Airway Pressure Therapy

Continuous positive airway pressure (CPAP) therapy is a form of inhalation therapy that mechanically provides positive pressure throughout the respiratory cycle to assist the patient with ventilation. The result of this therapy is increased functional residual capacity while reducing the effort to breathe. CPAP therapy is delivered using a mask or nasal cannula. CPAP therapy is typically administered by a respiratory therapist.
CPAP therapy can be used instead of

- Mechanical ventilation

- Intubation

CPAP therapy is used for

- Bronchiolitis

- Pneumonia

- Respiratory distress syndrome

- Atelectasis

- Pulmonary embolus

- Pulmonary edema

During CPAP therapy monitor the patient for

- Nausea and vomiting, as patient is at risk for aspiration

- Swallowing air, as the patient might experience gastric distress

- Decreased cardiac output

### 4.4.4 Endotracheal Rapid Sequence Intubation

Endotracheal rapid sequence intubation is an emergency procedure that ensures a patent airway by the insertion of a tube through the mouth between the vocal cords and into the trachea (orotracheal intubation). This prevents aspiration and enables the emergency medical team to suction secretions while providing a stable airway for respiratory resuscitation.

Endotracheal tubes are measured in millimeters; 8 mm is common for men and 7.5 mm for women (see Figure 4.3).

The endotracheal tube (A) is inserted into the trachea (C). The tube (B) is inflated to hold the endotracheal tube in position. Be careful not to insert the endotracheal tube into the esophagus (D).

Here are the steps for endotracheal rapid sequence intubation:

- Establish IV access to administer fluids and medication.

- Monitor vital signs continually.

- Administer 100% oxygen using a partial rebreathing face mask for 3 minutes prior to intubation, if time permits.

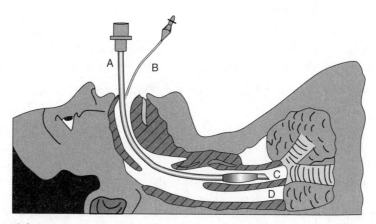

Figure 4.3 Use the appropriately sized endotracheal tube to ensure proper airway.

- Administer a sedative (see 4.3.3 Sedatives), if the patient is conscious.

- Administer

  - Atropine to maintain cardiac output

  - Ancetine to reduce the likelihood of facial muscle twitching

  - Lidocaine to reduce the likelihood of increased intracranial pressure

  - A neuromuscular blocking medication (see 4.3.4 Neuromuscular Blocking Medication), if the patient is conscious

- Remove dentures, if present.

- Insert the endotracheal tube.

- Inflate the endotracheal tube cuff.

- Verify placement of the endotracheal tube.

  - **Observation:** the stomach does not inflate. The patient displays normal respirations.

  - **Auscultation:** normal respirations are heard over the lung areas. There is absence of sounds in the stomach/abdomen.

  - **End-tidal carbon dioxide:** normal end-tidal carbon dioxide values are seen (see 4.2.3 End-tidal Carbon Dioxide Monitor).

  - **Chest x-ray:** the endotracheal tube is seen in the trachea (see 4.2.5 Chest X-Ray).

- Secure the endotracheal tube with tape.

- Administer mechanical ventilation (see 4.4.5 Mechanical Ventilation).

- Continually monitor the patient's vital signs, respiration, and arterial blood gas (see 4.2.2 Arterial Blood Gas).

- Maintain therapeutic levels of sedation and neuromuscular blocking medication until the endotracheal tube is removed.

Common complications of endotracheal tube intubation are

- **Infection:** coughing helps reduce infection. The patient is unable to cough while the endotracheal tube is in place.

- **Spasm:** insertion of the endotracheal tube may stimulate nerves to cause bronchospasm or laryngospasm.

- **Injury:** intubation may damage teeth, vocal cords, mouth, or pharynx.

- **Aspiration:** stomach contents, blood, and other secretions may enter the respiratory system if the endotracheal tube is not in the proper position or if the endotracheal tube becomes dislodged. The patient's normal coughing response is unavailable to expel this content.

- **Cardiac arrhythmias:** insertion of the endotracheal tube may stimulate nerves to cause an abnormal heartbeat.

- **Hypoxemia:** decreased oxygenation of the blood can occur if intubation is not performed rapidly. During intubation, respiratory resuscitation stops.

If there is trauma to the mouth that prevents insertion of the endotracheal tube, then insert the endotracheal tube through the nose (nasal intubation). Nasal intubation is also used for elective intubation because this route is more comfortable for the patient, there is less risk of displacement of the endotracheal tube, and there is less risk of tissue damage.

## 4.4.5  Mechanical Ventilation

Mechanical ventilation is a procedure where a handheld or automated device is used to administer positive or negative pressure to move air into or out of the patient's lungs. The mechanical ventilator is connected to the endotracheal tube or tracheostomy tube depending on which is used with the patient.

- **Handheld device:** the handheld device is a resuscitation bag that is manually operated by squeezing the bag and forcing air into the patient's lungs. The resuscitation bag can be connected to an oxygen supply (see 4.4.1 Oxygen Therapy). The handheld device is used for temporary ventilation during transportation and whenever the automated mechanical ventilator is unavailable. When using a handheld device:

  - Be sure to deliver breaths when the patient inhales and release the bag when the patient exhales.

  - Monitor respirations by observing the rise and fall of the patient's chest, indicating proper ventilation is occurring.

  - Make sure that the handheld device remains properly attached to the tube.

  - Fully squeeze the bag and allow the bag to fully inflate to ensure that the patient is properly ventilated.

  - Document the date and time when the patient was manually ventilated.

- **Automated device:** an automated device is a mechanical ventilator that uses an electrical pump and other electromechanical components to move air into and out of the patient's lungs.

  - There are several types of automated ventilators:

    - Volume-cycled ventilator: the volume-cycled ventilator delivers a specific volume of air to the patient regardless of resistance by the patient's lungs.

    - Time-cycled ventilator: a time-cycled ventilator delivers air for a specified respiratory cycle.

    - Pressure-cycled ventilator: the pressure-cycled ventilator delivers air until a specific pressure is reached. The pressure is resistance by the patient's lungs.

  - Automated mechanical ventilators are typically implemented and maintained by a respiratory therapist. However, the nurse must remember that the patient's life depends on the proper functioning of the ventilator.

  - Be sure that the ventilator alarms are operational at all times. These alarms signal when there is a problem with the ventilator.

  - Make sure that a therapeutic level of sedation and neuromuscular blocking medication is maintained while the patient is on the ventilator.

  - Monitor vital signs, including auscultation of the respiratory system, every two hours.

  - Be sure that the patient and the patient's family understand that the paralysis of natural breathing is temporary.

## 4.4.6  Tracheotomy

A tracheotomy is a surgical procedure where an opening is made into the patient's trachea and an indwelling tube is inserted in the opening to maintain the patient's airway.

- In an emergency, the tracheotomy is performed if there is an obstruction in the airway above the trachea, such as with swelling related to anaphylactic reaction or from a foreign body. In this situation, the tracheotomy tube is open to the environment and the patient is able to breathe normally.

- An elective tracheotomy is performed if the patient requires extended use of an automated mechanical ventilator. If the patient is on an automated mechanical ventilator (see 4.4.5 Mechanical Ventilation), then the tracheotomy tube is cuffed to prevent backflow and the automated mechanical ventilator is connected to the tracheotomy tube.

Make sure that

- The patient and family members realize that the patient will not be able to speak normally until the tracheotomy tube is removed.
- A respiratory assessment including arterial blood gas (see 4.2.2 Arterial Blood Gas) is done before and after the tracheotomy to ensure that the patient's respiration has improved because of the procedure.
- Tracheotomy tube assessment and care such as suctioning and cleaning are performed as scheduled.
- The patient is monitored for secretions that must be suctioned.
- The patient is monitored for bleeding around the surgical site.
- Documentation is made of all secretions suctioned from the patient.

### 4.4.7   Chest Tube

Insertion of a chest tube into the pleural space is an emergency surgical procedure used to drain fluid, blood, or air from the pleural space, restoring negative pressure and enabling the lung to reinflate. The chest tube is typically positioned in the fourth intercostal space.
    Chest tubes are used to treat

- Chylothorax: lymphatic fluid accumulated in the pleural cavity
- Empyema: pus accumulated in the pleural cavity
- Hemothorax: blood accumulated in the pleural cavity
- Pleural effusion: fluid accumulated in the pleural cavity
- Pneumothorax: air accumulated in the pleural cavity

    The chest tube is connected to a water-seal chamber. The water rises on inspiration and decreases on expiration. If the patient is on an automated ventilator providing positive pressure, then water rises on expiration and decreases on inspiration.
    Fluid is collected in a collection chamber. Document the amount of drainage and the type of drainage. Drainage should not exceed 200 ml/hr. If it does, then notify the practitioner because the patient might be bleeding. Empty the collection chamber by double-clamping the chest tube close to the insertion site and then remove the collection chamber. Replace the collection chamber and then remove the clamps.
    When using a drainage system

- Make sure the drainage system is below the patient's chest to prevent backflow into the chest tube.
- Don't clamp the chest tube for more than one minute; otherwise, the patient may experience a tension pneumothorax.
- Monitor the patient's vital signs and respiration for signs of respiratory distress.
- Monitor for chest tube leaks. Bubbles in the water-seal chamber indicate a leak between the patient and the drainage system. Bubbles should stop once the site of the leak is found.

○ Tighten and seal loose connections. If the bubbles continue, begin clamping the chest tube.

○ Clamp the chest tube close to the patient. If the bubbles continue, then the leak is at the insertion site or inside the patient. Notify the practitioner.

○ Clamp the chest tube farther away from the patient until the bubbles stop. If the bubbles stop, then there is a leak in the tube. Notify the practitioner.

○ Clamp the chest tube close to the drainage device. If the bubbles continue, then the drainage device needs to be replaced.

### 4.4.8   Oropharyngeal Suctioning

- Administer 100% oxygen before suctioning.

- Measure the catheter before suctioning. The suctioning catheter should be the distance from the tip of the patient's nose to the earlobe.

- Insert the suctioning catheter into the oropharynx beyond the tongue.

- Apply suction by covering the opening in the suctioning catheter.

- Rotate the suctioning catheter when suctioning.

- Limit suctioning to less than 10 seconds.

- Administer 100% oxygen after removing the suctioning catheter.

### 4.4.9   Endotracheal Suctioning

- Use a sterile technique.

- Administer 100% oxygen before suctioning.

- Insert the suctioning catheter into the endotracheal tube.

  ○ Don't insert the tip of the suctioning catheter beyond the tip of the endotracheal tube.

  ○ Don't cover the opening in the suctioning catheter when inserting the suctioning catheter into the endotracheal tube.

- Apply suction by covering the opening in the suctioning catheter only when withdrawing the suctioning catheter.

- Rotate the suctioning catheter when suctioning.

- Limit suctioning to less than 10 seconds.

- Administer 100% oxygen after removing the suctioning catheter.

## 4.5   Acute Respiratory Distress Syndrome (ARDS)

Shock, trauma, or sepsis causes fluid and protein to build up in the alveoli from an inflammatory response, resulting in alveolar collapse and impaired gas exchange.

### 4.5.1   Signs and Symptoms

- Dyspnea

- Pulmonary edema

- Tachypnea

- Rales (crackles)

- Hypoxemia

- Accessory muscle used for respiration

- Decreased breath sounds

- Cyanosis

- Rhonchi

- Anxiety

- Tachycardia

- Restlessness due to decreased oxygen levels

### 4.5.2  Medical Tests

- Arterial blood gases shows respiratory acidosis.

- Pulse oximetry shows lowered oxygen levels.

- Chest x-ray shows infiltrates within lung.

### 4.5.3  Treatment

- Monitor and maintain airway, breathing, and circulatory status.

- Administer positive end-expiratory pressure (PEEP) mechanical ventilation.

- Administer continuous positive airway pressure (CPAP) mechanical ventilation.

- Administer endotracheal intubation.

- Administer
  - Analgesic to decrease pain
    - Morphine
  - Diuretics to decrease fluid
    - Lasix (furosemide); Edecrin (ethacrynic acid); Bumex (bumetanide)
  - Anesthetic during endotracheal intubation
    - Diprivan (propofol)
  - Neuromuscular blocking agent during mechanical ventilation
    - Pavulon (pancuronium); Norcuron (vecuronium)
  - Proton pump inhibitor to decrease risk of aspiration and gastric stress ulcer
    - Zantac (ranitidine); Pepcid (famotidine); Axid (nizatidine); Prilosec (omeprazole)
  - Anticoagulant to decrease coagulation
    - Heparin; Coumadin (warfarin); Fragmin (dalteparin); Lovenox (enoxaparin)

- Steroids to decrease inflammation
  - Hydrocortisone; Medrol (methylprednisolone)
- Exogenous surfactant
  - Survanta (beractant)

## 4.5.4   Intervention

- Prescribe bed rest.
- Record intake and output of fluid.
- Monitor for fluid overload.
- Weigh daily.
- Tell the patient no overexertion.
- Instruct the patient
  - Practice coughing and deep-breathing exercises.
  - Call healthcare provider at first sign of respiratory distress.

## 4.6   Asthma

An allergen or non-allergen factor triggers inflammation of the airway and/or bronchospasm, resulting in dyspnea. There are two types of asthma:

- Atopic (extrinsic) asthma caused by allergens
- Non-atopic (intrinsic) asthma caused by a non-allergic factor such as cold air, humidity, or respiratory tract infection.

### 4.6.1   Signs and Symptoms

- Asymptomatic between asthma attacks
- Dyspnea
- Bronchoconstriction
- Tachypnea
- Wheezing on expiration, but can also occur on inspiration
- Cough
- Use of accessory muscles to breathe
- Tachycardia
- Anxiety
- Sweating (diaphoresis)
- Hyperresonance on percussion related to hyperinflation

## 4.6.2  Medical Tests

- Arterial blood gas shows respiratory acidosis.

- Chest x-ray shows hyperinflated lungs.

- Pulse oximetry shows decreased $O_2$.

- CBC shows eosinophils increase.

- Sputum shows positive eosinophils.

- Pulmonary function test shows decreased force on expiration during attack.

## 4.6.3  Treatment

- Administer 3 liters of fluid daily to liquefy any secretions.

- Remove allergens and triggers.

- Administer
  - Beta$_2$-adrenergic bronchodilators
    - Salmeterol, formoterol, albuterol, pirbuterol, metaproterenol, terbutaline, levalbuterol
  - Leukotriene anti-inflammatory modulators
    - Zafirlukast, zileuton, montelukast
  - Anticholinergics to reduce bronchospasm
    - Ipratropium inhaler, tiotropium inhaler
  - Antacids
    - Aluminum hydroxide/magnesium hydroxide, calcium carbonate
  - H2 blockers
    - Ranitidine, famotidine, nizatidine, cimetidine
  - Proton pump inhibitors
    - Omeprazole, lansoprazole, esomeprazole, rabeprazole, pantoprazole
  - Mast cell stabilizers
    - Cromolyn, nedocromil
  - Steroids to decrease inflammation
    - Hydrocortisone, Medrol (methylprednisolone), prednisolone
  - Methylxanthines for bronchodilation
    - Aminophylline, theophylline

## 4.6.4  Intervention

- Place patient in high Fowler's position for comfort.

- Administer oxygen therapy 1 to 2 liters per minute.

- Monitor oxygen saturation.

- Monitor vital signs.

- Instruct the patient

  - Avoid allergen.

  - Identify signs of asthma attack.

  - Use inhaler properly.

## 4.7   Atelectasis

In atelectasis, a lung collapses due to airway obstruction, pleural space infusion, tumor, anesthesia, immobility, or no deep-breathing exercises postoperatively, resulting in decreased gas exchange.

### 4.7.1   Signs and Symptoms

- Decreased breaths

- Diaphoresis

- Dyspnea

- Hypoxemia

- Tachypnea

- Tachycardia

- Cyanosis

- Anxiety

- Use of accessory muscles for breathing

### 4.7.2   Medical Tests

- Chest x-ray shows shadows in collapsed area.

- CT scan shows collapsed area.

### 4.7.3   Treatment

- Administer

  - Beta$_2$-adrenergic bronchodilators

    - Salmeterol, formoterol, albuterol, pirbuterol, metaproterenol, terbutaline, levalbuterol

  - Mucolytics to loosen secretions

    - Acetylcystine (inhaled), guaifenesin (oral)

### 4.7.4   Intervention

- Administer oxygen therapy 1 to 2 liters per minute.

- Provide humidified air.

- Monitor breathing.

- Instruct the patient
  - Use the incentive spirometer properly.
  - Cough and practice deep breathing exercise every 2 hours.

## 4.8   Bronchiectasis

The bronchi become obstructed with excessive mucus due to abnormal dilation of bronchi and bronchioles related to infection and inflammation. Patient may develop atelectasis and bronchitis.

### 4.8.1   Signs and Symptoms

- Hemoptysis
- Dyspnea
- Cyanosis
- Cough when lying down
- Foul-smelling cough
- Crackles on inspiration
- Rhonchi on inspiration
- Bronchial infections
- Weight loss
- Anemia

### 4.8.2   Medical Tests

- Pulmonary function test show decreased vital capacity.
- Chest x-ray shows shadows.
- CT scan shows bronchiectasis.
- Culture and sensitivity of sputum identifies microorganism and medication.

### 4.8.3   Treatment

- Bronchoscopy removes excessive secretions.
- Postural drainage uses gravity to move mucus from lungs to throat.

- Administer
  - Beta$_2$-adrenergic bronchodilators
    - Salmeterol, formoterol, albuterol, pirbuterol, metaproterenol, terbutaline, levalbuterol
  - Antibiotics to treat infection

### 4.8.4   Intervention

- Administer oxygen therapy 1 to 2 liters per minute.
- Chest percussion loosens secretions.
- Monitor vital signs.
- Instruct the patient's family
  - To perform chest percussion
  - To check postural drainage

## 4.9   Bronchitis

Infection or airborne irritants cause increased mucus production leading to blocked airways and decreased gas exchange.

- Acute bronchitis is reversible within 10 days.
- Chronic bronchitis is not reversible and is classified as chronic obstructive pulmonary disease (COPD)

### 4.9.1   Signs and Symptoms

- Productive cough (acute bronchitis)
- Chronic productive cough for three months (chronic bronchitis) annually, for at least two years
- Cough due to mucus production and irritation of airways
- Dyspnea
- Wheezing
- Use of accessory muscles to breathe
- Fever
- Weight gain due to edema from right-sided heart failure (chronic bronchitis)
- Chest discomfort
- Fatigue

### 4.9.2   Medical Tests

- Arterial blood gases shows respiratory acidosis.
- Hemoglobin increases.

- Chest x-ray shows infiltrate related to infection.
- Pulmonary function testing shows
  - Forced vital capacity decreased
  - Forced expiratory volume in one second (FEV1) decreased
  - Residual volume (RV) increased

### 4.9.3 Treatment

- Administer
  - Beta$_2$-adrenergic bronchodilators
    - Salmeterol, formoterol, albuterol, pirbuterol, metaproterenol, terbutaline, levalbuterol
  - Steroids to decrease inflammation
    - Hydrocortisone, Medrol (methylprednisolone), prednisolone
  - Methylxanthines for bronchodilation
    - Aminophylline, theophylline
  - Diuretics to decrease fluid
    - Lasix (furosemide), Edecrin (ethacrynic acid), Bumex (bumetanide)
  - Proton pump inhibitor to decrease risk of aspiration and gastric stress ulcer
    - Zantac (ranitidine), Pepcid (famotidine), Axid (nizatidine), Prilosec (omeprazole)
  - H2 blockers
    - Ranitidine, famotidine, nizatidine, cimetidine
  - Antacid
    - Aluminum hydroxide/magnesium hydroxide, calcium carbonate
  - Expectorant to liquefy secretions
    - Guaifenesin
  - Anticholinergic to reduce bronchospasm
    - Ipratropium inhaler, tiotropium inhaler

### 4.9.4 Intervention

- Use incentive spirometer.
- Implement high Fowler's position for comfort.
- Administer 3 liters of fluid daily to help liquefy secretions.
- Implement oxygen therapy 1 to 2 liters per minute via nasal cannula.
- Monitor vital signs.
- Weigh patient daily. Notify healthcare provider of weight gain of 2 lbs in one day.
- Monitor sputum changes.
- Monitor intake and output.
- Increase fluids to keep mucus thinner and easier to expel.

- Instruct the patient
  - To administer oxygen
  - To turn, cough, and practice deep-breathing exercises
  - To increase calories and protein in diet
  - To increase vitamin C intake

## 4.10 Cor Pulmonale

Right-sided heart failure results from chronic obstructive pulmonary disease (COPD), leading to pulmonary hypertension and enlargement of the right ventricle.

### 4.10.1 Signs and Symptoms

- Productive cough
- Edema
- Weight gain
- Orthopnea
- Dyspnea
- Tachycardia
- Cyanosis
- Fatigue
- Tachypnea
- Wheezing

### 4.10.2 Medical Tests

- Pulse oximetry shows lowered oxygen levels.
- Hemoglobin is increased.
- Arterial blood gas shows respiratory acidosis.
- Chest x-ray shows enlarged right ventricle and enlarged pulmonary arteries.
- Echocardiograph shows enlarged right ventricle.
- Pulmonary artery catheterization shows increased pulmonary artery and right ventricular pressure.

### 4.10.3 Treatment

- Administer
  - Calcium channel blockers to decrease blood pressure and heart rate
    - Isoptin (verapamil); Cardizem, Tiazac (diltiazem); Procardia (nifedipine); Cardene (nicardipine); Norvasc (amlodipine)

- Potassium channel activator to dilate pulmonary artery
  - Diazoxide, hydralazine, nitroprusside
- Angiotensin-converting enzyme inhibitor
  - Captopril, enalapril
- Diuretics to decrease fluid
  - Lasix (furosemide), Edecrin (ethacrynic acid), Bumex (bumetanide)
- Anticoagulant to decrease coagulation
  - Heparin, Coumadin (warfarin), Fragmin (dalteparin), Lovenox (enoxaparin)
- Cardiac glycoside
  - Digitalis (digoxin)

### 4.10.4 Intervention

- Place patient on bed rest.
- Monitor vital signs.
- Weigh patient daily. Notify healthcare provider of weight gain of 2 lbs in one day.
- Instruct patient to avoid overexertion.
- Administer oxygen therapy 1 to 2 liters per minute via nasal cannula.
- Monitor digoxin level to avoid toxic effect.
- Monitor serum potassium levels if patient is given ACE inhibitors and diuretics.
- Instruct the patient
  - Follow a low-sodium diet.
  - Limit fluid to 2 liters each day.

## 4.11  Emphysema

Chronic inflammation of the lungs results in decreased flexibility of the alveoli walls and loss of elastic recoil leading to overdistention of the alveolar walls and trapped air, causing decreased gas exchange. Emphysema is linked to smoking and can also be caused by inherited alpha-1 antitrypsin deficiency—but this is less frequent.

### 4.11.1  Signs and Symptoms

- Difficulty breathing (dyspnea)
- Use of accessory muscles to breathe
- Barrel-chested
- Loss of weight
- Diminished breath sounds
- Expiratory wheezing
- Hyperresonance

## 4.11.2   Medical Tests

- Pulmonary function test shows increased residual volume.

- Arterial blood gas shows respiratory acidosis.

- Chest x-ray shows flattened diaphragm and overinflated lungs.

## 4.11.3   Treatment

- Administer
  - Beta$_2$-adrenergic bronchodilators
    - Salmeterol, formoterol, albuterol, pirbuterol, metaproterenol, terbutaline, levalbuterol
  - Anticholinergic to reduce bronchospasm
    - Ipratropium inhaler, tiotropium inhaler
  - Methylxanthines for bronchodilation
    - Aminophylline, theophylline
  - Steroids to decrease inflammation
    - Hydrocortisone, Medrol (methylprednisolone), prednisolone
  - Antacid
    - Aluminum hydroxide/magnesium hydroxide, calcium carbonate
  - H2 blockers
    - Ranitidine, famotidine, nizatidine, cimetidine
  - Proton pump inhibitor
    - Omeprazole, lansoprazole, esomeprazole, rabeprazole, pantoprazole
  - Expectorant to liquefy secretions
    - Guaifenesin
  - Diuretics to decrease fluid
    - Lasix (furosemide), Edecrin (ethacrynic acid), Bumex (bumetanide)
  - Select treatment based on results of culture and sensitivity study or given empirically.
  - Administer alpha-1 antitrypsin therapy for patients with deficiency.
  - Teach patient use of the incentive spirometer to encourage deep breathing and to enhance coughing and expelling of mucus.
  - Teach patient use of flutter valve to increase the expiration force.
  - Administer nocturnal negative-pressure ventilation for hypercapnic (elevated $CO_2$ levels) patients.

## 4.11.4   Intervention

- Administer oxygen therapy of 1 to 2 liters per minute via nasal cannula.

- Administer 3 liters of fluid daily to help liquefy secretions.

- Monitor sputum changes.

- Use incentive spirometer.
- Place patient in high Fowler's position for comfort.
- Monitor intake and output.
- Monitor vital signs.
- Weigh patient daily. Notify healthcare provider of weight gain of 2 lbs in one day.
- Instruct the patient
  - Use oxygen.
  - Turn, cough, and practice deep-breathing exercises.
  - Avoid infection.
  - Stop smoking.
  - Perform abdominal diaphragmatic breathing exercise with pursed-lip breathing.
  - Avoid pollutants and irritants.

## 4.12   Pleural Effusion

The pleural sac fills with serous fluid, blood (hemothorax), or pus (empyema) restricting lung expansion, displaying lung tissue, and interfering with gas exchange. Causes include postoperative complication, congestive heart failure, renal failure, pulmonary infarction, embolus, infection, trauma, lupus erythematosis, or cancer.

### 4.12.1   Signs and Symptoms

- Dyspnea
- Decreased breath sounds
- Increased respiration
- Increased pulse
- Decreased BP (hemothorax)
- Chest pain if inflamed
- Fever (empyema)
- Dullness on percussion over the affected area
- Cough
- Pleural friction rub

### 4.12.2   Medical Tests

- Pulse oximeter shows decreased oxygen saturation.
- Chest x-ray shows pleural effusion.
- Chest CT scan shows pleural effusion.
- Chest ultrasound shows pleural effusion.

### 4.12.3   Treatment

- Thoracentesis to remove fluid
- Chest tube to drain fluid
- Antibiotics (empyema)

### 4.12.4   Intervention

- Administer oxygen therapy 2 to 4 liters per minute.
- Monitor chest tube drainage and patency.
- Monitor vital signs.
- Instruct the patient to turn, cough, and practice deep-breathing exercises.

## 4.13   Pneumonia

Inhalation of bacteria, viruses, parasites, irritating agents, or aspirated liquids or foods leads to infection and inflammation resulting in increased mucus production, thickening of alveolar fluid, and decreased gas exchange.

### 4.13.1   Signs and Symptoms

- Dyspnea
- Crackles
- Rhonchi
- Discolored, blood-tinged sputum
- Cough
- Fever
- Chills
- Pain on respiration
- Tachypnea
- Tachycardia
- Muscle pain (myalgia)
- Hypoxemia
- Sweating (diaphoresis)
- Wheezing

### 4.13.2   Medical Tests

- Pulse oximeter shows decreased oxygen saturation.
- Chest x-ray shows infiltration.

- WBC is elevated.
- Arterial blood gas shows respiratory acidosis.
- Culture and sensitivity of the sputum must be performed.

### 4.13.3   Treatment

- Chest x-ray
- Blood culture
- Sputum culture
- Administer
  - Antipyretics when fever is >101°F, for patient comfort
    - Tylenol (acetaminophen); Advil, Motrin (ibuprofen)
  - Brochodilators
    - Albuterol, metaproterenol, levalbuterol
  - Antibiotics for bacterial infection
    - Azithromycin, clarithromycin, levofloxacin, moxifloxacin, amoxicillin/clavulanate, cefotaxime, ceftriaxone, cefuroxime axetil, cefpodoxime, ampicillin/sulbactam, telithromycin

### 4.13.4   Intervention

- Administer oxygen therapy 2 to 4 liters per minute.
- Have patient use incentive spirometer every two hours.
- Monitor intake and output.
- Monitor vital signs.
- Monitor sputum characteristics.
- Place patient in high Fowler's position for comfort.
- Indicate bed rest.
- Increase fluids for hydration (by oral intake or IV).
- Instruct the patient
  - Add 3 liters of fluid daily to help liquefy secretions.
  - Use incentive spirometer every two hours.
  - Use nebulizer bronchodilator as needed.

## 4.14   Pneumothorax

Air enters the pleural space from an opening in the lung or chest, leading to partial or complete collapse of the lung. Types of pneumothorax are:

- Open pneumothorax (penetrating chest wound)
- Closed pneumothorax (blunt trauma)

- Spontaneous pneumothorax (caused by underlying disease—e.g., emphysema)

- Tension pneumothorax (displacement of the mediastinum causes unaffected lung to collapse)

### 4.14.1  Signs and Symptoms

- Sharp chest pain aggravated by coughing

- Tracheal deviation toward the unaffected side with tension pneumothorax

- Subcutaneous emphysema

- Absent breath sounds over the affected area

- Tachypnea

- Tachycardia

### 4.14.2  Medical Tests

- Pulse oximeter shows decreased oxygen saturation.

- Chest x-ray shows infiltration.

- Arterial blood gas shows respiratory acidosis.

### 4.14.3  Treatment

- A small-bore chest tube is inserted to the upper chest and connected to a standard water-seal chamber or into a Heimlich valve of a suction device to re-expand lung.

- Administer analgesic such as morphine.

### 4.14.4  Intervention

- Place patient in high Fowler's position.

- Indicate bed rest.

- Adminster oxygen therapy 2 to 4 liters per minute.

- Monitor chest tube drainage and patency.

- Monitor vital signs.

- Instruct the patient to turn, cough, and practice deep-breathing exercises.

## 4.15  Respiratory Acidosis

Blood becomes more acidic as a result of acute or chronic respiratory disease, hypoventilation, asphyxia, or central nervous system disorders. Carbon dioxide (acid) increases, resulting in increased respiration and retention of bicarbonate and sodium. This causes the kidneys to compensate by excreting hydrogen ions.

### 4.15.1   Signs and Symptoms

- Dyspnea

- Hypoxemia

- Headache

- Irritability

- Confusion

- Restlessness

- Cardiac arrhythmia

### 4.15.2   Medical Tests

- Arterial blood gas:
  - Carbon dioxide ($Paco_2$) >50 mm Hg
  - pH of blood <7.35

### 4.15.3   Treatment

- Treat underlying cause.

- Implement mechanical ventilation.

- Administer
  - Brochodilators such as albuterol, metaproterenol, levalbuterol

### 4.15.4   Intervention

- Implement oxygen therapy, 2 to 4 liters per minute

- Monitor vitals.

- Monitor blood chemistry.

- Instruct the patient to turn, cough, and practice deep-breathing exercises

## 4.16   Tuberculosis

A lung infection caused by *Mycobacterium tuberculosis*, tuberculosis is transmitted by coughing, sneezing, or talking and can infect other organs.

- Primary tuberculosis occurs when the patient is initially infected with *Mycobacterium tuberculosis*.

- Secondary tuberculosis is a reactivation of *Mycobacterium tuberculosis* from a previous infection.

- When exposure to *Mycobacterium tuberculosis* results in negative test results and no symptoms, patient may or may not have tuberculosis.

- Latent tuberculosis results in positive test results and no symptoms.

### 4.16.1   Signs and Symptoms

- Low-grade fever
- Productive cough persisting for two weeks
- Blood-tinged sputum (hemoptysis)
- Fatigue
- Night sweats
- Chills
- Anorexia
- Weight loss
- Shortness of breath

### 4.16.2   Medical Tests

- Mantoux (PPD) skin test is positive.
- Sputum test is positive for *Mycobacterium tuberculosis*.
- Chest x-ray shows areas of granuloma or cavitation

### 4.16.3   Treatment

- Administer antitubercular agents such as
  - Isoniazid, rifampin, pyrazinamide, ethambutol, streptomycin

### 4.16.4   Intervention

- Indicate respiratory isolation.
- Increase carbohydrate, protein, and vitamin C in patient's diet.
- Monitor vitals.
- Monitor intake and output.
- Instruct the patient
  - Take in 3 liters of fluid daily to help liquefy secretions.
  - Follow scheduled rest periods.
  - Learn how to prevent spread of tuberculosis.

## 4.17   Acute Respiratory Failure

Insufficient ventilation reduces adequate gas exchange in the lungs, resulting in increased carbon dioxide and decreased oxygen in blood. Acute respiratory failure occurs due to depression of the central nervous system resulting from medication or trauma or decompensation from a respiratory illness.

### 4.17.1 Signs and Symptoms

- Dyspnea
- Orthopnea
- Tachypnea
- Coughing
- Fatigue
- Diminished breath sounds
- Hemoptysis
- Diaphoresis
- Crackles
- Rhonchi
- Cyanosis

### 4.17.2 Medical Tests

- Arterial blood gas:
  - Oxygen ($Pao_2$) <60 mmHg
  - Carbon dioxide ($Paco_2$) >50 mm Hg
  - Oxygen saturation ($Sao_2$) <90%
  - pH of blood <7.30
- Pulse oximeter shows decreased oxygen saturation.
- WBC is increased.

### 4.17.3 Treatment

- Treat underlying cause.
- Implement mechanical ventilation.
- Administer
  - Brochodilators
    - Albuterol, metaproterenol, levalbuterol
  - Anticholinergic to reduce bronchospasm
    - Ipratropium inhaler, tiotropium inhaler
  - Anesthetic to ease intubation
    - Propofol
  - Neuromuscular blocking agent to ease mechanical ventilation
    - Pancuronium, vecuronium, atracurium
  - Steroids to decrease inflammation
    - Hydrocortisone, methylprednisolone, prednisone

- ○ Anticoagulant to decrease coagulation
  - ▪ Heparin, Coumadin (warfarin), Fragmin (dalteparin), Lovenox (enoxaparin)
- ○ Antacid
  - ▪ Aluminum hydroxide/magnesium hydroxide, calcium carbonate
- ○ H2 blockers
  - ▪ Ranitidine, famotidine, nizatidine, cimetidine
- ○ Proton pump inhibitor
  - ▪ Omeprazole, lansoprazole, esomeprazole, rabeprazole, pantoprazole
- ○ Analgesic for discomfort and to decrease myocardial oxygen demand
  - ▪ Morphine

### 4.17.4 Intervention

- Place patient in high Fowler's position.
- Administer oxygen therapy 2 to 4 liters per minute.
- Monitor vitals.
- Change patient's position every two hours.
- Monitor intake and output.
- Instruct the patient to turn, cough, and practice deep-breathing exercises.

## 4.18 Pulmonary Embolism

Gas exchange is impaired because of alveoli collapse due to an obstruction of blood flow in the lungs caused by thrombus, air emboli, or fat emboli. A small area of atelectasis self-resolves. A large area of atelectasis is fatal. Most common pulmonary embolisms result from a thrombus that breaks loose from a deep vein in the legs or pelvis.

### 4.18.1 Signs and Symptoms

- Sudden dyspnea
- Chest pain
- Tachypnea
- Tachycardia
- Crackles at site of emboli
- Coughing
- Hemoptysis
- Anxiety
- Leg pain
- Leg swelling

- Hypotension
- Decreased level of consciousness
- Fainting (syncope)

### 4.18.2 Medical Tests

- Lung scan shows ventilation/perfusion mismatch.
- Chest x-ray shows dilated pulmonary artery.
- Pulmonary angiography shows clot.
- Helical CT scan shows clot in pulmonary arteries.
- Arterial blood gas shows respiratory acidosis.
- D-dimer is positive when a thromboembolic event has occurred.
- Pulse oximeter shows decreased oxygen saturation.
- Ultrasound of the lower extremities shows thrombus.

### 4.18.3 Treatment

- Surgical insertion of a vena cava filter
- Surgical removal of the emboli
- Administer
  - Anticoagulant to decrease coagulation
    - Heparin, Coumadin (warfarin), Fragmin (dalteparin), Lovenox (enoxaparin)
  - Analgesic for discomfort and to decrease myocardial oxygen demand
    - Morphine
  - Thrombolytics to remove clot within 3 to 12 hours of blockages
    - Urokinase, alteplase

### 4.18.4 Intervention

- Prescribe bed rest.
- Place patient in high Fowler's position.
- Administer oxygen therapy 2 to 4 liters per minute.
- Monitor oxygen saturation levels.
- Monitor vitals.
- Instruct the patient
  - Turn, cough, and practice deep-breathing exercises.
  - Do not cross legs.

○   Do not sit or stand for too long.

○   Call healthcare provider at first sign of bleeding.

○   Call healthcare provider at first sign of respiratory increase.

## 4.19   Influenza

Influenza is a viral infection of the upper layer of cells in the respiratory tract transmitted by inhaling droplets or by direct contact with virus containing droplets. This can lead to a secondary bacterial infection.

### 4.19.1   Signs and Symptoms

- Myalgia
- Fever $>101°$ F
- Malaise
- Diaphoresis
- Nonproductive cough
- Abrupt onset of symptoms
- Headache
- Watery discharge
- Sore throat

### 4.19.2   Medical Tests

- Nasopharyngeal viral culture identifies virus.
- Rapid diagnostic test is positive for virus.

### 4.19.3   Treatment

- Administer
  ○   Antipyretics when fever $>101°$ F, for patient comfort
    ▪   Tylenol (acetaminophen); Advil, Motrin (ibuprofen)
  ○   Antiviral medications
    ▪   Zanamivir, oseltamivir, amantadine, rimantadine

### 4.19.4   Intervention

- Monitor vital signs.
- Instruct the patient
  ○   Increase fluid intake.
  ○   Increase electrolyte intake.

## 4.20   Respiratory Arrest

Respiratory arrest occurs when gas exchange is ineffective because the patient's respiratory system has failed. The patient has a pulse indicating his or her cardiovascular system is functioning, although the patient's heart will stop once oxygen level decreases and the patient becomes hypoxic.

If you realize the patient is in respiratory arrest, then perform the following procedures:

- Try arousing the patient by stimulating the upper sternum with your fingers while calling the patient by his or her first name.
- Call for assistance and call a code immediately.
- Stay with the patient.
- Open the airway:
    - Head tilted and chin lifted
    - Jaw lifted, without head extension if the patient's neck is immobilized
- Look for the rise and fall of the chest.
- Listen for escaping air during exhalation.
- Feel for the flow of air against your cheek.
- If no respirations are felt, then begin rescue breathing.
- Give two breaths each 1 second long.
- Monitor the carotid pulse for 5 seconds. Remember that respiratory arrest quickly becomes cardiac arrest if respirations are not restored.
- If patient has a pulse, then the patient is not in cardiac arrest. Don't begin cardiac compressions. Focus on restoring the patient's respiration.
- Insert an airway or intubate to ensure airway is patent if the patient is unconscious.
- Use a bag mask to ventilate the patient. Compress the bag once every 5 seconds to provide 10 breaths per minute.
- Monitor end-tidal carbon dioxide (see 4.2.3 End-Tidal Carbon Dioxide Monitor) to assess expired gas in the patient's breath.
- Open intravenous access.
- Attach ECG.
- Monitor pulse oximetry (see 4.2.1 Pulse Oximetry). Administer supplementary oxygen if oxygen saturation falls below 90%.
- Identify and treat underlying cause.

## Solved Problems

**4.1**   What is respiratory arrest?

Respiratory arrest occurs when there is inadequate gas exchange as a result of failure of the patient's respiratory system.

**4.2**   Why isn't a patient's pulse oximetry measured if the patient has carbon monoxide poisoning?

Carbon monoxide adheres to hemoglobin and is recorded as oxygen by the pulse oximetry device.

**4.3**   What is the purpose of end-tidal carbon dioxide monitoring?

End-tidal carbon dioxide monitoring uses infrared light to measure carbon dioxide concentration in gas expired from the patient's breath. This is used to assess if the patient is breathing.

**4.4**   What might be indicated if the patient has rusty sputum?

Pneumonia may be indicated.

**4.5**   If a sputum sample that is bubbly and frothy is collected what would the healthcare provider do?

The sample is likely saliva and not sputum. Ask the patient to give another sample and show the patient how to cough deeply to retrieve the new sample.

**4.6**   Why is a thoracic CT scan ordered?

This is ordered to provide a three-dimensional image of the respiratory system, enabling the practitioner to identify normal and abnormal structures.

**4.7**   If a practitioner suspects a lung tumor, what imaging test would the practitioner likely order?

A thoracic MRI scan that is able to assess fluid-filled soft tissue and tumors within the thoracic area is ordered.

**4.8**   What is the purpose of a ventilation scan?

A ventilation scan determines the ability of air to reach all parts of the lung.

**4.9**   What is the purpose of a perfusion scan?

A perfusion scan determines how well blood circulates within the lungs.

**4.10**   Why would the healthcare provider keep Benadryl and Deltasone available during a ventilation perfusion scan?

The ventilation and perfusion scan uses contrast material that is hyperallergenic especially for patients who are allergic to iodine and shellfish. Benadryl is an antihistamine that reverses the allergic reaction. Deltasone is cortisone that reduces the immune system's effect during an allergic reaction.

**4.11**   What is the purpose of administering a bronchodilator?

A bronchodilator relaxes smooth muscles that surround the bronchi, resulting in dilation of the bronchi and enabling an increased flow of air through the bronchi.

**4.12**   What is the purpose of administering anti-inflammatory medication when a patient has respiratory distress?

Respiratory distress can be the result of narrowing of the bronchi caused by tightening of smooth muscles around the bronchi and the swelling of blood vessels around the bronchi in response to an allergic reaction. Anti-inflammatory medication decreases the immune response and thereby reduces the swelling of blood vessels around the bronchi.

**4.13**   Why are sedatives given to a patient who is on an automated mechanical ventilation device?

An automated mechanical ventilation device takes over the spontaneous breathing for the patient. A neuromuscular blocking medication is used to stop the patient's own spontaneous breathing. However, the patient's level of consciousness remains unchanged. The patient is fully aware that his or her natural breathing is paralyzed, which is distressful. Sedatives are used to decrease the patient's anxiety.

**4.14    Why is two liters of oxygen the maximum given to a patient who has COPD?**

A COPD patient's urge to breathe is stimulated by the patient's carbon dioxide level. If the patient's carbon dioxide level decreases, so will the patient's urge to breathe. The administration of two liters of oxygen helps to maintain an adequate carbon dioxide level. Increasing oxygen beyond two liters decreases the patient's carbon dioxide level, leading to a decreased stimulation to breathe.

**4.15    What is the purpose of CPAP therapy?**

The purpose of this therapy is to increase functional residual capacity while reducing the effort to breath.

**4.16    What does it mean when bubbles are present in the water-seal chamber of a chest tube collection device?**

There is a leak in the tube.

**4.17    What should the healthcare provider do before performing endotracheal suctioning?**

He or she should administer 100% oxygen to the patient.

**4.18    What is intrinsic asthma?**

Asthma caused by a non-allergic factor such as cold air, humidity, or a respiratory tract infection is intrinsic asthma.

**4.19    What is atelectasis?**

Atelectasis is a lung collapse.

**4.20    What is acute bronchitis?**

Bronchitis that is resolved within 10 days is acute bronchitis.

**4.21    What is cor pulmonale?**

Cor pulmonale is right-sided heart failure resulting from chronic obstructive pulmonary disease (COPD) and leading to pulmonary hypertension and enlargement of the right ventricle.

**4.22    What is emphysema?**

Emphysema is a chronic inflammation of the lungs that results in decreased flexibility of the alveoli walls and leads to overdistention of the alveolar walls and trapped air, causing decreased gas exchange. It is linked to smoking. It can also be caused by inherited alpha-1 antitrypsin deficiency, but this is less frequent.

**4.23    What is pleural effusion?**

The pleural sac fills with serous fluid, blood (hemothorax), or pus (empyema), restricting lung expansion, displacing lung tissue, and interfering with gas exchange.

**4.24    What is the cause of a pneumothorax?**

Air entering the plural sac is the cause of pneumothorax.

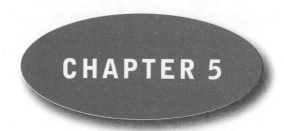

# CHAPTER 5

# *Neurological Emergencies*

## 5.1 Define

- A neurological emergency is a condition that alters the neurologic system, resulting in a temporary or permanent disability that may be life threatening to the patient.

- A neurological emergency is considered life threatening until proven otherwise.

- Subtle changes in the patient's presentation can indicate deterioration of the patient's neurologic system.

- Focus on neurological problems after the patient's airway, breathing, circulation, and cervical spine are stabilized.

- The first sign of a neurological emergency is the patient's altered mental status (AMS). Level of consciousness (LOC) is the most important indicator of neurologic function.

- A neurological emergency requires immediate intervention.

### 5.1.1 Goal of Treating Neurological Emergencies

- The goal of the emergency-department staff is to identify the neurological emergency and stabilize the patient's respiration. Treatment of the underlying condition occurs in follow-up care.

- An unstable airway and unstable breathing and circulation can be caused by an unstable neurological condition; however, stabilize the airway, breathing, and circulation first as if there is no underlying neurological problem.

- Diagnose the acute problem. For example, a neurological problem might cause decreased respiration leading to ineffective gas exchange. The acute problem is decreased respiration and ineffective gas exchange.

- Establish as baseline the patient's mental status upon arrival in the emergency department. Reassess the patient's mental status during the patient's stay, comparing the results to the baseline to determine if the patient's mental status has changed.

- Assess the patient completely before beginning treatment. For example, administering medication may mask a sign or symptom that indicates a neurological emergency.

- Refer the patient to follow-up care to treat the underlying cause(s) of the problem.

## 5.1.2   Neurological Assessment

- Begin with a head-to-toe examination.

- Assess for the causes of altered mental status.

  - AEIOU

    - **A**lcohol, arrhythmia

    - **E**ndocrine/exocrine, electrolytes, encephalopathy

    - **I**nsulin

    - **O**xygen, opiates

    - **U**remia

  - TIPS

    - **T**rauma, temperature disorders

    - **I**nfection

    - **P**sychiatric, porphyria, poisons

    - **S**hock, seizure, stroke, subarachnoid hemorrhage, space-occupying lesion

- A patient who has a neurological impairment may present as

  - Alert and oriented and reporting signs of neurological impairment

    - Focus your interview on the patient.

  - Disoriented and in an altered mental state and unable to report signs of neurological impairment

    - Focus your interview on first responders, family, and friends who accompanied the patient to the hospital or who can provide information about the patient's condition via phone interview.

- The neurological assessment interview begins with open-ended questions.

  - Why did you come to the hospital today?

  - What makes you feel that something is wrong?

- Next, gather more information about each sign reported by the patient.

  - Describe what you are feeling.

  - When did you first notice it?

  - What were you doing when you first noticed it?

  - Has this ever happened before today?

- Next ask about the patient's health history.

  - Are you being treated for any illness?

  - Were you treated for any illness in the past?

  - Were your injured recently, or in the past?

  - Do you have any allergies?

  - Have you had any surgeries?

- Next ask about the patient's lifestyle.

  - What is your occupation?

  - Were you ever exposed to toxic chemicals?

  - Do you or people around you use recreational drugs?

  - Do you smoke?

  - Do you drink alcohol?

  - Do you have any hobbies that may have exposed you to toxic chemicals?

- Assess the patient's altered mental status.

  - **Alert:** the patient responds to stimuli with little or no delay.

  - **Oriented:** the patient is oriented to time, person, and place.

    - What day is this?

    - What is your name?

    - Where are you?

  - **Sleepy:** the patient is arousable to a normal level of awareness.

  - **Lethargic:** the patient is drowsy and sluggish.

  - **Stupor:** the patient is sleepy but can be aroused to a seminormal level of awareness using noxious stimuli.

  - **Coma:** the patient cannot be aroused.

  - **Delirium:** the patient is acutely confused, showing psychomotor excitement and impaired memory and perception. The patient may experience hallucinations.

  - **Dementia:** a gradual deterioration of mental function is evident.

- Assess for mental impairment using the Abbreviated Mental Test Score (AMTS). Each answer is valued at 1 point. A score of 6 or less suggests mental impairment that requires further testing.

  - What is your age?

  - What is the time to the nearest hour?

  - What year is this?

  - What is the name of this hospital?

  - Do you know who I am? Do you know who this person is? (The patient is expected to recognize two people who are in the room by name or title.)

  - When was Pearl Harbor attacked? (Or ask about any important historical event.)

  - Who is the president of the United States?

  - Count backward from 20 to 1.

  - Mention an address to the patient, then ask the patient to repeat the address.

- Develop the patient's baseline mental status using the Glasgow Coma Scale (see Chapter 1, 1.7.1 Assessment).

- Assess breath odor.
  - **Alcohol:** might indicate alcohol intoxication as a cause for neural impairment. However, don't assume that alcohol is the underlying cause of neural impairment just because the patient's breath smells of alcohol. Rule out other possible causes.
  - **Acetone:** might indicate diabetic ketoacidosis as a cause for neural impairment that can be reversed by administering insulin and fluids.
- Assess cardiac effectiveness.
  - **Cardiac arrhythmia:** may result in decreased circulatory function leading to decreased oxygenation and neural impairment.
- Assess respiratory effectiveness.
  - **Respiratory disorder:** may result in ineffective gas exchange leading to decreased oxygenation and neural impairment.

### 5.1.2.1  Signs and Symptoms

Neurological assessment in an emergency situation requires the nurse to recognize common signs and symptoms of underlying causes and then prepare for the anticipated treatment that the practitioner is likely to order.
  Commonly seen signs and symptoms:

- Changes in pupils
  - Pinpoint, bilateral, nonreactive to light may indicate:
    - Lesion in the pons resulting from a hemorrhage
    - Drug intoxication (heroin, opiates)
  - Dilated bilateral, fixed, nonreactive to light may indicate:
    - Cerebral ischemia
    - Anticholinergic toxicity
    - Severe brain damage
    - Hypoxia
    - Drug (sympathomimetic) intoxication (cocaine, methamphetamines, amphetamines, ecstasy, bath salts, stimulants)
  - Small, unilateral, nonreactive to light may indicate:
    - Spinal cord lesion
  - Dilated, unilateral fixed, nonreactive to light may indicate:
    - Normal, if patient has a history of severe eye injury
    - Increased intracranial pressure
    - Subdural hematoma or epidural hematoma
    - Brain stem compression
    - Brain herniation leading to oculomotor nerve damage
  - Midsize, bilateral, fixed, nonreactive to light may indicate:
    - Contusion
    - Brain edema

- Brain hemorrhage
- Laceration of the brain
- Infarction in the brain
- Abnormal cranial nerve function
  - There are 12 cranial nerves responsible for motor and sensory pathway to the brain.
  - Table 5.1 shows how to assess the cranial nerves.

TABLE **5.1  Assessment of Cranial Nerves**

| CRANIAL NERVE | FUNCTION | EXAMINE |
|---|---|---|
| I. Olfactory | Smell | Test each nostril with scents such as peppermint, coffee, and vanilla. |
| II. Optic | Vision | Test eyes with Snellen eye chart. |
| III. Oculomotor | Eye movement<br>Constricting pupils<br>Raising eyelid | Check pupil size.<br>Check pupil shape.<br>Check pupil response to light. |
| IV. Trochlear | Moving eyes down and in | Ask the patient to move her eyes down and in. |
| V. Trigeminal | Sensation for face and scalp<br>Chewing<br>Corneal reflex | Ask the patient to look up and out. Touch a piece of cotton to the side of one eye. Both eyes should blink.<br><br>Ask patient to close both eyes. Randomly press a sharp and blunt object to the patient's forehead, jaw, and cheek. Ask the patient if he feels anything, and, if so, to describe the feeling as sharp or dull.<br><br>Ask the patient to open his mouth and clench his teeth. |
| VI. Abducens | Moving eyes laterally | Ask the patient to move her eyes laterally. |
| VII. Facial | Taste<br>Moving mouth, eyes, and forehead to show expression<br>Tears (lacrimation), salivation | Ask the patient to raise and lower eyebrows.<br>Ask him to smile showing teeth.<br>Ask him to puff cheeks.<br>Ask patient to wrinkle forehead. |
| VIII. Acoustic | Balance<br>Hearing | Stand an arm's length away from the patient's ear and rub two fingers. Ask if the patient hears anything. Repeat the test on the other ear.<br><br>Conduct the Weber's test by placing a vibrating fork on the patient's forehead, asking, "Where do you hear sound coming from?" The response should be midline. |

*(Continued)*

**TABLE 5.1  Assessment of Cranial Nerves (*Continued*)**

| CRANIAL NERVE | FUNCTION | EXAMINE |
|---|---|---|
| | | Conduct the Rinne's test. Place a vibrating fork on the mastoid bone behind the ear. Ask the patient when he stops hearing it. Then move the fork to the patient's ear so the patient can hear the tone. The patient should hear better with the fork by the ear rather than on the mastoid bone. |
| IX. Glossopharyngeal | Taste<br>Swallowing<br>Gag reflex<br>Salivating | Ask the patient to swallow. |
| X. Vagus | Gag reflex<br>Swallowing<br>Heart rate<br>Peristalsis<br>Talking<br>Abdominal function<br>Thoracic functions | Ask the patient to talk.<br>Check the gag reflex by touching the back of the tongue with the tongue blade.<br>Ask the patient to open her mouth and say, "Ah." Uvula should be midline and soft palate should appear symmetrically upward. |
| XI. Accessory | Rotation of head<br>Moving shoulder | Ask the patient to shrug, and press down on his shoulders. The shrug should be bilaterally equal.<br>Apply resistance to the side of the patient's head while the patient rotates his head against the resistance. Repeat on the other side of the head. |
| XII. Hypoglossal | Moving tongue | Ask the patient to stick out her tongue. The tongue should be midline.<br>Ask the patient to say, "Round the rugged rock that ragged rascal ran." The patient should show little problem articulating. Results are dependent on the patient's cognitive ability.<br>Ask the patient to push her tongue against her cheek. Apply resistance to the cheek. The tongue should be symmetrical. |

- Motor function
  - Ask the patient to push against your hands. There should be equal pressure from both arms.
  - Ask the patient to close his eyes then extend both arms palms up for 20 seconds. Both arms should remain in position without any drift.
  - Ask the patient to sit at the edge of the bed and raise both legs against your hands. There should be equal pressure from both legs.

○ Ask the patient to push her feet against your hands. There should be equal pressure from both legs.

○ Ask the patient to stand. The patient should stand without assistance or support.

○ Ask the patient to sit. The patient should sit without assistance or support.

○ Ask the patient to walk. The patient's gait should be steady.

  ▪ Bias toward one side may indicate a cerebellar lesion on that side.

  ▪ Unsteady gait may indicate abnormal cerebellar functioning.

○ Ask the patient to touch his nose with an extended finger one hand at a time. The patient should be able to perform this action without hesitation.

○ Ask the patient to touch your extended finger as you move your finger. The patient should be able to perform this action without hesitation.

○ Ask the patient to touch each finger with her thumb on her same hand. Repeat the test on the other hand. The patient should be able to perform this action without hesitation.

  ▪ Inability to perform this exercise quickly may indicate alcohol toxicity, cerebellar disorder, or stroke.

- Reflexes

  ○ **Tactile stimulation:** stroke the patient's skin. The more you stroke, the less of a reflex response should be noticed.

  ○ **Plantar reflex:** use a tongue blade and slowly stroke from the patient's heel to the great toe. Toes should flex. The Babinski's reflex (fanning of the smaller toes and upward movement of the great toe) is abnormal unless the patient is two years of age or younger.

  ○ **Abdominal reflex:** stroke one side of the abdomen with the handle of the reflex hammer. Abdominal muscles should contract and the umbilicus should deviate toward the same side. Repeat this on the opposite side.

## 5.2   Neurological Tests and Procedures

Neurological tests are designed to assess the effectiveness and the capability of the nervous system to function. Emergency-department practitioners order neurological tests to collect objective data to further assess and assist in stabilizing the patient. Once stabilized, the patient is transferred or referred for follow-up care designed to treat the underlying cause of the current episode and which may require additional neurological tests. Neurological procedures are performed to stabilize the patient.

The following are neurological tests and procedures commonly ordered by the emergency department's practitioners.

### 5.2.1   Spinal X-Ray

During a spinal x-ray, x-ray particles are beamed through the front, back, and side of the patient onto a photographic film or to a computer. Dense structures such as bone block x-ray particles, causing those structures to appear white. Less-dense structures such as lesions and deteriorated bone block some x-ray particles, causing those structures to appear gray. Spinal tissue that does not block x-ray particles appears dark.

The practitioner typically orders a spinal x-ray to assess for:

- Fractures

- Displacements

- Lesions

- Tumors

**Spinal X-Ray Procedure**

- Be sure the patient's spine is stabilized. Immobilize the spine, if necessary.

- Be sure the patient is not pregnant.

- Remove all jewelry in the area to be x-rayed, since jewelry may appear on the x-ray image.

- Assess if the patient has scars in the spinal area. If so, note the location of the scars since the scars may appear on the x-ray image.

- Instruct the patient to remove his clothes, assisting patient as needed. Provide the patient with a gown.

- The patient lies down on the x-ray table, and the x-ray plate is positioned below the table.

- The initial result, called a "wet read," provides a relatively superficial assessment of the image. A more thorough reading is taken hours or days later.

## 5.2.2   Brain and Spinal CT Scan

A brain CT scan provides a three-dimensional image of the brain using x-rays and enables the practitioner to visualize normal and abnormal structures within the brain. A spinal CT scan provides a three-dimensional image of the spine. A CT can be performed with or without a contrast agent. A contrast agent is iodine-based and enhances images of blood vessels and less-dense areas of the brain and spine.

The practitioner orders a brain CT scan to assess for:

- Inflammation

- Lesions

- Contusion

- Vascular anomalies

- Cerebral atrophy

- Blood clots

- Aneurysms

- Infarctions

- Calcifications

- Hydrocephalus

- Foreign bodies

The practitioner orders a spinal CT scan to assess for:

- Fractures

- Dislocation

- Herniated disk

- Tumors

- Spinal stenosis

**CT Scan Procedure**

- Ask the patient if he is allergic to iodine or shellfish if the patient is undergoing a CT scan with contrast. Patients who are allergic to iodine or shellfish have a high likelihood to experience an allergic reaction to the contrast agent.

- Administer diphenhydramine (Benadryl) and prednisone (Deltasone) before the CT scan to reduce the risk of an allergic reaction to the contrast agent, if the contrast agent is ordered.

- Administer the contrast agent through an IV. The patient may feel flushed and have a salty or metallic taste in his mouth.

- Explain to the patient that the contrast material typically discolors the urine for upward of 24 hours following the CT scan. The patient should increase fluid intake after the CT scan to flush the contrast agent from his body, if the contrast agent is used for the CT scan.

- Assess if the patient is claustrophobic, as the patient will be placed in an enclosed space during the test.

- Assess if the patient can remain still for 30 minutes during the CT scan. The CT scanner encircles the patient for up to 30 minutes.

## 5.2.3   Central Nervous System (CNS) MRI

A central-nervous-system magnetic resonance imaging (MRI) provides a three-dimensional view of the central nervous system using radio waves, a strong magnet, and a computer. An MRI is particularly useful to assess fluid-filled soft tissue and to identify tumors from other structures within the central nervous system.

**Central Nervous System MRI Procedure**

- All metal must be removed from the patient.

- No metal must enter the room containing the MRI scanner. The MRI scanner's magnet is always activated.

- Assess if the patient is claustrophobic. If so, then ask the healthcare provider if an open MRI scanner should be used for the test or if the patient should be sedated before the scan begins.

- The CNS MRI scan takes about 30 minutes.

- The CNS MRI scan is noninvasive, and the patient will not feel any discomfort.

## 5.2.4   Cerebral Angiograph

A cerebral angiograph is a test that enables the practitioner to examine blood vessels in the brain. Radiopaque contrast medium is injected into the brachial artery or femoral artery. The contrast medium highlights blood vessels on the image.

The practitioner orders a cerebral angiograph to assess for:

- Hematoma
- Cerebral edema
- Displaced vessels
- Aneurysms
- Stenosis
- Occlusion
- Arteriovenous malformations
- Circulation

**Cerebral Angiograph Procedure**

- Assess if the patient is allergic to iodine or shellfish. Patients who are allergic to iodine or shellfish have a high likelihood of experiencing an allergic reaction to the contrast agent.
- Administer diphenhydramine (Benadryl) and prednisone (Deltasone) before the cerebral angiograph to reduce the risk of an allergic reaction to the contrast agent.
- Explain to the patient that the contrast material typically discolors the urine for upward of 24 hours following the cerebral angiograph. The patient should increase fluid intake after the cerebral angiograph to flush the contrast agent from her body.
- Asses renal function (serum creatinine and BUN) before the procedure to ensure that the patient is able to void the contrast medium.
- Assess coagulation (PT, PTT, INR, platelet count) before the procedure to ensure that there will not be excessive bleeding following the procedure.
- Use a FemoStop device to maintain pressure on the injection site following the procedure.
- Monitor the patient for neurologic changes during and after the procedure.

## 5.2.5 Lumbar Puncture

A lumbar puncture is a procedure where the practitioner takes a sample of the patient's spinal fluid. A sterile needle is inserted into a subarachnoid space between the third and fourth lumbar vertebrae while the patient lies on his side and is held by staff. The sample is then sent to the laboratory for analysis.

The practitioner orders a lumbar puncture to assess for:

- Bacteria
- Blood
- Relative intracranial pressure

**Lumbar Puncture Procedure**

- Assess if the patient has a lumbar spinal deformity; if so, the procedure is not performed.
- Explain that the patient may feel discomfort.
- Administer a local anesthetic at the injection site.
- Assess the patient for back spasms, headache, or seizures following the procedure.

## 5.3   Neurological Medication

There are several categories of medication commonly used in neurological emergencies. These are used to counter conditions that make the patient's neurologic system unstable. Each medication can cause adverse side effects; therefore, the patient must be monitored carefully following administration of these medications.

### 5.3.1   Anticonvulsants

Anticonvulsant medication is used to treat seizures, which are episodes of disturbed brain activity that can affect muscular capability and behavior. Seizures can be caused by epilepsy or head trauma. Anticonvulsant medications can sometimes increase intracranial pressure and cause cerebral edema in addition to causing bradycardia.

- Fosphenytoin (Cerebyx)
- Phenytoin (Dilantin)

### 5.3.2   Anticoagulants

Anticoagulant medication is used to prevent an embolism following a cerebrovascular accident (CVA). Anticoagulant medication increases the risk of bleeding.

- Heparin

### 5.3.3   Antiplatelets

Antiplatelet medication is used to reduce coagulants following a CVA or a transient ischemic attack. Antiplatelet medication increases the risk of low platelet count (thrombocytopenia) and low white blood cell count (agranulocytosis).

- Aspirin
- Ticlopidine (Ticlid)

### 5.3.4   Barbiturates

Barbiturates are used to reduce the patient's irritability and agitation. In addition, barbiturates are used to treat seizures, except for febrile seizures and absence seizures. Barbiturates increase the risk of respiratory depression and bradycardia.

- Phenobarbital (Luminal)

### 5.3.5   Benzodiazepines

Benzodiazepines are used to reduce the patient's anxiety and agitation. In addition, benzodiazepines are used to treat seizures and muscle spasms. Benzodiazepines increase the risk of respiratory depression and bradycardia and can cause the patient to experience withdrawal symptoms.

- Diazepam (Valium)
- Lorazepam (Ativan)

## 5.3.6   Calcium Channel Blockers

Calcium channel blockers are used to reduce vasoconstriction caused by vasospasm that occurs after the rupture of an aneurysm. Calcium channel blockers increase the risk of edema and tachycardia related to hypotension.

- Nimodipine (Sular)

## 5.3.7   Corticosteroids

Corticosteroids are used to reduce inflammation and cerebral edema. Corticosteroids increase the risk of pancreatitis, heart failure, and thromboembolism.

- Dexamethasone (Dexone)
- Methylprednisolone (Solu-Medrol)

## 5.3.8   Diuretics

Diuretics are used to reduce cerebral edema and intracranial pressure. Diuretics increase the risk of seizures, electrolyte imbalance, renal failure, heart failure, and dehydration.

- Furosemide (Lasiz)
- Mannitol (Osmitroil)

## 5.3.9   Opioid Analgesics

Opioid analgesics are used to reduce pain. Opioids increase the risk of respiratory depression, bradycardia, sedation, and constipation.

- Oxycodone (OxyContin)
- Morphine (Duramorph)

## 5.3.10   Thrombolytics

Thrombolytics are used to remove a blood clot following an acute ischemic CVA. Thrombolytics medication increases the risk of bleeding.

- Alteplase (Activase)

## 5.3.11   Serotonin Inhibitors

Serotonin inhibitors are used to treat migraine headaches. Serotonin inhibitors increase the risk of unstable blood pressure.

- Sumatriptan (Imitrex)

## 5.4 Cerebral Hemorrhage

Bleeding occurs within the brain, the layers covering the brain, or between the skull and the dura mater. It can occur at the time of the injury or hours or days later. Types of cerebral hemorrhages are:

- **Epidural hematoma:** bleeding occurs from an artery, with blood accumulating between the dura and skull.

- **Subdural hematoma:** bleeding occurs from a vein in the area between the dura mater and the arachnoid mater, resulting in slow, chronic bleeding.

- **Subarachnoid hemorrhage:** bleeding occurs between the brain and the tissue covering the brain.

- **Intracerebral hemorrhage:** bleeding occurs within brain tissue caused by shearing or tearing of small vessels within the brain and between the cerebrum and brain stem.

- **Concussion:** blunt force trauma thrusts the brain against the inside of the skull resulting in bruising.

- **Cerebral contusion:** blunt force trauma thrusts the brain against the inside of the skull resulting in cerebral edema, cerebral hemorrhage, and loss of consciousness longer than that in a concussion.

- **Coup injury:** blunt force trauma thrusts the brain against the inside of the skull at the point of the blunt force trauma.

- **Countrecoup injury:** blunt force trauma causes the head to recoil, thrusting the brain against the inside of the skull at a point opposite of the blunt force trauma.

- **Cerebral edema:** fluid within the skull moves to the third space, resulting in increased cranial pressure.

### 5.4.1 Signs and Symptoms

- Nausea
- Vomiting
- Disorientation
- Headache
- Unequal pupil size
- Diminished or absent pupil reaction
- Cognitive changes
- Speech changes
- Motor movements changes
- Decreased level of consciousness or loss of consciousness
- Amnesia
- Unilateral paralysis
- Facial weakness or droop

### 5.4.2 Medical Tests

- CT scan shows cerebral edema and hemorrhage.
- MRI shows edema and hemorrhage.

### 5.4.3 Treatment

- Craniotomy
  - Stop bleeding surgically.
  - Debride wound and tissue necrosis.
  - Decompress cerebral pressure by drilling burr holes into the skull and surgically removing the hematoma.
- Intubation to open airway
- Supplemental oxygen
- Mechanical ventilation to assess breathing
- Administer
  - Osmotic diuretics to decrease cerebral edema
    - Mannitol
  - Loop diuretics to decrease edema and circulating blood volume
    - Lasix (furosemide)
  - Analgesics
    - Acetaminophen (Tylenol)
  - Antibiotics (open head wound) to prevent infection
  - Antihypertensives
    - Nitroprusside (Nipride)
  - Opioids (low dose) for restlessness, agitation, and pain (if on ventilator)
    - Morphine sulfate, fentanyl citrate

### 5.4.4 Intervention

- Administer supplemental oxygen.
- Follow seizure precautions.
- Monitor vital signs.
- Monitor signs of increased intracranial pressure: widening pulse pressure, increased blood pressure, slow pulse.
- Indicate high-protein, high-calorie, high-vitamin diet.
- Monitor intake and output.
- Monitor for diabetes insipidus due to injury to the pituitary gland.
- Monitor neurologic status (Glasgow Coma Scale; see 1.7.1 Assessment).
- Instruct the patient
  - Call the healthcare provider if patient becomes lethargic, changes in personality, or feels drowsy.
  - Be aware of seizure precautions.

## 5.5 Bell's Palsy

Bell's palsy is facial paralysis of the seventh cranial nerve affecting one side of the face related to inflammation and common in diabetics. Bell's palsy leads to the patient's inability to close the eyelid, smile, or raise the eyebrow. Patient may have change in taste and pain around the ear. This disorder is self-resolving in most patients.

### 5.5.1 Signs and Symptoms

- Unilateral facial paralysis
- Change in taste
- Ear and jaw pain

### 5.5.2 Medical Tests

- Electromyogram (EMG) used to assess recovery time

### 5.5.3 Treatment

- Administer
  - Corticosteroids to decrease inflammation
    - Prednisone
  - Artificial tears to moisten eyes

### 5.5.4 Intervention

- Monitor for eye irritation.
- Provide meals in private.
  - Instruct the patient on how to properly apply artificial tears.

## 5.6 Brain Abscess

Pus collects within the brain as a result of infection from the ear, sinuses, systemic circulation, or from within the brain, leading to cerebral edema. The cause is streptococci, staphylococci, anaerobes, or mixed organism infections.

### 5.6.1 Signs and Symptoms

- Seizures
- Headache
- Drowsiness
- Confusion
- Ataxia (loss of coordination)

- Widened pulse pressure

- Nystagmus (involuntary eye movement)

- Aphasia (inability to use or understand language)

### 5.6.2 Medical Tests

- WBC is elevated.

- MRI shows abscess.

- CT shows abscess.

- Biopsy identifies organism.

### 5.6.3 Treatment

- Drain the abscess.

- Administer

  ○ Antibiotics

    ▪ Nafcillin sodium (penicillinase-resistant penicillin)

    ▪ Penicillin G benzathine

    ▪ Chloramphenicol

    ▪ Metronidazole

    ▪ Vancomycin

  ○ Corticosteroids

    ▪ Dexamethasone

  ○ Anticonvulsants

    ▪ Phenytoin

    ▪ Phenobarbital

  ○ Osmotic diuretics to decrease cerebral edema

    ▪ Mannitol

### 5.6.4 Intervention

- Monitor vital signs.

- Monitor mental status.

- Monitor fluid intake and output.

- Monitor movement.

- Monitor senses (taste, smell, hearing, sight, touch).

  ○ Instruct the patient to continue antibiotic treatments.

## 5.7   Brain Tumor

A brain tumor is characterized by a growth of abnormal cells within the brain, leading to increased intracranial pressure. Abnormal cells may be metastasized cancer cells from a site outside the brain (secondary).

- **Meningiomas:** benign tumor generated from the meninges
- **Gliomas:** malignant, rapid-growing tumor generated from neuroglial cells
- **Astrocytoma:** type of gliomas
- **Oligodendroglioma:** slower-growing gliomas
- **Glioblastoma:** differentiated gliomas

### 5.7.1   Signs and Symptoms

- Parietal lobe
  - Visual field defect
  - Sensory loss
  - Seizures
- Frontal lobe
  - Anosmia (loss of sense of smell)
  - Personality changes
  - Expressive aphasia
  - Slowing of mental activity
- Occipital lobe
  - Prosopagnosia
  - Impaired vision
- Cerebellum or brain stem
  - Ataxia
  - Lack of coordination
  - Hypotonia of limbs
- Temporal lobe
  - Receptive aphasia
  - Auditory hallucinations
  - Depersonalization
  - Seizures
  - Smell hallucinations
  - Emotional changes
  - Visual field defects

### 5.7.2  Medical Tests

- CT shows meningioma.
- MRI with contrast shows tumor.

### 5.7.3  Treatment

- Craniotomy to remove the tumor
- Radiation to decrease tumor size
- Administer
  - Glucocorticoid to decrease inflammation
    - Dexamethasone
  - Anticonvulsant to decrease seizure activity
    - Phenytoin, phenobarbital, carbamazepine, divalproex sodium, valproic acid, levetiracetam, lamotrigine, clonazepam, topiramate, ethosuximide
  - Osmotic diuretic to reduce cerebral edema
    - Mannitol
  - Proton pump inhibitors to decrease gastric irritation
    - Lansoprazole, omeprazole, esomeprazole, rabeprazole, pantoprazole
  - H2-receptor antagonists to decrease gastric irritation
    - Ranitidine, famotidine, nizatidine, cimetidine
  - Mucosal barrier fortifier to decrease gastric irritation
    - Sucralfate
  - Chemotherapeutic agents based on cell type
    - Carmustine, lomustine, procarbazine, vincristine, temozolomide, erlotinib, gefitinib

### 5.7.4  Intervention

- Monitor neurologic function.
- Take precautions in case of seizures.
  - Instruct the patient on seizure precautions.

## 5.8  Cerebral Aneurysm

Weakening of a blood vessel wall in the brain results in ballooning of the vessel wall that may lead to a rupture and intracranial bleeding. This can be caused by congenital malformation, infection, lesion on the blood vessel wall, trauma, or atherosclerosis.

### 5.8.1   Signs and Symptoms

- Asymptomatic unless rupture occurs
- Decreased level of consciousness
- Headache due to hemorrhage and increased intracranial pressure

### 5.8.2   Medical Tests

- CT shows the aneurysm.
- Single photon emission computed tomography (SPECT) shows the aneurysm.
- Angiogram shows the aneurysm.
- Digital subtraction angiography shows the aneurysm.
- Diffusion/perfusion MRA (magnetic resonance angiography) shows the aneurysm.

### 5.8.3   Treatment

- Surgical resection of the aneurysm
- Administer
  - Glucocorticoid to decrease inflammation
    - Dexamethasone
  - Anticonvulsant to decrease seizure activity
    - Phenytoin, phenobarbital, carbamazepine, divalproex sodium, valproic acid, levetiracetam, lamotrigine, clonazepam, topiramate, ethosuximide
  - Stool softener to decrease need to strain
    - Colace (Docusate sodium)

### 5.8.4   Intervention

- Elevate head of bed 30 degrees.
- Indicate bed rest.
- Monitor level of consciousness.
- Monitor vital signs for indication of increased intracranial pressure (widened pulse pressure and bradycardia).
  - Instruct the patient to report any headache immediately to the healthcare provider.

## 5.9   Encephalitis

Encephalitis is an inflammation of the brain in response to an infection by a virus (common), bacteria, fungus, or protozoa.

### 5.9.1   Signs and Symptoms

- Fever
- Stiff neck
- Headache
- Nausea and vomiting
- Drowsiness
- Lethargy
- Seizure

### 5.9.2   Medical Tests

- Blood cultures and sensitivity

### 5.9.3   Treatment

- Administer
  - Glucocorticoid to decrease inflammation
    - Dexamethasone
  - Anticonvulsant to decrease seizure activity
    - Phenytoin, phenobarbital, carbamazepine, divalproex sodium, valproic acid, levetiracetam, lamotrigine, clonazepam, topiramate, ethosuximide
  - Diuretic to reduce cerebral edema
    - Mannitol, Lasix (furosemide)
  - Antipyretics to reduce fever
    - Tylenol (acetaminophen)

### 5.9.4   Intervention

- Monitor vital signs for indication of increased intracranial pressure (widened pulse pressure and bradycardia).
- Monitor neurological changes.
- Monitor fluid input and output.
- Monitor electrolyte levels.
- Provide a quiet environment.
- Indicate range-of-motion exercises—active or passive.
- Turn and position patient every two hours if the patient is unable to move by himself.
- Instruct the patient to turn himself, if he is able, every two hours.

## 5.10   Guillain-Barré Syndrome

An autoimmune reaction damages the myelin surrounding the axon on the peripheral nerves resulting in an acute, progressive weakness and paralysis of muscles. This occurs a few weeks following a viral infection, acute illness, or surgery. Damage may be permanent if nerve cells are damaged. Damage may be temporary if axons are damaged.

- **Ascending Guillain-Barré:** the damage begins at the distal lower extremities and moves upward.
- **Descending Guillain-Barré:** the damage begins with muscles in the face and throat and moves downward, resulting in paralysis of the diaphragm and intercostal muscles and leading to respiratory compromise.

### 5.10.1   Signs and Symptoms

- Acute illness or infection within the past several weeks
- Absence of deep tendon reflexes
- Burning or prickling feeling
- Symmetrical weakness
- Flaccid paralysis
- Fluctuating blood pressure
- Cardiac dysrhythmias
- Facial weakness
- Difficulty swallowing (dysphagia)

### 5.10.2   Medical Tests

- Nerve-conduction studies show slowed velocity (speed of neural conduction).
- Pulmonary function tests show diminished tidal volume and vital capacity.
- Lumbar puncture shows increased protein in cerebrospinal fluid.

### 5.10.3   Treatment

- Use plasmapheresis to remove antibodies from blood.
- Employ endotracheal intubation if necessary.
- Monitor respiration and support ventilation if necessary.
- Administer immunoglobulin IV.

### 5.10.4   Intervention

- Monitor airway, breathing, and circulation.
- Monitor vital signs.
- Monitor for progression of change.

- Monitor gag reflex.

- Insert NG tube if dysphagia is present.

- Develop nonverbal communication method (e.g., call bell).

- Instruct the patient to turn every two hours.

## 5.11   Meningitis

It is an infection of the meningeal coverings of the brain and spinal cord commonly caused by bacteria (*Streptococcus pneumoniae* [pneumococcal]), *Neisseria memingitides* (meningococcal), or *Haemophilus influenza*, but it can also be caused by a virus, fungus, protozoa, or toxic exposure. Bacterial meningitis is transmitted when people live in close quarters. Viral meningitis may follow a viral infection and is self-limiting. Fungal meningitis may occur in patients who are immunocompromised.

### 5.11.1   Signs and Symptoms

- Fever

- Nuchal rigidity (pain when flexing chin toward chest)

- Stiff neck

- Petechial rash on skin and mucous membranes

- Photophobia (sensitivity to light)

- Headache

- Malaise and fatigue

- Seizures

- Nausea and vomiting

- Myalgia (muscle aches)

- Chills

- Altered level of consciousness

### 5.11.2   Medical Tests

- Lumbar puncture to sample cerebrospinal fluid

- Polymerase chain reaction (PCR) test of cerebrospinal fluid for organisms

- Culture and sensitivity of cerebrospinal fluid and blood

- CT of brain to rule out lesion

### 5.11.3   Treatment

- Administer

  - Glucocorticoid to decrease inflammation

    - Dexamethasone

- Anticonvulsant to decrease seizure activity
  - Phenytoin, phenobarbital, carbamazepine, divalproex sodium, valproic acid, levetiracetam, lamotrigine, clonazepam, topiramate, ethosuximide
- Diuretic to reduce cerebral edema
  - Mannitol, Lasix (furosemide)
- Antipyretics to reduce fever
  - Tylenol (acetaminophen)
- Antibiotics for bacterial meningitis
  - Penicillin G, ceftriaxone, cefotaxime, Vancomycin plus ceftriaxone or cefotaxime, ceftazidime
- Antifungal medication for fungal infection
  - Amphotericin B, fluconazole, flucytosine

### 5.11.4   Intervention

- Indicate isolation for patient.
- Darken room.
- Take precautions for seizures.
- Indicate bed rest.
- Monitor fluid intake and output.
- Monitor neurologic function every two hours.
- Instruct the patient by explaining all restrictions.

## 5.12   Spinal Cord Injury

Pulling, twisting, compressing, or severing the spinal cord may result in damage to part (incomplete) or entire thickness (complete) of the spinal cord. Damage is assessed after inflammation related to trauma subsides. Spinal cord tissue does not regenerate. The level of damage to the spinal cord determines the degree of disability.

### 5.12.1   Signs and Symptoms

- Tingling (paresthesia)
- Reduced sensation (hypoesthesia)
- Increased sensation (hyperesthesia)
- Weakness (flaccid paralysis)
- Absence of reflexes
- Lack of bowel control
- Loss of bladder control
- Hypotension

- Hypothermia

- Bradycardia

- Loss of motor control below the level of the injury

### 5.12.2  Medical Tests

- CT scan shows injury.

- MRI shows injury.

### 5.12.3  Treatment

- Administer
  - Corticosteroid to decrease inflammation
    - Methylprednisolone, prednisone, dexamethasone
  - Plasma expander to increase circulation and oxygen to injured tissues
    - Dextran
  - H2 receptor antagonists to protect formation of stress ulcer
    - Cimetidine, ranitidine, famotidine, nizatidine
  - Gastric mucosal protective agent to protect formation of stress ulcer
    - Sucralfate
  - Surgical decompression or repair of fracture

### 5.12.4  Intervention

- Position patient flat on rotating bed to prevent pressure ulcers.

- Prohibit flexion.

- Immobilize spinal cord with traction to decrease irritation.

- Monitor traction to prevent skin irritation.

- Monitor for spinal shock (loss of reflexes below injury, bradycardia, hypotension, paralytic ileus, flaccid paralysis).

- Monitor vital signs.

- Monitor intake and output.

- Monitor mental status.

- Monitor neurologic status.

- Monitor skin for pressure ulcers.

- Indicate care of cervical traction pin sites.

- Instruct the patient on
  - Proper transfer from wheelchair to bed
  - Need for regular bowel movements and urination
  - Need to use the incentive spirometer
  - Need to turn and reposition

## 5.13   Cerebrovascular Accident (CVA)

Interruption of blood supply to the brain results in infarction (necrosis) in the affective tissue. Patients with high cholesterol, diabetes mellitus, smoking habit, obesity, oral contraceptive use, or atrial fibrillation have a high risk for cerebrovascular accident. There are three types of cerebrovascular accidents. These are:

- **Ischemic stroke** (accounts for 88% of all strokes) is an interruption of arterial blood flow by an obstruction (clot) by the thrombus or embolus.

- **Hemorrhagic stroke** is an interruption of blood flow by rupture or leakage of a blood vessel into brain tissues and ventricles.

- **Transient ischemic attack** (TIA) is a temporary interruption of blood flow that resolves in a few hours with no permanent neurologic deficit.

### 5.13.1   Signs and Symptoms

- Difficulty speaking (aphasia)
- Personality changes
- Confusion
- Sensory changes
- Numbness
- Weakness
- Severe headache
- Seizure
- Difficulty with gait and coordination
- Facial droop
- Altered vision

### 5.13.2   Medical Tests

- Single photon emission computed tomography (SPECT) shows decreased perfusion.
- Magnetic resonance angiography (MRA) shows abnormal vessels.
- CT scan shows bleeding.
- MRI shows ischemic vessels.

### 5.13.3   Treatment

- Carotid artery endarterectomy to remove plaque from carotid artery (ischemic)
- Surgical implantation of a stent in the carotid artery (ischemic)
- Surgical correction of bleeding (hemorrhagic)
- Administer
    - Thrombolytic agent within three hours of onset of symptoms (ischemic)
        - TPA

- Anticoagulants after TPA (ischemic)
  - Heparin, warfarin, Lovenox, aspirin
- Antiplatelet medications to decrease platelet adhesiveness (ischemic)
  - Clopidogrel, ticlopidine hydrochloride, dipyridamole
- Corticosteroid to decrease inflammation
  - Dexamethasone (Decadron)

### 5.13.4 Intervention

- Indicate bed rest.
- Monitor vital signs.
- Monitor neurological status.
- Monitor for increased intracranial pressure (decreased level of consciousness, restlessness, confusion, headaches, nausea, and vomiting).
- Develop nonverbal communication method (e.g., call bell).
- Prescribe physical therapy to maintain muscle tone.
- Indicate speech therapy to assist swallowing and speech.
- Indicate occupational therapy to regain independent living.
- Instruct the patient on
  - Proper transfer from wheelchair to bed
  - Effects of CVA on activities of daily living

## 5.14  Seizure Disorder

Sudden, uncontrolled discharge of neurons in the brain results in abnormal behavior caused by metabolic disorder, intracranial pressure, tumor, cerebrovascular accident, medication, or seizure disorder. Prior to the seizure (pre-ictal stage) the patient may experience alterations in sight, sound, or smell. After the seizure (post-ictal stage) the patient is fatigued, confused, and may not recall the seizure.

### 5.14.1  Signs and Symptoms

**Generalized Seizures**

| | |
|---|---|
| Tonic/clonic | First tonic (limb rigidity) loss of consciousness |
| | Then clonic (rhythmic jerking) |
| Tonic | Limb rigidity, loss of consciousness |
| Clonic | Rhythmic jerking |
| Absence | Staring and brief loss of consciousness |
| Myoclonic | Brief rhythmic jerking |
| Atonic | Loss of muscle tone |

**Partial Seizures**

| | |
|---|---|
| Simple partial | No loss of consciousness, unusual sensation, unusual movement, begins with aura |
| Complex partial | Lip smacking, patting, picking, loss of consciousness |

### 5.14.2   Medical Tests

- CT scan of brain rules out tumor or bleed.

- MRI of brain rules out tumor or bleed.

- Electroencephalogram (EEG) shows abnormal electrical activity in brain.

### 5.14.3   Treatment

- Treat underlying cause.

- Surgically remove seizure focal area.

- Implant vagal nerve stimulator to decrease frequency of seizures.

- Administer

  - Antiepileptic medication

    - Carbamazepine (Tegretol), phenytoin (Dilantin), phenobarbital (Solfoton), clonazepam (Klonopin), valproic acid (Depakote), lamotrigine (Lamictal), gabapentin (Neurontin), levetiracetam (Keppra), oxcarbazepine (Trileptal), primidone (Mysoline), tiagabine (Gabitril), topiramate (Topamax)

### 5.14.4   Intervention

- Take precautions for seizures.

- During seizure:

  - Place patient on his side to decrease risk of aspiration.

  - Remove objects from around patient to prevent injury.

  - Note duration and patient's actions during seizure.

  - Monitor for status epilepticus (prolonged seizures or repeated seizures).

  - Do not insert anything in patient's mouth during seizure.

- Instruct the patient

  - Explain seizure precautions to family and friends.

  - Instruct family and friends what to do during a seizure.

  - Explain importance of taking medications as prescribed.

## 5.15   Concussion

Head trauma causes the brain to move within the skull, resulting in neural dysfunction. There is no bruising of brain tissue. The patient typically loses consciousness for a few minutes but not more than six hours. The patient experiences a headache for months. Full recovery occurs within 48 hours of the head trauma.

### 5.15.1   Signs and Symptoms

- Vomiting
- Lethargy
- Unusual behavior
- Headache
- Temporary amnesia related to traumatic event
- Dizziness
- Blurry vision
- Not thinking clearly

### 5.15.2   Medical Tests

- CT scan shows absence of bruising of brain tissue.
- MRI shows absence of bruising of brain tissue and evidence of head trauma.

### 5.15.3   Treatment

- Indicate bed rest.
- Apply cold pack wrapped in thin cloth for up to 20 minutes on any swelling.
- Administer
  - Analgesic
    - Acetaminophen (Tylenol)
    - Ibuprofen (Advil, Motrin)

### 5.15.4   Intervention

- Monitor vital signs.
- Monitor neurological status.
- Monitor for increased intracranial pressure (decreased level of consciousness, restlessness, confusion, headaches, nausea, and vomiting).
- Instruct the patient
  - Refrain from activities that are physically or mentally demanding.
  - Refrain from alcohol or illegal drugs.

## 5.16   Contusion

A contusion is a bruise of the brain as a result of acceleration-deceleration brain trauma; a coup, where bruising occurs at the site of the impact such as in a force blow to the head; or a contrecoup, where bruising occurs at the opposite side of the impact such as when the head hits the windshield in a motor-vehicle accident.

### 5.16.1   Signs and Symptoms

- Difficulty breathing
- Disorientation
- Confusion
- Loss of consciousness
- Visible wound may or may not exist
- Agitation
- Unequal pupils
- Drowsiness
- Violent behavior
- Weakness on one side (hemiparesis)
- Abnormal posturing
- Nausea or vomiting
- Visual disturbance
- Difficulty speaking

### 5.16.2   Medical Tests

- CT scan shows bruising of brain tissue and evidence of head trauma.
- MRI shows bruising of brain tissue and evidence of head trauma.

### 5.16.3   Treatment

- Administer
  - Diuretic to reduce cerebral edema
    - Mannitol, Lasix (furosemide)
  - Antiepileptic
    - Carbamazepine (Tegretol), phenytoin (Dilantin), phenobarbital (Solfoton), clonazepam (Klonopin), valproic acid (Depakote), lamotrigine (Lamictal), gabapentin (Neurontin), levetiracetam (Keppra), oxcarbazepine (Trileptal), primidone (Mysoline), tiagabine (Gabitril), topiramate (Topamax)

### 5.16.4   Intervention

- Elevate head of bed.
- Monitor vital signs.
- Monitor neurological status.

- Monitor for increased intracranial pressure (decreased level of consciousness, restlessness, confusion, headaches, nausea, and vomiting).
- Instruct the patient
    - Refrain from activities that are physically or mentally demanding.
    - Refrain from alcohol or illegal drugs.

## 5.17  Subdural Hematoma

A subdural hematoma is blood (blood clot) that accumulates between the dura mater and arachnoid in what is called the subdural space and has the highest mortality and morbidity rate of all hematomas. Subdural hematomas can be caused by head trauma or occur as a result of a lumbar puncture or other procedures, administration of anticoagulants, or spontaneously. Bleeding is typically from veins in the venous sinus and cerebral cortex. There are three classifications of subdural hematoma, each of which can be bilateral or unilateral.

- **Acute:** less than 72 hours after an acute injury and considered a medical emergency requiring surgical intervention to prevent increased intracranial pressure from occurring
- **Subacute:** 48 hours to two weeks following an acute injury
- **Chronic:** 21 days or older following an acute injury

### 5.17.1  Signs and Symptoms

- Unequal pupils indicating increased intracranial pressure
- Severe headache that is worsening related to increased bleedings
- Decreased level of consciousness (acute)
- Confusion
- Weakness on one side of the body (hemiparesis) (acute)
- Fixed/dilated pupils (acute)

### 5.17.2  Medical Tests

- CT scan shows hematoma.
- MRI shows hematoma.
- Arteriography shows altered blood flow.
- Lumbar puncture shows cerebrospinal fluid is yellow and low in protein if chronic subdural hematoma.

### 5.17.3  Treatment

- Small subdural hematomas are monitored and typically are self-resolving.
- Hematoma is surgically removed.

- Administer
  - Antiemetic medication for nausea and vomiting
    - Reglan (metoclopramide)
    - Zofran (ondansetron)
    - Compazine (prochlorperazine)
  - Diuretic to reduce cerebral edema
    - Mannitol, Lasix (furosemide)

### 5.17.4   Intervention

- Indicate bed rest.
- Monitor vital signs.
- Monitor neurological status.
- Monitor for increased intracranial pressure (decreased level of consciousness, restlessness, confusion, headaches, nausea, and vomiting).
- Instruct the patient
  - Do not take aspirin.
  - Do not take anticoagulants (heparin, Coumadin, Plavix).

## 5.18   Diffuse Axonal Injury

A diffuse axonal injury is a traumatic injury to the brain resulting in axon damage (white matter) in the brain stem, cerebral hemispheres, and corpus callosum, leading to axon disconnection and swelling. Diffuse axonal injuries are classified as:

- **Mild:** patient returns to baseline neurologic function within 24 hours of the injury.
- **Moderate:** patient is in a coma for a few days.
- **Severe:** patient is in a coma for weeks.

### 5.18.1   Signs and Symptoms

- Loss of consciousness
- Abnormal posturing
- Coma
- Dysautonomia (dysfunction of the autonomic nervous system)

### 5.18.2   Medical Tests

- CT scan shows cerebral edema and cerebral tissue damage.
- MRI shows cerebral edema and cerebral tissue damage.

### 5.18.3 Treatment

- Administer
  - ○ Polyethylene glycol to seal the membrane and prevent severe calcium influx
  - ○ Diuretic to reduce cerebral edema
    - ▪ Mannitol, Lasix (furosemide)
  - ○ Corticosteroid to decrease inflammation
    - ▪ Dexamethasone (Decadron)

### 5.18.4 Intervention

- Indicate bed rest.
- Total care is required. The patient is typically in a coma.
- Monitor vital signs.
- Monitor neurological status.
- Instruct the patient
  - ○ The patient may experience amnesia when he or she returns to baseline neurologic function.
  - ○ The patient may require rehabilitation therapy.

## 5.19 Skull Fracture

A skull fracture is breakage of bones in the skull caused by blunt-force head trauma. Common skull fractures are:

- **Linear:** breakage transverses the thickness of the skull. No bone displacement occurs.
- **Comminuted:** bone is crushed, broken, and splintered.
- **Depressed:** breakage causes bone to be displaced inward, leading to increased intracranial pressure.
- **Basilar:** breakage occurs at the base of the skull.
- **Diastatic:** breakage occurs at a suture line.
- **Compound:** breakage causes the bone to tear the epidermis, meninges, paranasal sinuses, or middle ear.

### 5.19.1 Signs and Symptoms

- Asymptomatic
- Bleeding from nose, ears, eyes, or site of wound
- Pupils unequal and not reactive to light
- Visual disturbances
- Drainage of clear fluid (cerebral spinal fluid) from the ears or nose
- Bruising behind the ears (Battle sign) or under the eyes (raccoon eyes)

- Loss of smell
- Confusion
- Irritability
- Nausea or vomiting
- Confusion
- Restlessness
- Headache
- Seizure

## 5.19.2 Medical Tests

- CT scan shows fracture, hemorrhage, and swelling.
- MRI shows fracture, hemorrhage, and swelling.

## 5.19.3 Treatment

- Linear fractures: no treatment is indicated.
- Observe overnight.
- Do not probe wound.
- Stabilize head and neck.
- Perform surgical repair (nonlinear fractures).
- Administer
  - Antibiotic (compound fracture)
  - Diuretic to reduce cerebral edema
    - Mannitol, Lasix (furosemide)
  - Corticosteroid to decrease inflammation
    - Dexamethasone (Decadron)
  - Antiepileptic
    - Carbamazepine (Tegretol), phenytoin (Dilantin), phenobarbital (Solfoton), clonazepam (Klonopin), valproic acid (Depakote), lamotrigine (Lamictal), gabapentin (Neurontin), levetiracetam (Keppra), oxcarbazepine (Trileptal), primidone (Mysoline), tiagabine (Gabitril), topiramate (Topamax)

## 5.19.4 Intervention

- Indicate bed rest.
- Monitor vital signs.
- Monitor neurological status.

- Monitor for increased intracranial pressure (decreased level of consciousness, restlessness, confusion, headaches, nausea, and vomiting).

- Instruct the patient

  ○ Do not take aspirin.

  ○ Do not take anticoagulants (heparin, Coumadin, Plavix).

## 5.20  Intracerebral Hematoma

An intracerebral hematoma is blood (blood clot) that accumulates in the cerebrum related to shear-force brain trauma leading to movement of the brain and surrounding nerve tissue. This can also be caused by hypertension. Bleeding is typically from veins, leading to slower bleeding.

### 5.20.1  Signs and Symptoms

- Unequal pupils, indicating increased intracranial pressure
- Severe headache worsening related to increased bleedings
- Decreased level of consciousness
- Confusion
- Nausea or vomiting
- Memory loss
- Impaired language ability (aphasia)

### 5.20.2  Medical Tests

- CT scan shows hematoma.
- MRI shows hematoma.

### 5.20.3  Treatment

- Surgical removal of the hematoma
- Administer

  ○ Antiemetic nausea and vomiting medication

    ▪ Reglan (metoclopramide)

    ▪ Zofran (Ondansetron)

    ▪ Compazine (prochlorperazine)

  ○ Diuretic to reduce cerebral edema

    ▪ Mannitol, Lasix (furosemide)

  ○ Antiepileptic

    ▪ Carbamazepine (Tegretol), phenytoin (Dilantin), phenobarbital (Solfoton), clonazepam (Klonopin), valproic acid (Depakote), lamotrigine (Lamictal), gabapentin (Neurontin), levetiracetam (Keppra), oxcarbazepine (Trileptal), primidone (Mysoline), tiagabine (Gabitril), topiramate (Topamax)

### 5.20.4   Intervention

- Indicate bed rest.

- Monitor vital signs.

- Monitor neurological status.

- Monitor for increased intracranial pressure (decreased level of consciousness, restlessness, confusion, headaches, nausea, and vomiting).

- Instruct the patient

    ○ Do not take aspirin.

    ○ Do not use anticoagulants (heparin, Coumadin, Plavix).

## 5.21   Subarachnoid Hemorrhage

A subarachnoid hemorrhage is bleeding into the area between the arachnoid membrane and the pia mater surrounding the brain, called the subarachnoid space, and is commonly caused by rupture of a cerebral aneurysm. It is often seen in elderly patients who have fallen and hit their head.

### 5.21.1   Signs and Symptoms

- Asymptomatic

- Thunderclap headache

- Low level of consciousness

- Vomiting

- Seizures

- Neck stiffness

- Drowsiness

- Coma

- Confusion

- Bleeding into the eyeball (Terson syndrome [intraocular hemorrhage])

### 5.21.2   Medical Tests

- CT scan shows bleeding.

- MRI scan shows bleeding.

- Cerebral angiography shows altered blood flow.

- Arteriography shows altered blood flow.

- Lumbar puncture indicates cerebrospinal fluid containing elevated number of red blood cells.

### 5.21.3 Treatment

- Surgical repair of bleeding

- Administer

  - Antiemetic for nausea and vomiting

    - Reglan (metoclopramide)

    - Zofran (Ondansetron)

    - Compazine (prochlorperazine)

  - Diuretic to reduce cerebral edema

    - Mannitol, Lasix (furosemide)

  - Antiepileptic

    - Carbamazepine (Tegretol), phenytoin (Dilantin), phenobarbital (Solfoton), clonazepam (Klonopin), valproic acid (Depakote), lamotrigine (Lamictal), gabapentin (Neurontin), levetiracetam (Keppra), oxcarbazepine (Trileptal), primidone (Mysoline), tiagabine (Gabitril), topiramate (Topamax)

### 5.21.4 Intervention

- Indicate bed rest.

- Monitor vital signs.

- Monitor neurological status.

- Monitor for increased intracranial pressure (decreased level of consciousness, restlessness, confusion, headaches, nausea, and vomiting).

- Instruct the patient

  - Do not take aspirin.

  - Do not use anticoagulants (heparin, Coumadin, Plavix).

## Solved Problems

**5.1**    How should a neurological emergency be approached?

A neurological emergency is considered life threatening until proven otherwise.

**5.2**    What is the initial focus in a neurological emergency?

Focus is on neurological problems after the patient's airway, breathing, circulation, and cervical spine are stabilized.

**5.3**    What is the first sign of a neurological emergency?

The first sign of a neurological emergency is the patient's altered mental status (AMS).

**5.4**    Why is it important to establish a baseline of the patient's mental status upon arrival in the emergency department?

It is a reference for later assessments of the patient's mental status, enabling the healthcare provider to know if the patient's mental status has changed.

**5.5**   What should the healthcare provider do if the patient presents as disoriented and unable to report signs of neurological impairment?

Focus the interview on first responders, family, and friends who accompanied the patient to the hospital or who can provide information about the patient's condition via phone.

**5.6**   How would the healthcare provider determine if a drowsy patient is sleeping?

A sleepy patient is arousable to a normal level of awareness.

**5.7**   How would the healthcare provider determine if a sleepy patient is in a stupor?

The patient is sleepy and can be aroused to a seminormal level of awareness using noxious stimuli.

**5.8**   How would the healthcare provider assess for mental impairment?

He or she would use the Abbreviated Mental Test Score (AMTS).

**5.9**   How would the healthcare provider develop the patient's baseline mental status?

He or she would use the Glasgow Coma Scale.

**5.10**   What would the healthcare provider suspect if the patient presents in an altered mental status and has the odor of acetone on his breath?

This may indicate diabetic ketoacidosis as a cause for neural impairment that can be reversed by administering insulin and fluids.

**5.11**   Why would the healthcare provider assess the patient's cardiac effectiveness in a neurological emergency?

Cardiac ineffectiveness may result in decreased circulatory function, leading to decreased oxygenation and neural impairment.

**5.12**   Why would the healthcare provider assess the patient's respiratory effectiveness in a neurological emergency?

Respiratory ineffectiveness may result in ineffective gas exchange, leading to decreased oxygenation and neural impairment.

**5.13**   What might pinpoint bilateral pupils that are nonreactive to light indicate?

- Lesion in the pons resulting from a hemorrhage may be indicated.

- Drug intoxication (heroin, opiates) may be indicated.

**5.14**   What might dilated bilateral fixed pupils that are nonreactive to light indicate?

- Cerebral ischemia

- Anticholinergic toxicity

- Severe brain damage

- Hypoxia

- Drug (sympathomimetic) intoxication (cocaine, methamphetamine, amphetamines, ecstasy, bath salts, stimulants)

**5.15** How would the healthcare provider test Cranial Nerve II?

Cranial Nerve II is involved in vision and can be tested using the Snellen eye chart.

**5.16** What is the easiest way to test Cranial Nerve X?

Ask the patient to talk.

**5.17** What is a cerebral angiograph?

A cerebral angiograph is a test that enables the practitioner to examine blood vessels in the brain.

**5.18** What are common reasons to perform a lumbar puncture?

The practitioner orders a lumbar puncture to assess for

- Bacteria
- Blood
- Relative intracranial pressure

**5.19** Why would a patient be administered barbiturates?

Barbiturates are used to reduce patient irritability and agitation. In addition, barbiturates are used to treat seizures, except for febrile seizures and absence seizures.

**5.20** What would a prescriber order for migraine headaches?

Serotonin inhibitors (Sumatriptan [Imitrex]) are used to treat migraine headaches. Serotonin inhibitors increase the risk of unstable blood pressure.

**5.22** What is a subdural hematoma?

A subdrual hematoma is bleeding from a vein in the area between the dura mater and the arachnoid mater resulting in slow, chronic bleeding.

**5.23** What is a countercoup?

Blunt-force trauma causes the head to recoil, thrusting the brain against the inside of the skull at a point opposite the blunt-force trauma.

**5.24** What causes increased intracranial pressure?

Cerebral edema, when fluid within the skull moves to the third space, causes increased intracranial pressure.

**5.25** What is a brain abscess?

Pus collects within the brain as a result of infection from the ear, sinuses, systemic circulation, or from within the brain, leading to cerebral edema. The cause is streptococci, staphylococci, anaerobes, or mixed organism infections.

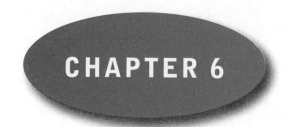

# CHAPTER 6

# *Gastrointestinal Emergencies*

## 6.1 Define

- A gastrointestinal emergency is a condition that alters ingestion, digestion, or fecal elimination, resulting in the patient becoming unstable.

- Gastrointestinal physiology can be disrupted by an obstruction, inflammation, infection, or trauma.

- A gastrointestinal emergency is considered life threatening until proven otherwise.

- Subtle changes in the patient's presentation can indicate deterioration of the patient's gastrointestinal system.

- The healthcare provider focuses on gastrointestinal problems after the patient's airway, breathing, circulation, cervical spine, and neurological system are stabilized.

- A gastrointestinal emergency requires immediate intervention.

### 6.1.1 Goal of Treating Gastrointestinal Emergencies

- The goal of the emergency-department staff is to identify the gastrointestinal emergency and stabilize the patient—not to treat the underlying cause of the gastrointestinal emergency, except in cases where the emergency department staff is able to resolve the problem. For example, a patient with an impacted stool might have the stool removed and is then discharged with a prescription for stool softener and intstructions to follow up with the patient's primary healthcare provider.

- Thoroughly assess the patient before beginning treatment. Administering medication may mask a sign or symptom that indicates a gastrointestinal emergency.

- Diagnose the acute problem.

- Stabilize the patient by relieving pain and treating the acute problem.

- Refer the patient to follow-up care to treat the underlying cause of the problem.

### 6.1.2 Gastrointestinal Assessment

- Be sure to follow the order of the gastrointestinal assessment:
  - Inspection
  - Auscultation

- ○ Percussion
- ○ Palpation
- The gastrointestinal assessment interview includes
  - ○ Open-ended questions:
    - Why did you come to the hospital today?
    - What makes you feel that something is wrong?
  - ○ Looking for clues for underlying cause of the gastrointestinal emergency:
    - Do you have allergies?
      - □ What allergies?
      - □ What allergic reactions do you experience?
    - Have you taken any medications or herbal supplements recently? (Medication can cause gastrointestinal problems such as nausea and vomiting, diarrhea, or constipation.)
      - □ What medications or herbal supplements have you taken?
      - □ When did you take them?
    - Have you undergone any medical procedure recently?
      - □ What medical procedure?
      - □ When was the medical procedure performed?
    - Have you eaten recently?
      - □ What did you eat?
      - □ When did you eat it?
      - □ Was there any immediate reaction?
    - What happened prior to your noticing this problem?
    - Do you have irregular bowel movements?
      - □ Describe the frequency and consistency of your bowel movements.
    - Is there blood in your stool?
      - □ How much blood?
    - Have there been changes in the appearance of your stool?
      - □ What changes did you notice?
      - □ When did you first notice the changes?
    - Have you recently traveled out of the country?
      - □ What country did you visit?
      - □ When did you travel?
      - □ What did you ingest while you were traveling?
      - □ Did you notice this problem when you were traveling?
      - □ Did you receive any vaccinations prior to traveling?
  - ○ Follow-up questions to help probe further into the presenting gastrointestinal problem:
    - When did this problem start?
    - How long have you had this problem?

- Can you describe the problem?

- How much does the problem bother you?

- Where do you feel uncomfortable?

- Is the problem spreading, or does the problem remain in one place?

- Does anything make the problem worse?

- Does anything make the problem better?

  - Questions about the patient's lifestyle:

    - Do you drink alcohol?

      - How much alcohol do you drink?

      - When did you start drinking alcohol?

      - Have you ever been treated for alcoholism?

    - Do you use recreational drugs or prescription drugs that are not prescribed to you?

      - What drugs?

      - How much do you use?

      - When did you start using drugs?

      - Have you ever been treated for drug abuse?

    - Do you use laxatives?

      - How frequently?

      - Are you able to have a bowel movement without using laxatives?

    - What stressors are in your life?

    - What is your occupation?

    - Do you have any dental problems or problems chewing food?

    - Do you have any dietary restrictions?

    - Do you exercise?

    - Do you use tobacco?

    - Have you been diagnosed with any medical condition?

      - What medical condition?

      - Are you being treated for the medical condition?

        - What is the treatment?

        - Who is treating you?

  - Questions about the patient's family history:

    - Does anyone in your family have colon cancer or a history of colon cancer?

    - Does anyone in your family have Crohn's disease or a history of Crohn's disease?

    - Does anyone in your family have ulcerative colitis or a history of ulcerative colitis?

- Inspection

  - Eyes

    - Abnormal: yellowing of the sclera

- Mouth
  - Abnormal: acetone, unusual odor
- Jaw
  - Abnormal: asymmetrical, swollen
- Bite
  - Abnormal: overbite or underbite
- Teeth
  - Abnormal: broken, missing
- Dentures
  - Abnormal: existing, improperly fitting
- Gums
  - Abnormal: swelling, bleeding, ulceration, exudate
- Lips
  - Abnormal: swelling, bleeding, ulceration, exudate
- Tongue
  - Abnormal: swelling, bleeding, ulceration
- Pharynx
  - Abnormal: lesions, uvular deviation, plaque, exudate, abnormal tonsils
- Abdomen
  - Skin
    - Abnormal: striated (pink, blue, silvery white), dilated veins, scars
  - Surface
    - Abnormal: asymmetrical, masses, bulges, peristalsis waves, pulsation
- Auscultation
  - Abdomen
    - Turn off suction to abdominal tube or nasogastric tube before auscultating the abdomen.
    - Listen for at least 2 minutes in each quadrant (Figure 6.1).
    - Use the diaphragm of the stethoscope to listen for bowel sounds.
    - Use the bell of the stethoscope to listen for vascular sounds.
    - No vascular sounds should be heard in a normal abdomen.
    - Right lower quadrant
      - Abnormal: hypoactive bowel sounds, hyperactive bowel sounds
    - Right upper quadrant
      - Abnormal: hypoactive bowel sounds, hyperactive bowel sounds
    - Left upper quadrant
      - Abnormal: hypoactive bowel sounds, hyperactive bowel sounds
    - Left lower quadrant
      - Abnormal: hypoactive bowel sounds, hyperactive bowel sounds

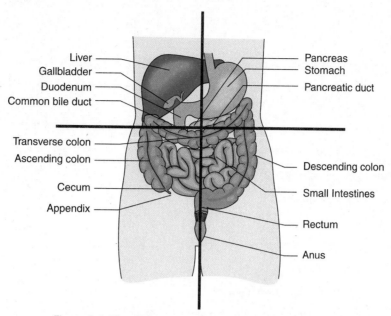

Figure 6.1 The abdomen is divided into four quadrants.

- Percussion
  - Abdomen
    - Don't percuss the abdomen if the patient received a transplanted abdominal organ.
    - Don't percuss the abdomen if you hear a bruit, venous hum, or friction rub over the abdomen.
    - Direct percussion: strike your finger over the abdomen.
    - Indirect percussion: rest your finger on the abdomen and strike the finger with the middle finger of your dominant hand.
    - Determine the location and size of abdominal organs.
      - Tympany sound (clear, hollow sound) indicates no organ or hollow organ.
      - Dull sound indicates organ or solid mass.
    - Percuss right lower quadrant.
    - Percuss right upper quadrant.
    - Percuss left upper quadrant.
    - Percuss left lower quadrant.
  - Liver
    - Begin percussing below the umbilicus at the right, mid-clavicular line.
      - Initial sound is tympany.
    - Move upward.
      - Dullness indicates the edge of the liver. Mark this position with a felt-tip pen.
    - Move downward from above the nipple along the right, mid-clavicular line.
      - The sound should be from tympany over the lungs to dullness near the 5th to 7th intercostal space. Mark this position with a felt-tip pen.
    - Measure the distance between these two marks to estimate the size of the liver.

- Palpation
  - Abdomen
    - **Light palpation:** press fingertips lightly into the abdomen ½ inch to ¾ inch
    - **Deep palpation:** press fingertips of both hands into the abdomen 1½ inches, moving in a circular motion over structures within the abdomen.
      - Rebound tenderness may occur when fingertips are withdrawn from the abdomen.
    - Palpate right lower quadrant
    - Palpate right upper quadrant
    - Palpate left upper quadrant
    - Palpate left lower quadrant
  - Spleen
    - Ask the patient to stand.
    - Stand to the right side of the patient.
    - Place your hand on the back left of the patient's lower rib cage.
    - Ask the patient to take a deep breath.
    - Place your right hand on the patient's abdomen.
    - Press your right hand up to the spleen
    - Stop palpating if you feel the spleen, as continuing to palpate risks rupturing the spleen.
      - A normal spleen is not palpable.
  - Liver
    - Begin at the lower left quadrant.
    - Ask the patient to take and hold a deep breath.
    - Ask the patient to exhale while you move your hands upward to the margin of the liver.
      - A normal liver is not palpable.

### 6.1.2.1   Signs and Symptoms

Gastrointestinal assessment in an emergency situation requires the nurse to recognize common signs and symptoms of underlying causes and then prepare for the treatment that the practitioner is likely to order.

Commonly seen signs and symptoms:

- Rebound tenderness is caused by aggravation of the parietal layer of the peritoneum by stretching or moving.
  - Place patient in the supine position.
  - The patient needs to relax abdominal muscles.
  - Place hand on the right lower quadrant between the umbilicus and the anterior superior iliac spine (McBurney's point).
  - Dip fingers deeply into the abdomen.

- ○ Release pressure quickly.
- ○ If pain:
  - ▪ Rebound tenderness is present (appendicitis).
  - ▪ Assessment should not be repeated (risk of rupturing appendix).
- • Obturator sign (Cope sign) indicates irritation of the obturator internus muscle.
  - ○ Place patient in the supine position.
  - ○ Flex right leg 90 degrees.
  - ○ Hold leg at ankle and above the knee.
  - ○ Rotate leg laterally.
  - ○ Rotate leg medially.
  - ○ If pain in hypogastric region:
    - ▪ Obturator sign is positive (irritation of the obturator muscle).
- • Iliopsoas sign (Psoas sign) indicates irritation to the iliopsoas group or hip flexors in the abdomen.
  - ○ Place patient in the left side position.
  - ○ Keep legs straight.
  - ○ Exert pressure as the patient raises his right leg.
  - ○ Exert pressure as the patient raises his left leg.
  - ○ If abdominal pain:
    - ▪ Iliopsoas sign is positive (irritation of psoas muscle).
- • Vomiting
  - ○ Projectile vomiting (hypertrophic pyloric stenosis)
- • Diarrhea
  - ○ 300 g within 24 hours (viral infection, bacterial infection, ulcerative colitis)
- • Constipation
- • Bleeding
  - ○ Vomiting red blood (hematemesis), possibly from gums, teeth, esophageal varices
  - ○ Vomiting dark blood resembling coffee grounds, indicating possible peptic ulcer
  - ○ Severe retching and coughing up blood (Mallory-Weiss syndrome, gastroesophageal laceration syndrome)
  - ○ Low blood pressure
  - ○ Rapid heart rate
  - ○ Black tarry stool (melena), indicating possible GI bleed
  - ○ Bloody red stool, indicating possible hemorrhoids
- • Jaundice
  - ○ Yellowing of sclera (white of the eye)
  - ○ Yellowing of skin
  - ○ Pale stool
  - ○ Dark urine

- Abdominal pain/tenderness
  - Sudden abdominal pain with rigidity, and then pain subsidies (possible perforation)
  - Abdominal rigidity (possible peritonitis)
  - Acute right upper quadrant pain (possible acute cholecystitis)
  - Colicky abdominal pain (possible hernia, adhesion, or tumor)
  - Left iliac fossa pain (possible acute diverticulitis)
  - Right iliac fossa pain (possible appendicitis)
- Abdominal sounds
  - Vascular swishing sound or bruits (possible arterial obstruction or arterial stenosis)
  - Vascular hum (possible cirrhosis)
  - Vascular grating sound (possible inflammation)
  - Hypoactive sound or absence of sound (possible peritonitis or paralytic ileus)
  - High-pitched rushing with presentment of abdominal cramps (possible intestinal obstruction)
  - Hyperactive (possible early intestinal obstruction, hunger, or diarrhea)
  - High-pitched tinkling (air or fluid in the intestine)
- Fever
- Increased white blood cell count or leukocytosis (indicating infection)

## 6.2   Gastrointestinal Tests

Gastrointestinal tests are designed to assess the effectiveness and the capability of the gastrointestinal system to function. Emergency-department practitioners order gastrointestinal tests to collect objective data to further assess and assist in stabilizing the patient. Once stabilized, the patient is transferred or referred to follow-up care designed to treat the underlying cause of the current episode, which may require additional gastrointestinal tests. Gastrointestinal procedures are performed to stabilize the patient.

The following are gastrointestinal tests and procedures commonly ordered by the emergency department's practitioners.

### 6.2.1   Abdominal X-Ray

An abdominal x-ray is commonly called a kidney-ureter-bladder radiography. Besides the kidneys, ureter, and bladder, the x-ray also creates an image of other structures within the abdomen. At least two images are captured: one lying down and the other standing.

Dense structures such as bone block x-ray particles, causing those structures to appear white. Less-dense structures such as fat block some x-ray particles, causing those structures to appear gray. Air does not block x-ray particles and appears dark. An x-ray image cannot differentiate between fluid and air.

The practitioner commonly orders an abdominal x-ray to assess for:

- Intestinal rupture
- Lesions
- Tumors

**Abdominal X-Ray Procedure**

- Be sure the patient is not pregnant.

- Tell patient to remove all jewelry from the area to be x-rayed since jewelry may appear on the x-ray image.

- Assess if the patient has scars in the abdomen area. If so, note the location of the scars since the scars may appear on the x-ray image.

- Instruct the patient to remove his clothes. Provide the patient with a gown.

- The patient lies down on the x-ray table, and the x-ray plate is positioned below the table. Or, the patient stands in front of the x-ray table, and the x-ray plate is positioned behind the patient.

- The initial result, called a "wet read," provides a relatively superficial assessment of the image. A more thorough reading is taken hours or days later.

## 6.2.2   Abdominal CT Scan

An abdominal CT scan provides a three-dimensional image of the abdomen using x-rays and enables the practitioner to visualize normal and abnormal structures within the abdomen. A CT can be performed with or without a contrast agent. A contrast agent is iodine-based and enhances images of blood vessels and less-dense areas of the abdomen.

The practitioner commonly orders an abdominal CT scan to assess for:

- Inflammation

- Tumor

- Occult malignancy

- Cysts

- Pseudocysts

- Blood clots

- Abscesses

- Differentiation between nonobstructive and obstructive jaundice

- Pancreatitis

**CT Scan Procedure**

- Assess if the patient is allergic to iodine or shellfish if the patient is undergoing a CT scan with contrast. Patients who are allergic to iodine or shellfish have a high likelihood of experiencing an allergic reaction to the contrast agent.

- Administer diphenhydramine (Benadryl) and prednisone (Deltasone) before the CT scan to reduce the risk of an allergic reaction to the contrast agent, if a contrast agent is ordered.

- Administer the contrast agent through an IV. The patient may feel flushed and have a salty or metallic taste in his or her mouth.

- Explain to the patient that the contrast material typically discolors the urine for upward of 24 hours following the CT scan. The patient should increase fluid intake after the CT scan to flush the contrast agent from the patient's body, if a contrast agent is used for the CT scan.

- Assess if the patient is claustrophobic. The patient will be placed in an enclosure during the test.

- Assess if the patient can remain still for 30 minutes during the CT scan, as the CT scanner encircles the patient for up to 30 minutes.

### 6.2.3　Gastrointestinal MRI

A gastrointestinal magnetic resonance imaging (MRI) provides a three-dimensional view of the gastrointestinal system using radio waves, a strong magnet, and a computer. An MRI is particularly used to assess fluid-filled soft tissue and to identify tumors from other structures within the gastrointestinal system.

**Gastrointestinal MRI Procedure**

- The patient may need to be NPO (nothing by mouth) for up to 12 hours before the test depending on the site of the MRI.

- All metal must be removed from the patient, and no metal may enter the room containing the MRI scanner. The MRI scanner's magnet is always activated.

- Assess if the patient is claustrophobic. If so, then ask the healthcare provider if an open MRI scanner should be used for the test, or if the patient should be sedated before the scan begins.

- The gastrointestinal MRI scan takes about 30 minutes.

- The gastrointestinal MRI scan is noninvasive. The patient will not feel any discomfort.

### 6.2.4　Upper Gastrointestinal Endoscopy

An upper gastrointestinal endoscopy is also referred to as a gastroscopy and is used to visualize the pharynx, esophagus, lower esophageal sphincter, stomach, pyloric sphincter, and duodenum. An upper gastrointestinal endoscopy is performed to diagnose peptic, gastric, or duodenal ulcers and to obtain biopsies and specimens for H. pylori.

**Upper Gastrointestinal Endoscopy Procedure**

- The patient will be NPO (nothing by mouth) for up to 12 hours before the procedure.

- The patient signs an informed consent prior to any anesthesia.

- The patient receives intravenous conscious sedation during the procedure. The healthcare provider monitors vital signs to determine if the patient is tolerating the sedation.

- The healthcare provider assesses for loss of teeth.

- Dentures must be removed.

- The back of the throat is anesthetized to prevent the gag reflex.

- A thin, flexible tube (endoscope) is passed through the pharynx, the stomach, and into the upper part of the small intestine.

- The practitioner observes, photographs, and obtains biopsies and specimens during the procedure as necessary.

- Vital signs are monitored during and after the procedure, including oxygen saturation.

- The patient is placed flat on his side until the sedation wears off.

- The patient is monitored until the gag reflex returns.

- The patient should receive nothing by mouth until the gag reflex returns.

- The patient receives ice chips and then sips of water after the gag reflex returns. The patient's intake is gradually increased based on patient's tolerance.

- The practitioner assesses for laryngospasm, difficulty swallowing, spitting up blood, black tarry stools, pain, and fever. These can be signs of a perforation that may have occurred during the procedure.

## 6.2.5   Nasogastric (NG) Intubation

A nasogastric (NG) tube is inserted into the patient to remove stomach contents either by bulb syringe or suction in cases of intestinal obstruction, bleeding, or other gastrointestinal difficulties where the stomach content places the patient at risk. The nasogastric tube can also be used for feeding.

**Nasogastric Intubation Procedure**

- Instruct the patient to sit.

- Measure the length of the nasogastric tube:

  - Hold the tip of the tube at tip of the patient's nose

  - Extend the tube to the patient's earlobe and hold the tube by the patient's earlobe.

  - Extend the tube from the patient's earlobe to the xiphoid process. This is the length of the nasogastric tube.

  - Mark this length on the tube with tape. The tape is the point where you stop inserting the nasogastric tube.

- Assess the patency of each nostril.

- Lubricate the end of the nasogastric tube.

- Ask the patient to place his chin on his chest as you insert the nasogastric tube.

- Insert the nasogastric tube into the patient's patent nostril.

- Ask the patient to swallow as the nasogastric tube advances through the pharynx.

- Check placement of the nasogastric tube:

  - Attach a bulb syringe to the nasogastric tube.

  - Aspirate the stomach contents.

  - Place the stomach contents on a pH test strip. The pH test strip should report less than or equal to 6.

## 6.2.6   Gastric Lavage

Gastric lavage is a procedure used to treat gastric hemorrhage and to treat drug overdoses, depending on the nature of the drug. Irrigating fluid is instilled through a nasogastric (NG) tube into the upper gastrointestinal system, and the gastric content is aspirated through the NG tube.

**Gastric Lavage Procedure**

- Protect the airway from aspiration and have suction equipment available.

- Monitor vital signs and oxygen saturation every 5 to 10 minutes.

- Insert a large-bore nasogastric tube (see 6.2.5 Nasogastric (NG) Intubation).

- Lower the head of the bed 15 degrees.

- Position the patient on his left side.

- Fill a syringe with 50 ml of irrigating solution. The practitioner may order a vasoconstrictor added to the irrigating fluid to increase the irrigation performance.

- Instill the contents of the syringe into the NG tube. Continue until 250 ml of irrigating solution is instilled.

- Wait 30 seconds.

- Withdraw the irrigating solution using the syringe, or drain the NG tube into an emesis basin.

- Measure the amount of irrigating solution instilled and the volume of fluid withdrawn. If less fluid is withdrawn, then suspect abdominal distention that may result in vomiting.

- Continuously monitor the patient. There is a risk of vomiting, aspiration, bradycardia, electrolyte imbalance, fluid overload, and metabolic acidosis.

### 6.2.7 Nasogastric Decompression

Nasogastric decompression is a process used to aspirate intestinal contents and to assist in resolving an intestinal obstruction using a nasogastric decompression tube. Nasogastric decompression is also used to prevent nausea and vomiting and to reduce the risk of abdominal distention following gastrointestinal surgery.

A nasogastric decompression tube contains a balloon filled with water, air, or mercury located at the end of the tube that is inserted into the patient. The nasogastric decompression tube stimulates peristalsis, enabling passage into the intestine. There are four commonly used nasogastric decompression tubes. They are:

- **Cantor tube:** single-lumen tube, used for aspiration and to relieve bowel obstruction

- **Dennis tube:** three-lumen tube used to decompress the intestines for surgery

- **Harris tube:** single-lumen tube used to lavage the intestinal tract

- **Miller-Abbott tube:** two-lumen tube used for aspiration and to reduce bowel obstruction

**Nasogastric Decompression Procedure**

- Assess the patency of each nostril for septal deviation.

- Estimate the length of the tube by measuring from the tip of the nose, around the ear, and down just below the costal margin.

- Position the patient in an upright position with the neck partially flexed.

- Lubricate the end of the nasogastric tube.

- Ask the patient to place her chin on her chest as you insert the nasogastric tube.

- Insert the nasogastric tube into the patient's patent nostril along the floor of the nose. Advance the tube parallel to the nasal floor until the tube reaches the back of the nasopharynx where resistance will be encountered.

- Ask the patient to swallow as the nasogastric tube advances through the pharynx until the estimated length is reached.

- Confirm placement using an x-ray.

- Connect to suction per practitioner's order.

- Continuously monitor the patient. There is a risk of vomiting, aspiration, bradycardia, electrolyte imbalance, fluid overload, and metabolic acidosis.

- Monitor for nasogastric decompression tube obstruction. If the nasogastric decompression tube is obstructed:

  ○ Disconnect nasogastric decompression tube from suction.

  ○ Irrigate the nasogastric decompression tube with normal saline. Drain the normal saline with gravity flow.

- ○ Carefully pull the nasogastric decompression tube to remove any kinks in it.

- ○ Don't pull the nasogastric decompression tube if:

    - ■ The nasogastric decompression tube was difficult to insert.

    - ■ The nasogastric decompression tube was inserted during surgery.

## 6.2.8   Spleen-Liver Scan

A spleen-liver scan is used to identify abnormalities in the liver and spleen. A radioactive marker is infused intravenously into the patient. A normal liver absorbs most of the marker, and the rest is absorbed by the spleen. Lack of absorption indicates an abnormal liver or spleen, which is confirmed by other imaging tests.

**Spleen-Liver Scan Procedure**

- Insert an intravenous line into the patient.

- Instill the radioactive marker.

- Place the patient in the spleen-liver scan.

- Monitor for adverse reactions from the radioactive marker and report any adverse reactions to the practitioner.

    - ○ Difficulty breathing

    - ○ Fever

    - ○ Flush feeling

    - ○ Light-headedness

## 6.2.9   Liver Function Test

Liver function tests are assessments of hepatic function based on analysis of venous blood obtained through a venipuncture. Normal values for tests are determined by the laboratory that is analyzing the blood sample. Liver function tests include:

- **Alanine transaminase (ALT):** an enzyme found mainly in liver cells, ALT helps the body metabolize protein. When the liver is damaged, ALT is released into the bloodstream.

- **Aspartate transaminase (AST):** the enzyme AST plays a role in the metabolism of alanine, an amino acid. An increase in AST levels may indicate liver damage or disease.

- **Alkaline phosphatase (ALP):** ALP is an enzyme found in high concentrations in the liver and bile ducts, as well as some other tissues. Higher than normal levels of ALP may indicate liver damage or disease.

- **Albumin and total protein:** levels of albumin—a protein made by the liver—and total protein show how well the liver is making proteins the body needs to fight infections and perform other functions. Lower than normal levels may indicate liver damage or disease.

- **Bilirubin:** bilirubin is a red-yellow pigment that results from the breakdown of red blood cells. Normally, bilirubin passes through the liver and is excreted in stool. Elevated levels of bilirubin (jaundice) may indicate liver damage or disease.

- **Gamma-glutamyl transferase (GGT):** this test measures the amount of the enzyme GGT in the blood. Higher than normal levels may indicate liver or bile duct injury.

- **Lactate dehydrogenase (LDH):** LDH is an enzyme found in many body tissues, including the liver. Elevated levels of LDH may indicate liver damage.

- **Prothrombin time (PT):** this test measures the clotting time of plasma. Increased PT may indicate liver damage.

- **Hepatitis panel:** tests for acute viral hepatitis include HBsAg, anti-HAV, IgM anti-HBc, and anti-HCV. Tests for chronic hepatitis include HBsAg and anti-HCV. HAV is confirmed by detecting an IgM antibody to HAV (IgM anti-HAV); HBV by HBsAg and IgM anti-HBc (when HBeAg is detected, patient is highly infectious); HCV by ELISA-2 and RIBA-2; HDV by anti-HDV and serologic markers for HBV. For HEV, only research-based tests are available at this time.

## 6.2.10   Paracentesis

Paracentesis is a procedure of aspirating fluid from the peritoneal space to decrease intra-abdominal pressure, treat ascites, and assess for intra-abdominal bleeding. Aspiration is performed by insertion of a needle or cannula through the abdominal wall into the peritoneal space.

**Paracentesis Procedure**

- The patient must sign an informed consent.

- The patient's bladder must be emptied prior to the procedure either through urination or insertion of an indwelling urinary catheter.

- The patient's weight and abdominal area are measured.

- The patient is positioned in the supine position in bed.

- A local anesthetic is administered to the insertion site.

- The collection container is placed below the level of the patient.

- The needle or cannula is inserted.

- The head of bed is raised 45 degrees or the patient is asked to sit at the side of the bed.

- Fluid drains via gravity from the peritoneal space into the collection container.

- No more than 1,500 ml should be aspirated during the procedure.

- The patient should be monitored every 15 minutes for adverse side effects. If adverse side effects are noticed, then the collection container should be raised closer to the level of the needle or cannula and adverse side effects should be reported to the practitioner immediately.

  ○ Hypovolemic shock

  ○ Diaphoresis

  ○ Tachycardia

  ○ Hypotension

  ○ Pallor

  ○ Dizziness

- A dry sterile pressure dressing is applied to the site once the needle or cannula is removed from the patient.

  ○ The dressing is changed every 15 minutes for the first 60 minutes.

  ○ The dressing is changed every 30 minutes for the next two hours.

  ○ The dressing is changed every four hours for the next 24 hours.

- Vital signs are monitored.

- The patient is monitored for signs of shock and hemorrhage.

- The patient's weight and abdominal area are documented following the procedure.

- The peritoneal fluid is sent to the laboratory for analysis.

## 6.2.11   Lower Gastrointestinal Endoscopy

A lower gastrointestinal endoscopy is also referred to as a colonoscopy and is used to assess structures and disorders in the lower gastrointestinal tract. Lower gastrointestinal endoscopy procedure requires the lower bowels to be clean prior to the procedure.

### Gastrointestinal Endoscopy Procedure

- The patient must sign an informed consent.

- The patient should not eat or ingest liquids for six hours before the procedure, if possible. In emergencies, this may not be possible; however, assess the last time the patient ingested food or liquid.

- The practitioner may want to perform an electrolyte gastric lavage (see 6.2.6 Gastric Lavage) prior to the lower gastrointestinal endoscopy to decrease the risk of aspiration.

- The bowel is cleaned with a Fleet enema.

- Baseline vital signs are recorded.

- The practitioner may administer conscious sedation prior to and during the procedure.

- Oxygen is administered per the practitioner's order.

- The patient is instructed to breathe slowly and deeply as the scope is inserted.

- The patient's vital signs are monitored during the procedure.

- After the procedure

  ○ The patient's vital signs are monitored every 15 minutes for the first hour.

  ○ The patient's vital signs are monitored every 30 minutes for the next hour.

  ○ The patient is monitored for rectal bleeding (frank and occult).

## 6.2.12   Fecal Test

A fecal test is used to assess gastrointestinal problems. A fecal sample is taken and sent to the laboratory for analysis. The laboratory results might indicate gastrointestinal abnormalities. There are common findings:

- **Hard, solid stool:** constipation related to medication or diet

- **Loose stool:** diarrhea related to viral infection or spastic bowel disorder

- **Pasty stool:** high-fat content related to pancreatic disorder or intestinal malabsorption disorder

- **Greasy stool:** high-fat content related to pancreatic disorder or intestinal malabsorption disorder

- **Yellow stool:** prolonged diarrhea

- **Green stool:** prolonged diarrhea

- **Narrow, ribbon stool:** irritable bowel disorder, obstruction of the bowel or rectum, or spastic bowel disorder

- **Black stool:** gastrointestinal bleed, iron supplement ingested

- **Red stool:** rectal bleeding related to hemorrhoids or side effect of drugs or foods
- **White stool:** blockage of hepatic or gallbladder duct, or cancer
- **Mucus containing stool:** bacterial infection
- **Pus containing stool:** colitis.

## 6.3   Gastrointestinal Medication

There are six categories of medication commonly used in gastrointestinal emergencies. These are antacids, antiemetics, histamine-2 receptor antagonists, proton pump inhibitors, ammonia detoxicants, and antidiuretic hormones. Antacids decrease stomach acidity. Antiemetics prevent and treat nausea and vomiting. Histamine-2 receptor antagonists and proton pump inhibitors reduce the production of acid in the stomach. Ammonia detoxicants decrease ammonia levels in blood. Antidiuretic hormones decrease gastrointestinal bleeding.

### 6.3.1   Antacids

Antacids are medication that increases the pH level in the stomach, resulting in decreased stomach acidity. Antacids are prescribed for indigestion, heartburn, and peptic ulcer disorders. Commonly prescribed antacids are:

- **Aluminum hydroxide (Alu-Cap):** can also cause intestinal obstruction and constipation
- **Aluminum hydroxide and magnesium hydroxide (Maalox):** can also cause diarrhea and hypermagnesemia
- **Calcium carbonate (Caltrate):** can be used as a calcium supplement and can also cause hypercalcemia, nausea, and vomiting

### 6.3.2   Antiemetics

Antiemetics are medications used to prevent and treat nausea and vomiting associated with postoperative procedures and adjunct therapy for treatment such as chemotherapy. Commonly prescribed antiemetics are:

- **Ondansetron (Zofran):** can also cause diarrhea, pruritus, abnormal liver tests, and arrhythmias
- **Dolasetron (Anzemet):** can also cause diarrhea, pruritus, abnormal liver tests, and arrhythmias
- **Metoclopramide (Reglan):** can increase emptying of the stomach and can cause anxiety, suicidal ideation, depression, hypertension, restlessness, seizures, and bradycardia

### 6.3.3   H2-Receptor Antagonists

H2-receptor antagonists are medications used to block the action of histamine on the parietal cells in the stomach, reducing the production of acid. H2-receptor antagonists are prescribed for treating Zollinger-Ellison syndrome, gastric ulcers, gastroesophageal reflux disease (GERD), and duodenal ulcers. Commonly prescribed H2-receptor antagonists are:

- **Famotidine (Pepcid):** can also cause diarrhea, constipation, headache, and palpitations
- **Ranitidine (Zantac):** can also cause blurred vision, malaise, leukopenia, jaundice, depression, and confusion

## 6.3.4  Proton Pump Inhibitors

Proton pump inhibitors are medications used to block the action of the gastric proton pump of the parietal cells in the stomach, resulting in reduced gastric acid secretions. Proton pump inhibitors are prescribed for treating Zollinger-Ellison syndrome, gastric ulcers, gastroesophageal reflux disease (GERD), and duodenal ulcers. Commonly prescribed proton pump inhibitors are:

- **Omeprazole (Prilosec):** can also cause hyperglycemia, constipation, diarrhea, and dizziness
- **Lansoprazole (Prevacid):** can also cause hyperglycemia, constipation, diarrhea, and dizziness
- **Pantoprazole (Protronix):** can also cause hyperglycemia, constipation, diarrhea, and dizziness

## 6.3.5  Ammonia Detoxicants

Ammonia detoxicants are medications used to decrease the ammonia in blood and are prescribed for treating encephalopathy. The commonly prescribed ammonia detoxicants is:

- **Lactulose (Chronulac):** can also cause flatulence, diarrhea, and abdominal cramps

## 6.3.6  Antidiuretic Hormone

Antidiuretic hormone is used to decrease bleeding and is prescribed for treating gastrointestinal hemorrhage. The commonly prescribed antidiuretic hormone is:

- **Vasopressin (Pitressin):** can also cause arrhythmias, bronchospasms, cardiac arrest, angina, and small bowel infarction

## 6.4  Appendicitis

An obstruction in the vermiform appendix leads to the secretion of fluid by the mucosal lining of the appendix, increased pressure, and decreased blood flow to the appendix, resulting in gangrene and possible perforation (rupture) within 36 to 48 hours.

## 6.4.1  Signs and Symptoms

- Guarding of the abdomen
- Abdominal pain from periumbical to right lower quadrant
- Abdominal rigidity
- Rebound pain
- Right lower quadrant abdominal pain that decreases with right hip flexing (indicates perforation)
- Loss of appetite
- Fever
- Nausea and vomiting

### 6.4.2 Medical Tests

- Ultrasound shows enlarged appendix.
- CT scan shows enlarged appendix.
- Blood test
  - Increased WBC

### 6.4.3 Treatment

- Appendectomy
- Administer
  - Analgesics for pain
    - Meperidine
  - Antibiotics

### 6.4.4 Intervention

- Indicate NPO.
- Monitor vital signs.
- Monitor intake and output.
- Monitor bowel sounds.
- Assess pain level.
- Instruct the patient that he or she can expect to return to a normal lifestyle following treatment.

## 6.5 Cholecystitis

This is acute or chronic inflammation of the gallbladder related to cholelithiasis (gallstones). Acute cholecystitis occurs when blood flow to the gallbladder decreases, commonly from a blocked cystic duct by a gallstone, leading to difficulty filling and emptying the gallbladder. The gallbladder becomes inflamed, bile is retained, and the gallbladder becomes distended. Chronic cholecystitis occurs when there are recurrent episodes of cholecystitis that result in chronic inflammation of the gallbladder, leading to obstructive jaundice and an increased risk of gangrene and perforation.

### 6.5.1 Signs and Symptoms

- Pain in the upper right quadrant of the abdomen or epigastric area radiating to the right shoulder
- Positive Murphy's sign (upper right quadrant abdominal pain increases with palpation on inspiration resulting in the patient being unable to take a deep breath)
- Increased flatulence
- Increased eructation (belching)
- Clay-colored stool
- Foamy, dark urine

- Nausea and vomiting following ingestion of fatty foods
- Decreased appetite
- Fever
- Icterus
- Pruritis (itching)
- Jaundice

## 6.5.2   Medical Tests

- Blood test
  - Increased bilirubin direct (conjugated)
  - Increased bilirubin indirect (unconjugated)
  - Increased WBC
  - Increased alkaline phosphatase, aspartate aminotransferase (AST)
  - Increased lactate dehydrogenase (LDH)
- CT scan shows inflammation of the gallbladder or gallstones.
- Ultrasound of gallbladder shows inflammation of the gallbladder or gallstones.
- HIDA scan (hepatic iminodiacetic acid) shows blocked cystic duct.

## 6.5.3   Treatment

- Aspiration of gallstone
- Surgical removal of gallbladder
  - Laparoscopic cholecystectomy, open cholecystectomy
- Insertion of stent into gallbladder if surgery is not an option
- Administer
  - Antiemetics for nausea and vomiting
    - Prochlorperazine, trimethobenzamide
  - Replacement of fat-soluble vitamins
    - Vitamins A, D, E, K
  - Analgesics for pain
    - Meperidine, no morphine
  - Antibiotics

## 6.5.4   Intervention

- Monitor vital signs.
- Monitor bowel sounds.
- Assess pain level.
- Instruct the patient to eat a low-fat diet.

## 6.6 Cirrhosis

Chronic inflammation of the liver and necrosis of liver tissue leads to fibrosis and nodule formation resulting in the blockage of blood vessels and the bile duct, causing increased portal vein pressure, backup of venous blood to the spleen, enlarged liver and spleen, and decreased liver function. Common causes are chronic alcohol use, hepatitis, fatty liver (steatohepatitis), metabolic disorders (hemachromatosis), or cystic fibrosis.

### 6.6.1 Signs and Symptoms

- Asymptomatic
- Fatigue
- Weight loss
- Ecchymosis (bruises) related to decreased vitamin K absorption
- Petechiae
- Muscle cramps
- Nausea
- Pruritus (itching)
- Spider veins
- Peripheral edema
- Portal hypertension
- Jaundice
- Hepatomegaly (enlarged liver)
- Palmar erythema (red palms)
- Impotence
- Ascites
- Dyspnea
- Glossitis (inflammation of the tongue)
- Encephalopathy (asterixis, tremors, delirium, drowsiness, dysarthria, coma)

### 6.6.2 Medical Tests

- Blood test
  - Increased
    - Aspartate aminotransferase (AST)
    - Alanine aminotransferase (ALT)
    - Lactate dehydrogenase (LDH)
    - Bilirubin direct (conjugated)
    - Bilirubin indirect (unconjugated)

- MCV
- MCH
- Ammonia
- Prothrombin time
  - Decreased
    - Protein
    - Albumin
    - WBC
    - Platelet count
- Urine analysis
  - Increased bilirubin
- Fecal analysis
  - Decreased urobilinogen
- X-ray shows hepatomegaly.
- CT scan shows hepatomegaly and ascites.
- Ultrasound shows hepatomegaly, ascites, and portal-vein blood flow.
- Esophagogastroduodenoscopy (EGD) shows esophageal varices.
- Liver biopsy shows fibrosis and regenerative nodules, which is the gold standard for the diagnosis.

### 6.6.3   Treatment

- Paracentesis to remove ascitic fluid
- Shunt inserted to drain ascitic fluid and divert blood flow
- Gastric lavage
- Esophagogastric balloon tamponade to control esophageal variceal bleeding
- Sclerotherapy to control esophageal variceal bleeding
- Liver transplant
- Administer
  - Vitamins
    - Folic acid, thiamine, multivitamin
  - Diuretics to excrete fluids
    - Furosemide, spironolactone
  - Lactulose to remove ammonia
  - Antibiotics to kill flora that produces ammonia
    - Neomycin sulfate, metronidazole

### 6.6.4   Intervention

- Elevate head of bed 30 degrees or more.
- Elevate feet.
- Monitor signs of bleeding.
- Monitor mental status.
- Restrict fluid intake.
- Monitor intake and output.
- Monitor vital signs.
- Weigh daily.
- Measure abdominal girth.
- Monitor electrolytes for imbalance.
- Monitor PT, PTT, INR.
- Monitor for peripheral edema.
- Monitor heart and lung sounds for excess fluid.
- Instruct the patient
  - Follow a low-sodium diet.
  - Do not drink alcohol.

## 6.7   Crohn's Disease

Crohn's disease is an inflammatory bowel disease that has periods of inflammation of the GI tract commonly affecting the intestine (terminal ileum and ascending colon), resulting in transmural inflammation (below the superficial mucosal layer) leading to strictures and fistulas.

### 6.7.1   Signs and Symptoms

- Non-bloody diarrhea
- Fatigue
- Weight loss
- Postprandial bloating (after meals)
- Borborygmi (loud, frequent bowel sounds)
- Abdominal cramping
- Pain in the right lower quadrant of the abdomen
- Fever
- Abdominal mass

- Fistula formation
- Vomiting
- Abcesses

### 6.7.2   Medical Tests

- Blood tests
  - Decreased RBC
  - Decreased albumin
  - Increased erythrocyte sedimentation rate (during exacerbations)
  - Decreased electrolytes
- CT scan shows thickening of bowel and abscess formation.
- Barium x-ray shows fistula formation, stricture formation.

### 6.7.3   Treatment

- Surgical repair of stricture and fistulas
- Administer
  - Vitamins
    - $B_{12}$, folic acid
  - Aminosalicylates
    - Mesalamine, sulfasalazine, olsalazine, balsalazide
  - Glucocorticoids
    - Hydrocortisone, budesonide
  - Purine
    - Azathioprine, 6-mercaptopurine
  - Methotrexate
  - Antidiarrheal medications
    - Diphenoxylate hydrochloride and atropine sulfate

### 6.7.4   Intervention

- Indicate dietary restrictions.
- Monitor intake and output.
- Monitor vital signs.
- Instruct the patient on
  - Proper skin care for bowel-skin fistula
  - Importance of dietary restrictions
  - Importance of nutritional supplements

## 6.8 Diverticulitis

Diverticulitis is a digestive disease particularly found in the large intestine in which undigested food becomes trapped in out-pouches (diverticula) along the intestinal tract, leading to bacterial growth that results in inflammation of the intestine and risk for bleeding, intestinal perforation, and formation of a fistula within the abdomen.

### 6.8.1 Signs and Symptoms

- Asymptomatic
- Bloating
- Rectal bleeding
- Change in bowel habits
- Abdominal pain (most common symptom)
- Fever
- Nausea
- Vomiting
- Lower left quadrant pain
- Fever
- High WBC (leukocytosis)
- Diarrhea
- Constipation

### 6.8.2 Medical Tests

- Blood test
  - Increased WBC
- CT scan shows thickening of intestinal wall.
- Barium enema shows diverticula (not performed during acute inflammation where there is a risk of perforation).
- Colonoscopy shows diverticula (not performed during acute inflammation where there is a risk of perforation).

### 6.8.3 Treatment

- Surgical repair of intestine
- Administer antibiotics
  - Ciprofloxacin, metronidazole, trimethoprim-sulfamethoxazole

### 6.8.4 Intervention

- Indicate NPO to rest bowel.
- Monitor vital signs.

- Monitor intake and output.

- Assess abdomen for bowel sounds and distention.

- Instruct the patient

  - High-fiber diet when asymptomatic

  - Low-residue diet during acute inflammation

  - No lifting during acute inflammation

  - No laxatives

  - No enemas

## 6.9   Gastroenteritis

Inflammation of the gastrointestinal mucosa, gastroenteritis is caused by a viral (common), bacterial, parasitic, or protozoal infection or an allergic response to toxin exposure.

### 6.9.1   Signs and Symptoms

- Diarrhea

- Abdominal pain

- Nausea and vomiting

- Fever

- Malaise

- Headache

- Dehydration

- Abdominal distention

### 6.9.2   Medical Tests

- Blood tests

  - Increased BUN

  - Increased creatinine

  - Electrolyte imbalance

  - Increased eosinophil count

  - Increased WBC count

- Stool sample

- Positive for parasitic infection

### 6.9.3   Treatment

- Administer

  - Intravenous fluids for dehydration

- Antiemetic medication
  - Prochlorperazine, trimethobenzamide
- Antidiarrheal medications
  - Loperamide, diphenoxylate, kaolin pectin, bismuth subsalicylate
- Antimicrobials
  - Ciprofloxacin, metronidazole

### 6.9.4 Intervention

- Monitor vital signs.
- Monitor intake and output.
- Assess for dehydration.
- Replace fluids.
- Instruct the patient that vomiting and diarrhea are the mechanisms that the body uses to remove the infecting microorganism.

## 6.10 Gastroesophageal Reflux Disease (GERD)

Gastroesophageal reflux disease occurs when contents (acid) of the stomach enter into the esophagus causing pain (heartburn) because the lining of the esophagus is unprotected, resulting in damage to the mucosal layer of the esophagus. Pain worsens after eating and when lying down. Scarring may occur, leading to formation of strictures and resulting in difficulty swallowing.

- Barrett's esophagus: a premalignant esophageal growth resulting from chronic GERD

### 6.10.1 Signs and Symptoms

- Sour taste in mouth
- Hoarseness
- Epigastric burning
- Burping (eructation)
- Coughing
- Nausea
- Bloating
- Difficulty swallowing (dysphagia)

### 6.10.2 Medical Tests

- Barium x-ray shows reflux.
- Endoscopy shows irritation.
- Esophageal manometry indicates decreased lower esophageal sphincter tone.

### 6.10.3   Treatment

- Surgery to strengthen lower esophageal sphincter tone
- Administer
  - Antacids
    - Maalox, Mylanta, Tums, Gaviscon
  - H2-receptor antagonists
    - Ranitidine, famotidine, nizatidine, cimetidine
  - Proton pump inhibitors
    - Omeprazole, esomeprazole, pantoprazole, rabeprazole, lansoprazole

### 6.10.4   Intervention

- Monitor vital signs.
- Elevate head of bed.
- Instruct patient to sleep on left side to reduce nighttime GERD.
- Instruct the patient
  - Eat six small meals daily.
  - Refrain from acidic foods (citrus, vinegar, tomato) and peppermint, and do not drink caffeine or alcohol.
  - Don't lie down after eating.
  - Refrain from wearing clothing that is tight at the waist.

## 6.11   Gastrointestinal Bleeding

Bleeding from the upper or lower gastrointestinal tract leads to substantial blood loss. Common causes of upper gastrointestinal bleeding are neoplasms, ulcers, Mallory-Weiss tears related to vomiting, and esophageal varices. Common causes of lower gastrointestinal bleeding are ulcerations, polyps, diverticulitis, fissure formation, colon cancer, and hemorrhoids.

### 6.11.1   Signs and Symptoms

- Pallor
- Light-headedness
- Diaphoresis
- Orthostatic blood pressure
- Black, tarry stool (melena)
- Red or maroon rectal bleeding (hematochezia)

- Vomiting maroon, coffee-ground-like blood (hematemesis)
- Nausea
- Tachycardia

### 6.11.2 Medical Tests

- Fecal occult blood test is positive.
- Colonoscopy shows site of bleeding.
- Arteriography shows site of bleeding.
- Endoscopy assesses the esophagus.
- Blood test
  - Decreased hemoglobin
  - Decreased hematocrit
  - Decreased RBC

### 6.11.3 Treatment

- Endoscopy to stop bleeding
- Tamponade with Blakemore-Sengstaken tube for esophageal varices
- Administer
  - Isotonic IV fluids
  - Normal saline
  - Transfused packed RBCs
  - Fresh-frozen plasma
  - Albumin

### 6.11.4 Intervention

- Monitor vital signs.
- Monitor intake and output.
- Maintain large-bore IV (16–18 gauge) access.
- Instruct the patient that treatment will stop the bleeding.

## 6.12 Gastritis

Inflammation of the stomach lining, gastritis leads to malnutrition, gastric cancer, or lymphoma.

- **Erosive gastritis:** caused by stress or medication (NSAIDs)
- **Atrophic gastritis:** caused by H. pylori, pernicious anemia, and alcohol use

### 6.12.1  Signs and Symptoms

- Vomiting maroon, coffee-ground-like blood (hematemesis)
- Nausea
- Black, tarry stool (melena)
- Epigastric tenderness
- Anorexia
- Anemia
- Abdominal bloating
- Abdominal pain

### 6.12.2  Medical Tests

- Endoscopy shows inflammation.
- Gastroscopy
- Fecal occult blood test is positive.
- Blood tests
  - Decreased hemoglobin
  - Decreased hematocrit
  - Decreased RBC
- H. pylori is positive.

### 6.12.3  Treatment

- Administer
  - Antacids
    - Maalox, Mylanta, Tums, Gaviscon
  - Sucralfate
  - H2-receptor antagonists
    - Ranitidine, famotidine, nizatidine, cimetidine
  - Proton pump inhibitors
    - Omeprazole, esomeprazole, pantoprazole, rabeprazole, lansoprazole

### 6.12.4  Intervention

- Monitor stool for occult blood.
- Monitor vital signs.

- Monitor intake and output.

- Instruct the patient

  - No alcohol, caffeine, or acidic foods.

  - No NSAIDs.

  - No smoking.

## 6.13   Hepatitis

Hepatitis is an inflammation of the liver commonly caused by a viral infection or exposure to drugs and toxins. Types of hepatitis:

- **Hepatitis A:** transmitted orally and related to contaminated water or poor sanitation. It can be prevented by vaccine.

- **Hepatitis B:** transmitted percutaneously and related to sexual contact, IV drug use, mother-to-neonate transmission, and transfusion. It can be prevented by vaccine.

- **Hepatitis C:** transmitted percutaneously and related to IV drug use and sexual contact (less common). No vaccine is available.

- **Hepatitis D:** transmitted percutaneously. It needs hepatitis B to spread. No vaccine is available.

- **Hepatitis E:** transmitted orally and related to water contamination. Acute. No vaccine is available.

- **Hepatitis G:** transmitted percutaneously. It is associated with chronic infection, but not liver disease.

### 6.13.1   Signs and Symptoms

- Acute hepatitis

  - Tenderness in right upper quadrant of abdomen

  - Jaundice

  - Dark urine

  - Hepatomegaly

  - Diarrhea

  - Constipation

  - Malaise

  - Nausea and vomiting

  - Low-grade fever

  - Anorexia

  - Muscle and joint pain

- Chronic hepatitis

  - Asymptomatic

  - Bleeding

  - Enlarged spleen

- Cirrhosis
- Ascites
- Esophageal varices
- Encephalopathy
- Same symptoms as acute hepatitis

### 6.13.2   Medical Tests

- Liver biopsy shows hepatocellular necrosis.
- Urine analysis shows protein and bilirubin.
- Blood tests
  - AST is increased.
  - ALT is increased.
  - WBC count is normal to low.
  - IgG anti-HBc shows convalescent or past infection with hepatitis B.
  - IgM anti-HBc shows acute or recent infection with hepatitis B.
  - HBsAg shows current or past infection with hepatitis B.
  - IgM anti-HAV shows acute or early convalescent stage of hepatitis A.
  - IgG anti-HAV shows later convalescent stage of hepatitis A.
  - HBeAg shows current viral replication of hepatitis B and infectivity.
  - HBV DNA shows presence of hepatitis B DNA (most sensitive).
  - Anti-HCV shows hepatitis C infection.
  - HCV RNA shows hepatitis C infection.
  - Anti-HDV shows hepatitis D infection.

### 6.13.3   Treatment

- Liver transplantation
- Administer
  - Interferon or lamivudine (chronic hepatitis B)
  - Interferon and ribavirin (hepatitis C)
  - Prednisone (autoimmune hepatitis)

### 6.13.4   Intervention

- Remove drug that can cause liver toxin.
- Indicate activity as tolerated.

- Monitor intake and output.

- Monitor vital signs.

- Schedule rest periods (acute).

- Instruct the patient

  ○ Do not smoke (and avoid secondhand smoke).

  ○ Eat a high-calorie diet.

  ○ Eat more at breakfast (best-tolerated meal).

  ○ Do not take medications that are metabolized in the liver (e.g., acetaminophen).

  ○ Do not drink alcohol.

## 6.14  Hiatal Hernia (Diaphragmatic Hernia)

Hiatal hernia is a protrusion of a portion of the stomach through the diaphragm into the chest near the esophagus.

- **Sliding hiatal hernia:** the upper portion of the stomach and the lower esophageal sphincter move throughout the diaphragm. GERD present.

- **Rolling hiatal hernia:** the upper portion of the stomach, but not the lower esophageal sphincter, moves throughout the diaphragm. No GERD present.

### 6.14.1  Signs and Symptoms

- Sliding hernia

  ○ Chest pain

  ○ Palpitations

  ○ Heartburn

  ○ Eructation (burping)

  ○ Dysphagia (difficulty swallowing)

- Rolling hernia

  ○ Chest pain

  ○ Palpitations

  ○ Fullness after eating

  ○ Difficulty breathing after eating

### 6.14.2  Medical Tests

- Barium x-ray shows hiatal hernia.

### 6.14.3  Treatment

- Surgical repair

- Administer

- Antacids for patients
  - Maalox, Mylanta, Tums, Gaviscon
- H2-receptor antagonists
  - Ranitidine, nizatidine, famotidine, cimetidine
- Proton pump inhibitors to reduce the production of acid
  - Omeprazole, esomeprazole, pantoprazole, rabeprazole, lansoprazole

### 6.14.4    Intervention

- Elevate head of bed.
- Monitor vital signs.
- Instruct the patient
  - Eat small, frequent meals.
  - Do not lie down after eating.
  - Do not wear clothes that are tight at the waist.
  - Do not eat acidic foods (citrus, vinegar, tomato), and peppermint, or drink caffeine or alcohol.
  - Do not smoke.

## 6.15    Intestinal Obstruction and Paralytic Ileus

Blocked motility through the intestine is caused by a mechanical obstruction such as fecal impaction, tumor, or adhesion or by a paralytic ileus such as sepsis, diabetic ketoacidosis, or medication.

### 6.15.1    Signs and Symptoms

- Paralytic ileus
  - Diminished or absent bowel sounds
  - Vomiting
  - Constant abdominal pain
  - Abdominal distention
- Obstruction
  - Vomiting
  - Constipation
  - High-pitched bowel sounds
  - Abdominal tenderness
  - Abdominal cramping
  - Intermittent or constant abdominal pain
  - Abdominal distention

### 6.15.2 Medical Tests

- Abdominal x-ray shows small bowel dilation.

### 6.15.3 Treatment

- Administer
  - Antiemetics after NG tube insertion
    - Prochlorperazine, trimethobenzamide
  - IV fluid replacement
    - Isotonic solution

### 6.15.4 Intervention

- Indicate NPO.
- Insert NG tube to suction and remove stomach contents.
- Administer parenteral nutrition and vitamin supplements.
- Monitor vital signs.
- Monitor intake and output.
- Assess for abdominal tenderness.
- Assess bowel sounds.
- Instruct the patient that normal lifestyle will return after intestinal motility is restored.

## 6.16 Pancreatitis

Pancreatitis is an inflammation of the pancreas as a result of chronic alcohol use, elevated cholesterol, blockage of the pancreatic duct by gallstones, or surgical or abdominal trauma.

- **Acute:** autodigestion of the pancreas by pancreatic enzymes and development of fibrosis. Life threatening and a risk for pleural effusion.
- **Chronic:** fibrosis resulting in decrease in pancreatic function.

### 6.16.1 Signs and Symptoms

- Cullen's sign (bluish-gray discoloration of periumbilical area and abdomen)
- Turner's sign (bluish-gray discoloration of flank areas)
- Abdominal pain
  - **Acute:** radiates to back or left shoulder
  - **Chronic:** gnawing continuous pain

- Epigastric pain

- Knee-chest position reduces pain.

- Nausea

- Vomiting

- Fatigue

- Hyperglycemia

- Ascites

- Weight loss

- Fever

- Jaundice

### 6.16.2   Medical Tests

- CT scan shows inflammation.

- Abdominal ultrasound shows inflammation.

- Blood test
  - Increased
    - Amylase
    - Lipase
    - WBC
    - Cholesterol
    - Glucose
    - Bilirubin

### 6.16.3   Treatment

- Surgical removal of abscess or pseudocyst
- Administer
  - IV fluids
  - Total parenteral nutrition
  - Vitamin supplements
  - Patient-controlled or transdermal analgesia
  - Insulin (chronic)
- Do not use morphine, as it causes spasm of the sphincter of Oddi.

### 6.16.4   Intervention

- Indicate NPO (acute).
- Insert NG tube to suction and remove stomach contents if patient is vomiting.
- Monitor intake and output.

- Monitor vital signs.
- Monitor blood glucose.
- Monitor lung sounds for plural effusion.
- Assess abdomen for bowel sounds, tenderness, masses, ascites.
- Instruct the patient
  - Schedule rest periods.
  - Take pancreatic enzymes with meals.
  - Do not drink alcohol.
  - Do not drink caffeine.
  - Follow bland, low-fat, high-protein, high-calorie diet.
  - Eat small, frequent meals.
  - Monitor blood glucose.

## 6.17 Peritonitis

An acute inflammation of the peritoneum (lining of the abdominal cavity), peritonitis is commonly caused by a bacterial infection. It is a life-threatening disease that may lead to septicemia if infection enters the bloodstream.

### 6.17.1 Signs and Symptoms

- Abdominal rebound pain
- Abdominal distention
- Rigid abdomen
- Decreased bowel sounds
- Fever
- Tachycardia
- Nausea
- Vomiting
- Decreased urine output
- Decreased appetite

### 6.17.2 Medical Tests

- Abdominal x-ray shows whether free air is present.
- Ultrasound shows underlying cause.
- CT scan shows underlying cause.

- Peritoneal lavage culture and sensitivity identifies microorganism.
- Blood test
  - Increased WBC
  - Blood cultures to identify microorganism

### 6.17.3   Treatment

- Surgery to correct underlying cause
- Administer
  - Broad-spectrum antibiotics
  - IV fluids

### 6.17.4   Intervention

- Indicate NPO.
- Elevate head of bed.
- Monitor vital signs.
- Monitor intake and output.
- Weigh daily.
- Instruct the patient that normal lifestyle will return after inflammation is resolved.

## 6.18   Peptic Ulcer Disease (PUD)

Erosion of the mucosal layer of the stomach or duodenum allowing stomach acid to contact epithelial tissues commonly caused by H. pylori or by stress leading to bleeding, perforation, peritonitis, paralytic ileus, septicemia, shock, ischemia, or ulceration.

- **Gastric ulcer:** mucosal layer of the stomach is eroded, lessening the curvature of the stomach.
- **Duodenal ulcer:** mucosal layer of the duodenal is eroded, resulting in penetration to the muscular layer.

### 6.18.1   Signs and Symptoms

- Bloating
- Loss of appetite
- Epigastric pain
  - Worsens after eating (gastric ulcer)
  - Worsens one to three hours after eating or at night (duodenal ulcer)
- Weight change
  - Loss of weight (gastric ulcer)
  - Gain of weight (duodenal ulcer)

- Bleeding
  - Vomiting red or maroon blood (hematemesis or gastric ulcer)
  - Coffee-grounds-like emesis (gastric ulcer)
  - Tarry stool (melena or duodenal ulcer)
- Perforation
  - Sudden, sharp pain relieved with knee-chest position
  - Tender, rigid abdomen
  - Hypovolemic shock

## 6.18.2   Medical Tests

- Blood tests
  - Decreased RBC
  - Decreased hemoglobin
  - Decreased hematocrit
- Barium x-ray shows ulceration.
- Abdominal x-ray shows free air if perforated.
- Endoscopy shows ulceration.
- Stool occult blood test is positive.
- H. pylori test is positive.

## 6.18.3   Treatment

- Administer
  - Antacids
    - Maalox, Mylanta, Amphojel
  - H2-receptor antagonists
    - Famotidine, ranitidine, nizatidine
  - Proton pump inhibitors
    - Omeprazole, lansoprazole, rabeprazole, esomeprazole, pantoprazole
  - Mucosal barrier fortifiers
    - Sucralfate
  - Prostaglandin analogue
    - Misoprostol
  - H. pylori medication
  - Proton pump inhibitor plus clarithromycin plus amoxicillin, proton pump inhibitor plus metronidazole plus clarithromycin, bismuth subsalicylate plus metronidazole plus tetracycline

### 6.18.4 Intervention

- Monitor intake and output.
- Monitor vital signs.
- Monitor bowel sounds.
- Monitor abdomen for tenderness and rigidity.
- Instruct the patient
  - Eat small, frequent meals.
  - Do not drink caffeine.
  - Do not drink alcohol.
  - Do not eat acidic foods.
  - Do not take NSAIDs.
  - Do not smoke.

## 6.19 Ulcerative Colitis

Ulcerative colitis is inflammation of the mucosal layer of the large intestine beginning with the colon and rectum and spreading to adjacent tissues, leading to ulcerations and abscess formation. There are periods of exacerbation and remission. Symptoms increase with each exacerbation. There are risks for malabsorption, toxic megacolon, and perforation.

### 6.19.1 Signs and Symptoms

- Chronic bloody diarrhea with pus
- Tenesmus (spasms of the anal sphincter)
- Weight loss
- Abdominal pain

### 6.19.2 Medical Tests

- Double-contrast barium x-ray shows ulceration and inflammation.
- Endoscopy assesses ulceration and inflammation.
- Colonoscopy show ulcerations and bleeding.
- Stool culture
- Renal function tests
- Liver function tests
- Electrolyte test
- Complete blood tests
  - Decreased RBC
  - Decreased hemoglobin

- Decreased hematocrit
- Increased erythrocyte sedimentation rate

### 6.19.3 Treatment

- Surgical resection of affected area
- Administer
  - Antidiarrheal medications
    - Loperamide, diphenoxylate hydrochloride, atropine
  - Salicylate medications
    - Sulfasalazine, mesalamine, olsalazine, balsalazide
  - Corticosteroids during exacerbations
    - Prednisone, hydrocortisone
  - Anticholinergics
    - Dicyclomine

### 6.19.4 Intervention

- Indicate NPO during exacerbations.
- Monitor intake and output.
- Monitor stool output.
- Weigh daily.
- Monitor for toxic megacolon (distended, tender abdomen; fever; distended colon).
- Instruct the patient
  - Keep stool diary to identify irritating foods.
  - Follow low-fiber, high-protein, high-calorie diet.
  - Indicate skin care for perianal area.
  - Utilize sitz bath.
  - Use A & D ointment.
  - Apply barrier cream to skin.
  - Apply witch hazel to soothe sensitive skin.
  - Do not use fragranced products.

## 6.20 Abdominal Trauma

Abdominal trauma is an injury to the abdominal area commonly from a motor-vehicle accident or a penetrating wound. There are two classifications of abdominal trauma: blunt abdominal trauma and penetrating abdominal trauma.

Blunt abdominal trauma is an injury caused by pressure applied to the abdominal area from a motor-vehicle accident, a fall, or a fight with another person or animal resulting in damage to organs within the abdomen (liver, spleen, intestines, pancreas, stomach, or diaphragm) and to the peritoneum.

Penetrating abdominal trauma is an injury caused by an object (bullet, knife) puncturing the abdominal area and resulting in lacerations and focused injury to abdominal organs (liver, spleen, intestines, pancreas, stomach, or diaphragm).

### 6.20.1 Signs and Symptoms

- Cullen's signs (discoloration in the umbilicus area)
- Penetrating wound site
- Abdominal tenderness
- Abdominal rigidity
- Abdominal pain
- Turner's sign (discoloration along the side of the abdomen)
- Abnormal bowel sounds
- Pain in right shoulder (referral pain indicating liver injury)
- Kehr's sign (left shoulder pain related to injury to diaphragm)
- The patient guards the abdominal area.

### 6.20.2 Medical Tests

- Abdominal x-rays show injuries.
- Ultrasound shows injuries.
- CT scan shows injuries.
- Blood tests
  - Complete blood count
  - Blood type and crossmatch
  - Coagulation test
  - Electrolyte test

### 6.20.3 Treatment

- Stabilize the patient (airway, breathing, circulation).
- Assess for trauma signs.
- Assess for internal bleeding (see 6.11 Gastrointestinal Bleeding).
- Assess neurologic status.
- Monitor vital signs.
- Insert two large-bore intravenous lines.
- Prepare the patient for surgery, if necessary.

- Administer oxygen per practitioner's order.
- Administer
  - ○ Fluids per practitioner's orders to maintain hemodynamic status
    - ■ Normal saline
  - ○ Lactated Ringer's solution
  - ○ Pain medication per practitioner's orders upon diagnosis

## 6.20.4 Intervention

- Indicate nothing by mouth (NPO).
- Monitor intake and output.
- Monitor vital signs continually.
- Instruct the patient
  - ○ Tell the patient to be calm.
  - ○ Explain each procedure and why the procedure is being performed.

## Solved Problems

6.1 What is the order of the gastrointestinal assessment?
- Inspection
- Auscultation
- Percussion
- Palpation

6.2 What part of the stethoscope is used to listen for vascular sounds?
The bell of the stethoscope is used.

6.3 When would you not percuss the abdomen?
- Don't percuss the abdomen if the patient received a transplanted abdominal organ.
- Don't percuss the abdomen if a bruit, venous hum, or friction rub is heard over the abdomen.

6.4 What is rebound tenderness?
Rebound tenderness is pain when fingertips are withdrawn from the abdomen during palpation.

6.5 What is a common cause of projectile vomiting?
Hypertrophic pyloric stenosis is a common cause of projectile vomiting.

6.6 What might dark, coffee-grounds-like bloody emesis indicate?
Upper gastrointestinal bleed from peptic ulcer may be indicated.

**6.7** What is a common cause of bloody red stools?

Hemorrhoids are often the cause of bloody red stools.


**6.8** What would be suspected if the patient's sclera is yellow, and the patient reports pale stools?

Jaundice may be suspected.


**6.9** What would be suspected if the patient had sudden abdominal pain with rigidity and then the pain subsides?

Abdominal perforation may be suspected.


**6.10** What are common causes of hyperactive abdominal sounds?

Early intestinal obstruction, hunger, or diarrhea may cause hyperactive abdominal sounds.


**6.11** What is a gastric lavage?

Gastric lavage is a procedure used to treat gastric hemorrhage and to treat drug overdoses, depending on the nature of the drug. Irrigating fluid is instilled through a nasogastric (NG) tube into the upper gastrointestinal system, and the gastric content is aspirated through the NG tube.


**6.12** What is a nasogastric decompression?

Nasogastric decompression is a process used to aspirate intestinal contents and to assist in resolving an intestinal obstruction using a nasogastric decompression tube. Nasogastric decompression is also used to prevent nausea and vomiting and to reduce the risk of abdominal distention following gastro-intestinal surgery.


**6.13** What is alanine transaminase (ALT)?

An enzyme found mainly in liver cells, ALT helps the body metabolize protein. When the liver is damaged, ALT is released into the bloodstream.


**6.14** What is bilirubin?

Bilirubin is a red-yellow pigment that results from the breakdown of red blood cells. Normally, bili-rubin passes through the liver and is excreted in the stool. Elevated levels of bilirubin (jaundice) may indicate liver damage or disease.


**6.15** What is paracentesis?

Paracentesis is a procedure of aspirating fluid from the peritoneal space to decrease intra-abdominal pressure, treat ascites, and assess for intra-abdominal bleeding. Aspiration is performed by insertion of a needle or cannula through the abdominal wall into the peritoneal space.


**6.16** What is the purpose of performing a lower gastrointestinal endoscopy?

A lower gastrointestinal endoscopy is also referred to as a colonoscopy and is used to assess structures and disorders in the lower gastrointestinal tract.


**6.17** What might a pasty stool indicate?

High fat content related to pancreatic disorder or intestinal malabsorption disorder may be indicated.

**6.18**    What might a narrow, ribbon stool indicate?

Irritable bowel disorder, obstruction of the bowel or rectum, or spastic bowel disorder may be indicated.

**6.19**    How does an antacid work?

Antacids are medications that increase the pH level in the stomach resulting in decreased stomach acidity.

**6.20**    How does Reglan work?

Reglan increases the emptying of the stomach.

**6.21**    How do histamine-2 receptor antagonists work?

Histamine-2 receptor antagonists are medications used to block the action of histamine on the parietal cells in the stomach, reducing the production of acid.

**6.22**    Why is lactulose prescribed?

Lactulose decreases ammonia in the blood and is prescribed for treating encephalopathy.

**6.23**    What would be suspected if the patient has abdominal pain from the periumbilical to right lower quadrant with rebound pain and abdominal rigidity?

Appendicitis would be suspected.

**6.24**    What is cholecystitis?

Cholecystitis is acute or chronic inflammation of the gallbladder related to cholelithiasis (gallstones). Acute cholecystitis occurs when blood flow to the gallbladder decreases, commonly from a cystic duct blocked by a gallstone, leading to difficulty filling and emptying the gallbladder. The gallbladder becomes inflamed, bile is retained, and the gallbladder becomes distended.

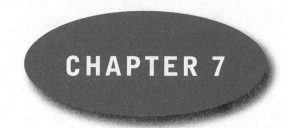

# CHAPTER 7

# *Musculoskeletal Emergencies*

## 7.1  Define

- A musculoskeletal emergency is a condition that alters muscles, tendons, ligaments, or bones, resulting in the patient becoming unstable.

- Musculoskeletal physiology can be disrupted by an inflammation, infection, or trauma.

- A musculoskeletal emergency is not life threatening.

- A musculoskeletal emergency can result in pain, disfigurement, and disability.

- The focus is on musculoskeletal problems after the patient's airway, breathing, circulation, cervical spine, and neurological system are stabilized.

- A musculoskeletal emergency requires immediate intervention.

### 7.1.1  Goal of Treating Musculoskeletal Emergencies

- The goal of the emergency-department staff is to identify the musculoskeletal emergency and stabilize the patient. This typically involves treating the underlying cause of the musculoskeletal emergency such as reducing a simple fracture.

- Thoroughly assess the patient before beginning treatment. Administering medication may mask a sign or symptom that indicates a musculoskeletal emergency.

- Diagnose the acute problem.

- Stabilize the patient by relieving pain and treating the acute problem.

- Refer the patient to follow-up care.

### 7.1.2  Musculoskeletal Assessment

- Focus on the five Ps of musculoskeletal injury from the head down to the feet.

  ○ Pain

  ○ Paralysis

  ○ Paresthesia

  ○ Pulse

  ○ Pallor

- Assess range of motion.
  - **Adduction:** moving the limb closer to the body (adding to the body)
  - **Abduction:** moving the limb away from the body (subtracting from the body)
- The musculoskeletal assessment interview
  - Open-ended questions:
    - Why did you come to the hospital today?
    - What makes you feel that something is wrong?
  - Clues for underlying cause of the musculoskeletal emergency
    - What happened prior to your noticing this problem?
    - Have you recently undergone any medical procedure?
      - What medical procedure?
      - When was the medical procedure performed?
  - Follow-up questions help probe further into the presenting musculoskeletal problem.
    - When did this problem start?
    - How long have you had this problem?
    - Can you describe the problem?
    - How much does the problem bother you?
    - Where do you feel uncomfortable?
    - Is the problem spreading, or does the problem remain in one place?
    - Does anything make the problem worse?
    - Does anything make the problem better?
    - Did you have this problem or a similar problem in the past?
      - Explain.
    - Have you been diagnosed with any medical condition?
      - What medical condition?
        - Are you being treated for the medical condition?
          - What is your treatment?
          - Who is treating you?
    - What medications do you use?
      - Prescribed
      - Over-the-counter
      - Cultural
      - Herbal
    - Do you use an assistive device?
      - Cane
      - Walker
      - Wheelchair

- Did you recently fall?

- Do you have a history of falling?

- Do you have any vision problems?

○ Ask about the patient's lifestyle.

- What is your occupation?

- Do you perform repetitive actions?

- Do you or did you exercise?

- Do you or did you play sports?

- Do you consume caffeine?

  □ How much caffeine do you consume?

  □ When did you start consuming caffeine?

- Do you drink alcohol?

  □ How much alcohol do you drink?

  □ When did you start drinking alcohol?

  □ Have you ever been treated for alcoholism?

- Do you use recreational drugs or prescription drugs that are not prescribed to you?

  □ What drugs?

  □ How much do you use?

  □ When did you start using drugs?

  □ Have you ever been treated for drug abuse?

- Do you use tobacco?

○ Ask about the patient's family history.

- Does anyone in your family have osteoarthritis or a history of osteoarthritis?

- Does anyone in your family have rheumatoid arthritis or a history of rheumatoid arthritis?

- Does anyone in your family have osteoporosis or a history of osteoporosis?

- Does anyone in your family have spondyloarthropathies or a history of spondyloarthropathies?

- Does anyone in your family have cancer or a history of cancer?

• Inspection

○ Ask the patient to walk, if possible, to assess the patient's gait.

- Does the patient have difficulty bearing weight?

- Is the patient guarding the site of the injury?

- Is there pain during movement or at rest? Assess facial expression for pain.

○ Muscles:

- Weakness

- Swelling

- Bruising

- ○ Bones:
    - ▪ Skin breakage
    - ▪ Deformed skeleton
    - ▪ Impaired range of motion (never force range-of-motion movement)
- • Auscultation
    - ○ Listen for abnormal sounds during the range-of-motion inspection.
        - ▪ Clicking
        - ▪ Crunching
        - ▪ Grating
- • Range-of-motion assessment
    - ○ Temporomandibular joint (TMJ)
        - ▪ Place first two fingers on patient's ear.
        - ▪ Ask patient to open and close his mouth.
        - ▪ Place fingers into the depression over the joint.
        - ▪ Ask patient to open and close his mouth.
        - ▪ The patient should easily open and close his mouth without pain or discomfort.
    - ○ Neck
        - ▪ Don't assess the neck until cervical spine injury is ruled out through imaging study.
        - ▪ Remove the cervical collar, if necessary.
        - ▪ Immobilize the neck with your hands.
        - ▪ Palpate the neck for pain, deformity, sensation, and crepitus.
        - ▪ If there is no suspected neck or spinal injury, ask the patient to
            - ▫ Touch right ear to right shoulder.
            - ▫ Touch left ear to left shoulder.
            - ▫ Touch chin to chest (45 degrees is normal).
            - ▫ Move head back and look at the ceiling (55 degrees is normal).
            - ▫ Turn head to each side.
            - ▫ Move head in a circle (70 degrees is normal).
    - ○ Spine
        - ▪ Don't assess the spine until spinal injury is ruled out through imaging study.
        - ▪ Use a log roll procedure with three staff members to keep the patient immobilized when turning the patient to assess the spine.
        - ▪ If there is no suspected neck or spinal injury, ask the patient to:
            - ▫ Bend at the waist.
            - ▫ Let arms hang at sides.
        - ▪ Palpate the spine with your fingers.
        - ▪ Palpate the spine with the side of your hands.
        - ▪ The spine should be symmetrical with no tenderness or swelling.

- Shoulders

  - Shoulders should be symmetric and not deformed.

  - Palpate the bony landmarks with your fingers.

  - Palpate shoulder muscles with your hand.

    - Muscles should be firm and symmetrical.

  - Palpate elbow and ulna.

  - Ask the patient to

    - Extend arms straight at your side (neutral position).

    - Lift arms straight to shoulder level.

    - Bend elbow at 90 degrees.

    - Extend arms out parallel to the floor, palms down, and fingers extended.

    - Extend forearms up with fingers pointed to the ceiling. Forearms should move 90 degrees.

    - Extend forearms down with fingers pointing to the floor. Forearms should move 90 degrees.

    - Extend arms straight at your side (neutral position).

    - Move arms forward and up over head.

    - Extend arms straight at your side (neutral position).

    - Move arms as far back as possible. Arms should bend 30 degrees.

    - Extend arms straight at your side (neutral position).

    - Move arms away from your body (abduction). Arms should move 180 degrees.

    - Extend arms straight at your side (neutral position).

    - Move arms across the front of your body (adduction). Arms should move 50 degrees.

    - Extend arms straight at your side (neutral position).

    - Flex elbows. Elbows should flex 90 degrees.

    - Place the sides of hands (thumbs facing up) on a flat surface.

    - Rotate the palms of hands down to the surface (pronation). The elbows should rotate 90 degrees.

    - Rotate the palms of hands upward from the surface (supination). The elbow should rotate 90 degrees.

- Wrists and hands

  - Examine the hands for

    - Deformities

    - Swelling

  - Feel bones in the fingers and wrist. Look for tenderness.

  - Ask the patient to

    - Rotate the wrist in a waxing motion. There should be 55 degrees of movement away from the body (lateral movement) and 20 degrees of movement toward the body (medial movement).

    - Move wrist backward with fingers pointing upward. The wrist should move 70 degrees.

    - Move wrist downward with fingers pointing to the floor. The wrist should move 90 degrees.

- □ Move only fingers toward the ceiling (extension). Fingers should move 30 degrees.

- □ Move only fingers toward the floor (flexion). Fingers should move 90 degrees.

- □ Touch little finger with thumb.

- □ Form a fist (adduction).

- □ Spread fingers (abduction).

- ■ Compare the length of the patient's arms. There should be no more than 1 cm difference in length.

- ○ Hips

  - ■ Examine the hips. Look for symmetry.

  - ■ Palpate the hips and note any tenderness.

  - ■ Assess the patient's hips one at a time.

    - □ **Flexion:** place your hand under the lumbar spine while the patient is lying down. Ask the patient to raise her knee to her chest. The patient's lumbar spine should touch your hand. The opposite thigh and hip should remain flat. Repeat the test with the other hip.

    - □ **Abduction:** press the superior iliac spine while the patient is lying down. Move the patient's leg by the ankle away from the other leg. You should feel movement of the iliac spine. The leg should move 45 degrees. Repeat the test with the other hip.

    - □ **Adduction:** press the superior iliac spine while the patient is lying down. Move the patient's leg by the ankle toward the other leg. You should feel movement of the iliac spine. The leg should move 30 degrees. Repeat the test with the other hip.

    - □ **Extension:** ask the patient to lie facedown. Ask the patient to raise her thigh upward. Repeat the test with the other hip.

    - □ **Internal and external rotation:** ask the patient to lie on her back and raise one leg while keeping the knee straight. Turn the patient's leg away from the other leg (external rotation) and then turn the patient's leg toward the other leg (internal rotation). The leg should turn 45 degrees. Repeat the test with the other hip.

- ○ Knees

  - ■ Ask the patient to stand.

  - ■ Examine the knees. Look for

    - □ Deformities

    - □ Swelling

    - □ Tenderness

  - ■ Ask the patient to

    - □ Bring his heel to his buttocks (flexion). The leg should move 120 degrees. If the patient is unable to stand, then ask the patient to lie down on his back and raise his knee to his chest. His thigh should touch his calf.

    - □ Bring his heel to the floor.

- ○ Ankles and feet

  - ■ Examine the ankles and feet. Look for

    - □ Deformities

    - □ Swelling

  - ■ Feel bones in the feet and ankles. Look for tenderness.

- Ask the patient to
    - Sit.
    - Point toes toward the floor (plantar flexion). The toes should move 45 degrees.
    - Point toes to the ceiling (dorsiflexion). The toes should move 20 degrees.
    - Turn feet inward (inversion). The feet should move 45 degrees.
    - Turn feet outward (eversion). The feet should move 20 degrees.
    - Clinch and release toes (metatarsophalangeal joints). Toes should move freely without tenderness.
- Compare the length of the patient's legs. There should be no more than 1 cm difference in length.
  - Muscles
    - Measure the circumference of the same muscle on each side of the body. Both should have relatively the same measurements.
    - Repeat the range-of-motion assessment (see above) except move the limb (passive range of motion). You should feel slight resistance to the motion (muscle tone).
    - The limb should return easily to the neutral position when you finish the range-of-motion assessment.
    - Ask the patient to extend arms with palms up for 30 seconds (strength of shoulder girdle).
    - Place your hands on patient's palms and press down. You should feel resistance.
    - Ask the patient to
        - Bend his arm. Pull down on the patient's arm (bicep strength). You should feel resistance. Repeat with other arm.
        - Bend his arm and then try to strengthen his arm as you push his forearm upward (triceps strength). You should feel resistance. Repeat with other arm.
        - Flex his wrist as you push against his wrist. You should feel resistance. Repeat with other wrist.
        - Extend his wrist as you push down on his wrist. You should feel resistance. Repeat with other wrist.
        - Squeeze your hand. You should feel resistance.
        - Lie on his back.
        - Raise both of his legs simultaneously. Both legs should raise to the same distance at the same time.
        - Lower his legs.
        - Raise each leg as you push down on the leg (quadricep strength). You should feel resistance.
        - Bend his knees as he places his feet on the bed.
    - Pull the patient's leg forward (lower leg strength). You should feel resistance.
    - Ask the patient to
        - Bend her knee as you push against the knee. You should feel resistance.
        - Push her foot down against your hand as you push her foot up (ankle strength). You should feel resistance.
        - Pull her foot up as you push her foot down. You should feel resistance.
    - Measure muscle strength by using the muscle grade.

| Grade | Description |
|-------|-------------|
| 0 | No muscle contraction |
| 1 | Muscle contraction is felt, but joint does not move |
| 2 | Complete range of motion with assistance (passive range of motion) |
| 3 | Complete range of motion against gravity |
| 4 | Complete range of motion against gravity with moderate resistance |
| 5 | Complete range of motion against gravity with full resistance |

### 7.1.2.1  Signs and Symptoms

Musculoskeletal assessment in an emergency situation requires the nurse to recognize common signs and symptoms of underlying causes and then prepare for the anticipated treatment that the practitioner is likely to order.

Commonly seen signs and symptoms:

- Unsteady gait
- Swelling (edema)
- Pain or tenderness, especially during movement
- Discoloration of skin
  - Pale (neurovascular problem)
  - Purple (ecchymosis)
- Skin temperature cool at site (neurovascular problem)
- Unstable joint(s)
- Difficulty with range of motion
- Loss of sensation (paresthesis) or abnormal sensation (neurovascular problem)
- Decrease or absence of pulse (reduced blood supply to site)
- Asymmetric skeletal structure
- Misaligned skeletal structure

## 7.2  Musculoskeletal Tests and Procedures

Musculoskeletal tests are designed to assess the effectiveness and the capability of the musculoskeletal system to function. Emergency-department practitioners order musculoskeletal tests to collect objective data to further assess and assist in stabilizing the patient. Once stabilized, the patient is transferred or referred to follow-up care designed to treat the underlying cause of the current episode, which may require additional musculoskeletal tests. Musculoskeletal procedures are performed to stabilize the patient.

The following are commonly ordered musculoskeletal tests and procedures by the emergency department's practitioners.

## 7.2.1 Musculoskeletal X-Ray

A musculoskeletal x-ray creates an image of the skeletal bones. The practitioner commonly orders one or multiple views. These are

- Anteroposterior
- Posteroanterior
- Lateral

Dense structures such as bone block x-ray particles, causing those structures to appear white. Less-dense structures such as fat block some x-ray particles, causing those structures to appear gray. Air does not block x-ray particles and appears dark. An x-ray image cannot differentiate between fluid and air.

The practitioner orders an abdominal x-ray typically to assess for:

- Fractures
- Dislocations
- Joint disorders
- Bone disorders

**Musculoskeletal X-Ray Procedure**

- Be sure that the patient's spine is stabilized. Immobilize the spine, if necessary.
- Be sure that the patient is not pregnant.
- Ask patient to remove all jewelry in the area since jewelry may appear on the x-ray image.
- Instruct the patient to remove clothes. Provide the patient with a gown.
- The patient lies down on the x-ray table and the x-ray plate is positioned below the table, or the patient stands in front of the x-ray table and the x-ray plate is positioned behind the patient.
- The initial result, called a "wet read," provides a relatively superficial assessment of the image. A more thorough reading is taken hours or days later.

## 7.2.2 Musculoskeletal CT Scan

A musculoskeletal CT scan provides a three-dimensional image of the musculoskeletal system using x-rays, enabling the practitioner to visualize normal and abnormal structures. A CT can be performed with or without a contrast agent. A contrast agent is iodine-based and enhances images of blood vessels and less-dense areas.

The practitioner typically orders a musculoskeletal CT scan to assess for:

- Inflammation
- Tumor
- Cysts
- Pseudocysts
- Fractures

- Dislocations
- Joint disorders
- Bone disorders

**CT Scan Procedure**

- Assess if the patient is allergic to iodine or shellfish if the patient is undergoing a CT scan with contrast. Patients who are allergic to iodine or shellfish have a high likelihood to experience an allergic reaction to the contrast agent.

- Administer diphenhydramine (Benadryl) and prednisone (Deltasone) before the CT scan to reduce the risk of an allergic reaction to the contrast agent, if a contrast agent is ordered.

- Administer the contrast agent through an IV. The patient may feel flushed and have a salty or metallic taste in his or her mouth.

- Explain to the patient that the contrast material typically discolors the urine for upward of 24 hours following the CT scan. The patient should increase fluid intake after the CT scan to flush the contrast agent from his or her body, if a contrast agent is used for the CT scan.

- Assess if the patient is claustrophobic, as the patient will be placed in an enclosure during the test.

- Assess if the patient can remain still for 30 minutes during the CT scan, as the CT scanner encircles the patient for up to 30 minutes.

### 7.2.3  Musculoskeletal MRI

A musculoskeletal magnetic resonance imaging (MRI) provides a three-dimensional view of the musculoskeletal system using radio waves, a strong magnet, and a computer. An MRI is particularly used to assess fluid-filled soft tissue and to identify tumors from other structures within the musculoskeletal system.

The practitioner typically orders a musculoskeletal MRI to assess for:

- Inflammation
- Tumor
- Cysts
- Pseudocysts
- Fractures
- Dislocations
- Joint disorders
- Bone disorders

**Musculoskeletal MRI Procedure**

- The patient may need to be NPO (nothing by mouth) for up to 12 hours before the test depending on the site of the MRI.

- All metal must be removed from the patient.

- No metal may enter the room containing the MRI scanner. The MRI scanner's magnet is always activated.

- Assess if the patient is claustrophobic. If so, then ask the healthcare provider if an open MRI scanner should be used for the test, or if the patient should be sedated before the scan begins.
- The musculoskeletal MRI scan takes about 30 minutes.
- The musculoskeletal MRI scan is noninvasive. The patient will not feel any discomfort.

## 7.2.4  Arthrocentesis

Arthrocentesis is a procedure that collects a sample of synovial fluid from a joint for analysis by the lab. This is also referred to as tapping synovial fluid. The appearance or color of the synovial fluid might indicate the underlying cause of swelling:

- **Crystals:** arthritis, gout (foot)
- **Cloudy:** infection (white blood cells)
- **Red:** bleeding (red blood cells), related to trauma

The practitioner typically orders an arthrocentesis to

- Assess for inflammation
- Assess for arthritis
- Assess for the underlying cause of swelling
- Relieve pressure and pain in the synovial joint

**Arthrocentesis Procedure**
- The patient is placed in a position that exposes the synovial joint.
- The site is cleaned with an antiseptic.
- A needle is inserted into the synovial joint.
- A syringe is used to aspirate the contents of the synovial joint.
- Cold packs are applied to the site following the procedure to reduce swelling related to the procedure.
- The patient may require an elastic bandage to strengthen the synovial joint temporarily, depending on the amount of fluid aspirated by the practitioner.

## 7.2.5  Immobilization

Immobilization is a treatment that requires the effected site to remain in position through the use of an immobilization device during the healing process. The immobilization device

- Maintains alignment
- Reduces pressure on the effected site
- Reduces pain
- Limits movement

Commonly used immobilization devices are

- Casts: used after a fracture is reduced

- Slings: used in injuries to arms and hands

- Braces: used in joint injuries

- Splints: used in dislocations

- Long spine boards: used to immobilize the spine

- Traction: used for fractures, muscle spasms, and dislocations

- Cervical collars: used for cervical injuries

The patient must

- Restrict activity

- Use assistive devices (i.e., crutches, walker, or cane) when prescribed to reduce pressure on the effected area

- Keep medical appointments, even if he or she feels no discomfort

- Not insert any device (i.e., metal coat hanger) between the cast and the skin, even if the patient feels itchiness at the effected site. That type of device can injure the skin and result in infection

- Contact the practitioner immediately if there are signs of:
  - Drainage
  - Pain
  - Swelling

- Know how to remove and replace a removable immobilization device

## 7.2.6   Closed Reduction

A closed reduction is a procedure used to realign a simple fracture and dislocated joint.

**Closed Reduction Procedure**
- The patient is administered sedation.
- The practitioner manipulates the effected area until realignment is achieved.
- An immobilization device holds the effected area in alignment.

## 7.2.7   Open Reduction

An open reduction is a procedure used to realign a fracture in surgery.

**Open Reduction Procedure**
- The patient is administered general anesthesia.
- The practitioner exposes the effected area in surgery.

- The effected area is realigned possibly using mechanical devices such as screws and plates.

- An immobilization device holds the effected area in alignment following surgery and remains in place until healing is completed.

## 7.3 Musculoskeletal Medication

Commonly used medications in musculoskeletal emergencies are skeletal muscle relaxants, nonsteroidal anti-inflammatory drugs, corticosteroids, and analgesics. These medications reduce pain and discomfort by preventing spasticity of skeletal muscles, reduce pressure on nerves caused by inflammation, and block neurological transmission.

### 7.3.1 Skeletal Muscle Relaxants

Skeletal muscle relaxants are used to reduce muscle tone and to treat muscle spasms and hyperreflexia by either interfering with neurological transmission to the muscle or by reducing the spasticity of the muscle. Muscle relaxants do not affect the central nervous system.

- Baclofen (Kemstro, Lioresal)
- Carisoprodol (Soma)
- Chlorphenesin (Maolate)
- Chlorzoxazone (Parafon Forte)
- Cyclobenzaprine (Flexeril)
- Metaxalone (Skelaxin)
- Methocarbamol (Robaxin)
- Orphenadrine (Norflex)

### 7.3.2 Nonsteroidal Anti-Inflammatory Drugs (NSAIDs)

Nonsteroidal anti-inflammatory drugs are medications that reduce swelling, pain, and stiffness without exposing the patient to the adverse side effects that occur when using corticosteroids.

- Aspirin (ASA)
- Ibuprofen (Motrin, Advil, Nuprin)
- Naproxen (Naprosyn, Aleve)
- Oxaprozin (Daypro)
- Ketoprofen (Orudis)
- Diclofenac sodium (Voltaren)
- Ketorolac (Toradol)
- Celecoxib (Celebrex)

### 7.3.3　Corticosteroids

Corticosteroids are used to reduce inflammation and cerebral edema. Corticosteroids increase the risk of pancreatitis, heart failure, and thromboembolism.

- Dexamethasone (Dexasone, Decadron)
- Methylprednisolone (Solu-Medrol)

### 7.3.4　Analgesics

Analgesics are used to reduce pain.

- Oxycodone (OxyContin)
- Morphine (Duramorph)

## 7.4　Carpal Tunnel Syndrome

Repetitive hand movement causes the median nerve in the anterior wrist to compress, causing pain and numbness to fingers. The median nerve passes through the carpal tunnel. This is more common in women.

### 7.4.1　Signs and Symptoms

- Weakness and pain in the hand
- Paresthesia in the hand
- Tingling in the hand
- Numbness in the hand

### 7.4.2　Medical Tests

- Electromyography (EMG) shows nerve dysfunction.
- Magnetic resonance imaging (MRI) shows swelling of the median nerve.
- Positive Tinnel's sign when tapping over the carpal tunnel area causes tingling, numbness, or pain in hand.
- Inflating the blood pressure cuff on the upper arm causes pain, tingling, or burning sensation in the wrist or hand.

### 7.4.3　Treatment

- Splint the wrist in a neutral or slightly extended position for two weeks to decrease compression.
- Utilize surgery to relieve pressure on the median nerve.

- Administer
  - NSAIDs to decrease inflammation
    - Ibuprofen (Motrin, Advil, Nuprin), naproxen (Naprosyn, Aleve), oxaprozin (Daypro), ketoprofen (Orudis), diclofenac sodium (Voltaren), ketorolac (Toradol), celecoxib (Celebrex)
  - Corticosteroids to decrease inflammation
    - Hydrocortisone (cortisol), methylprednisolone (Solu-Medrol), prednisone (Deltasone), dexamethasone (Dexasone, Decadron)

### 7.4.4   Intervention

- Check capillary refill, color, and sensation of fingers following surgery.
- Prescribe physical therapy.
- Instruct the patient on
  - Proper use of wrist splints
  - Use of ergonomic devices to reduce effects of repetitive motion
  - Exercises for fingers after surgery

## 7.5   Dislocations

A dislocation is a traumatic injury causing two or more bones in an articulated joint to move out of anatomical alignment. The dislocation may result in injury to nerves, soft tissue, and circulation. Common sites of dislocation are:

- **Shoulder:** resulting from a fall with the arm extended
- **Acromioclavicular separation:** resulting from blunt-force trauma to the shoulder
- **Elbow:** resulting from a fall with the arm extended
- **Wrist:** resulting from a fall with the hand extended
- **Finger:** resulting from blunt-force trauma to the fingertip or a fall with the hand extended
- **Hip:** resulting from blunt-force trauma to a bended knee (e.g., knee hitting the dashboard in a motor-vehicle accident)
- **Knee:** resulting from blunt-force trauma to the knee (e.g., sports injury)
- **Patella:** resulting from twisting the leg with the foot planted on the ground or blunt-force trauma to the knee
- **Ankle:** resulting from blunt-force trauma to the foot (e.g., pushing the brake pedal in a motor-vehicle accident)

### 7.5.1   Signs and Symptoms

- Pain or tenderness in the joint
- Deformity at the joint
- Reduced range of motion
- Swelling
- Enlargement of joint

### 7.5.2　Medical Tests

- X-ray shows dislocation.

- CT scan shows dislocation.

- MRI shows dislocation.

- Arteriogram shows circulation in the injured area.

### 7.5.3　Treatment

Reduction of the dislocation takes place at bedside in the emergency department or in surgery.

- Administer
  - Conscious sedation before reducing the dislocation
  - Analgesics:
    - Oxycodone (OxyContin)
    - Morphine (Duramorph)
    - Acetaminophen (Tylenol)
  - NSAIDs to decrease inflammation to aid in pain relief
    - Ibuprofen (Motrin, Advil)

### 7.5.4　Intervention

- Pain management
- Immobilization of the site
- Instruct the patient
  - Dislocation may take several months to heal.
  - Rehabilitation may be required.

## 7.6　Fractures

A fracture is a break in a bone due to trauma or excess stress, leading to hemorrhage, edema, and local muscle and tissue damage.

**Types of Fractures**

- **Incomplete fracture** is where the fracture is not completely through the bone.
- **Complete fracture** is where the fracture is completely through the bone, such as greenstick, spiral, comminuted, transverse, oblique, or impacted fracture.
- **Open fracture** is where the fracture penetrates the skin.
- **Closed fracture** is where the fracture does not penetrate the skin.

**Complications**

- Fat embolism is when yellow bone marrow releases fat into the blood stream resulting in emboli.

- Delayed union is a fracture that is not joined within six months.

- Compartment syndrome is a limb- and life-threatening condition when nerves, blood vessels, and muscles in a closed space caused by the facture are compressed, leading to tissue necrosis.

- Deep vein thrombosis (DVT) is when clots form as a result of immobility from fracture.

- Misalignment is when bone pieces are not anatomically aligned.

- Muscle wasting is the deterioration of muscle as a result of immobilization related to the fracture.

### 7.6.1   Signs and Symptoms

- Edema due to inflammatory reaction

- Abnormal range of motion

- Local bleeding

- Muscle spasms

### 7.6.2   Medical Tests

- CT scan shows fracture.

- X-ray shows fracture.

- Bone scan shows increased cellular activity in fracture.

### 7.6.3   Treatment

- Immobilize and splint the fracture.

- Reduce and cast the fracture.

- Administer pain medication.

### 7.6.4   Intervention

- Monitor vital signs.

- Monitor circulation in area of the fracture.

- Monitor signs of bleeding (increased pulse, increased respiration, decreased blood pressure).

- Perform range-of-motion exercises to maintain muscle tone.

- Instruct the patient not to insert objects into the cast. This can cause breakdown of skin.

## 7.7   Traumatic Amputation

A traumatic amputation is when there is a partial or total tearing away (avulsion) of a part of the body during a traumatic injury. There are two types of traumatic amputations:

- **Complete:** the body part is severed from the body. Tissue damage is minimal.

- **Incomplete:** a portion of the body part remains attached to the body as seen in a crushing or tearing traumatic injury. Severe tissue damage and collateral damage to other systems occurs.

### 7.7.1   Signs and Symptoms

- Missing all or a portion of the body part
- Severe bleeding
    - Red: arterial blood
    - Dark: venous blood

### 7.7.2   Medical Tests

- X-ray shows bone structure.
- Arteriogram shows circulation.
- Blood tests
    - Complete blood count (CBC) with differential
    - PT/INR/PTT

### 7.7.3   Treatment

- Assess and stabilize airway, breathing, circulation, and cervical spine.
- Control bleeding. Don't apply a tourniquet to the site unless patient is bleeding out (exanguination). When possible use point pressure to control bleeding.
- Immobilize the site.
- Gently clean and irrigate the site with normal saline.
- Place a sterile dressing to the site.
- Prepare the amputated body part:
    - Wrap the amputated body part in saline-moistened gauze.
    - Place body part in a sealed plastic bag.
    - Place the sealed plastic bag in an ice-water bath.
    - Make sure that the body part doesn't freeze by keeping it away from ice.
    - Take steps to prevent shock.
- Prepare the patient for surgery.
- Administer
    - Analgesics
        - Morphine (Duramorph)

### 7.7.4  Intervention

- Insert two IV lines, 18 gauge or larger.
- Instruct the patient
    - On the treatment
    - On upcoming surgery

## 7.8  Contusion

A contusion is a hemorrhage beneath the skin as a result of blunt trauma to the site, leading to discoloration and discomfort at the site of the injury. Blood beneath the skin appears dark at first, commonly referred to as a black-and-blue mark. Within 48 hours, the site will appear yellow-green as the blood is reabsorbed.

### 7.8.1  Signs and Symptoms

- Dark, black-and-blue mark beneath the skin at the site
- Yellow-green color at the site (48 hours after the trauma)
- Swelling
- Discomfort when the site is touched or with movement

### 7.8.2  Medical Tests

- X-ray shows no underlying abnormalities.

### 7.8.3  Treatment

- Ice the site 20 minutes on and 20 minutes off for the first 24 hours to reduce swelling.
- Administer
    - Analgesics
        - Acetaminophen (Tylenol)
    - NSAIDs to decrease inflammation and aid in pain relief
        - Ibuprofen (Motrin, Advil)

### 7.8.4  Intervention

- Assess if the patient is on aspirin or anticoagulant therapy that may affect bleeding.
- Assess if bleeding has stopped:
    - Outline the discolored site with a marker.
    - Reassess the discolored site in 15 minutes.
    - If the discoloration extends beyond the outline, then bleeding continues and the practitioner should be notified.

- Assess the underlying cause of the injury.
  - Physical abuse by spouse, parent, or friend (necessitates call to police)
  - Injury from poor eyesight or other disorders
- Instruct the patient
  - To contact his or her practitioner if the discoloration increases in size or is not resolved in a week
  - How to prevent further injury, especially if the practitioner suspects that an underlying disorder is the cause of the injury

## 7.9 Gout

Gout is a chronic metabolic disorder where purine-based proteins are not adequately metabolized, leading to uric-acid crystals accumulating in joints (e.g., big toe) and crystallization of uric acid in the kidneys leading to kidney stones. This is also secondary to treatment with thiazide diuretics and chemotherapy.

### 7.9.1 Signs and Symptoms

- Swollen joint
- Red, tender joint
- Joint pain especially at night
- Kidney stones (nephrolithiasis)

### 7.9.2 Medical Tests

- Arthrocentesis shows uric acid crystals.
- Erythrocyte sedimentation rate is increased.
- Serum uric acid level is increased.
- Urinary uric acid levels are increased.

### 7.9.3 Treatment

Do not use aspirin because aspirin retains uric acid.

- Administer
  - NSAIDs to decrease inflammation and to aid in pain relief
    - Indomethacin (Indocin), ibuprofen (Motrin, Advil), naproxen (Aleve, Midol)
  - Xanthine oxidase inhibitor to reduce uric acid level
    - Allopurinol (Zyloprim)
  - Colchicine for acute episode
  - Uricosuric to reduce uric acid level
    - Probenecid (Benemid), sulfinpyrazone (Anturane)

### 7.9.4   Intervention

- Monitor serum uric acid levels.

- Immobilize joint.

- Don't touch joint.

- Instruct the patient

  ○ Drink 3 liters of fluid per day to avoid crystallization of uric acid.

  ○ Avoid fructose-sweetened drinks.

  ○ Follow low-fat, low-cholesterol diet.

  ○ Avoid foods high in purine proteins such as turkey, organ meats, sardines, smelts, mackerel, anchovies, herring, and bacon.

  ○ Avoid alcohol, which inhibits renal excretion of uric acid.


## 7.10   Compartment Syndrome

Compartment syndrome is decreased circulation to a body part caused by increased pressure, resulting in damage to nerves, capillaries, and muscles at that site. There are two classifications of compartment syndrome:

- **Internal:** decreased circulation is caused by pressure of a buildup of blood in muscle or beneath the skin (contusion), frostbite, infiltration of an IV, snake bite, or fracture.

- **External:** decreased circulation is caused by pressure of an immobilization device such as a cast or dressing.

### 7.10.1   Signs and Symptoms

- Swelling

- Decreased pulse or pulseless

- Decreased temperature at site

- Numbness or tingling (paresthesia)

- Pain disproportionate to the underlying injury

- Pallor

- Paralysis

### 7.10.2   Medical Tests

- X-ray: shows no underlying abnormalities

- Pulse oximeter: if finger or toe, shows low oxygen level and decreased pulse

### 7.10.3   Treatment

- Remove immobilizing device if external compartment syndrome.

- Stabilize site.

- Apply ice to the site 20 minutes on, 20 minutes off.
- Surgical intervention is necessary in severe cases.
- Administer
  - Analgesics
    - Acetaminophen (Tylenol)

### 7.10.4   Intervention

- Pain management
- Instruct the patient
  - How to recognize the signs of compartment syndrome. Once the compartment syndrome resolves, the immobilization device may be reapplied.
  - On the cause of the compartment syndrome

## 7.11   Osteoarthritis

Osteoarthritis is a degenerative joint disease that results in the destruction of the articular cartilage through wear that leads to bones rubbing and injuring bone tissue. Regrowth of bone tissue results in bone spurs that project into joints and soft tissue, causing pain on movement.

### 7.11.1   Signs and Symptoms

- Crepitus
- Joint pain on movement, relieved with rest
- Stiff joints for short time in morning, usually 15 minutes or less
- Heberden's nodes
- Enlargement of joint

### 7.11.2   Medical Tests

- X-ray shows bone spurs.
- C-reactive protein tests positive.
- Erythrocyte sedimentation rate increases.
- Rheumatoid factor is negative.
- Cyclic citrullinated peptide antibody is negative.

### 7.11.3   Treatment

- Administer
  - NSAIDs to decrease inflammation and aid in pain relief
    - Indomethacin (Indocin), ibuprofen (Motrin, Advil), naproxen (Aleve, Midol)

- Analgesics to decrease pain
  - Acetaminophen (Anacin, Tylenol)
- Capsaicinoids to decrease pain
  - Capsaicin cream

### 7.11.4   Intervention

- Pain management
- Joint-replacement surgery
- Instruct the patient
  - Exercise to maintain mobility.
  - Reduce weight to decrease stress on joints.

## 7.12   Osteomyelitis

Trauma or an acute infection results in a secondary bone infection commonly caused by Staphylococcus aureus. This condition is more common in adolescents and children and also has been seen in patients who have recently undergone antibiotic treatment.

### 7.12.1   Signs and Symptoms

- Pain
- Malaise
- Fever
- Chills

### 7.12.2   Medical Tests

- WBC is increased.
- Bone scan shows increased cellular activity at site of infection.
- X-ray shows location of decreased bone density (osteolytic lesions).
- Bone biopsy is performed to collect tissue sample.
- Culture and sensitivity is used to identify microorganism and medication.

### 7.12.3   Treatment

- Debride.
- Drain infection.
- Immobilize bone.

- Amputate if gangrene.

- Administer

  ○ Analgesics to decrease pain

    ■ Acetaminophen (Anacin, Tylenol); ibuprofen (Advil, Motrin); naproxen (Aleve, Naprosyn); oxycodone (OxyContin, Roxicodone), hydrocodone (Vicodin)

  ○ Antibiotics orally (6 to 8 weeks) or parenterally (4 to 6 weeks)

    ■ Nafcillin, vancomycin, penicillin G, piperacillin, ticarcillin/clavulanate, ampicillin/sulbactam, pipercillin/tazobactam, clindamycin, cefazolin, linezolid, ceftazidime, ciprofloxacin

### 7.12.4   Intervention

- Monitor site for signs of infection.

- Monitor vital signs.

- Monitor IV site for patency.

- Instruct the patient to take antibiotics for the full length of time that the medication is prescribed.

## 7.13   Osteoporosis

Osteoporosis is a disease of the bone resulting in decreased bone density as the rate of replacement bone is exceeded by bone reabsorption. This leads to brittle bones and increased risk of fractures particularly in the hip, vertebrae, pelvis, and distal radius. This condition is caused by age, decreased physical activity, prolonged periods of immobility, medication (steroids, anticonvulsants), and poor nutrition and is secondary to underlying disease.

### 7.13.1   Signs and Symptoms

- Asymptomatic

- Decreased height

- Kyphosis

- Unexplained fractures

- Back pain

### 7.13.2   Medical Tests

- Dual energy x-ray absorptiometry (DEXA) shows decreased bone density, which is the gold standard for diagnosis.

- X-ray shows demineralization.

### 7.13.3   Treatment

- Administer

  ○ Selective estrogen receptor modulator for patients who were postmenopausal to prevent osteoporosis

  ○ Raloxifene (Evista)

- Bisphosphonate inhibits bone reabsorption.
  - Alendronate (Fosamax); ibandronate (Boniva); pamidronate (APD, Aredia); zoledronate (Zometa, Aclasta); etidronate (Didronel); clodronate (Bonefos, Loron); risedronate (Actonel)
- Forteo (teriparatide) stimulates collagenous bone.
  - Calcium 1000–1500 mg per day to enhance absorption
- Vitamin D enhances the absorption of calcium.

### 7.13.4  Intervention

- Bisphosphonates:
  - Take on an empty stomach.
  - Take first thing in the morning with a full glass of water.
  - Don't lie down for 30–60 minutes.
- Explain to the patient
  - Importance of weight-bearing activity
  - Importance of range-of-motion exercises

## 7.14  Sprain and Strain

A sprain is a traumatic injury resulting in stretching of ligaments (connect bone to bone) in a joint. A strain is a traumatic injury resulting in a muscular tear. Sprains and strains are classified by degree (see Table 7.1).

### 7.14.1  Signs and Symptoms

- Swelling
- Bruise (ecchymosis)
- Pain caused by movement
- Spasms
- Loss of function (third degree)

**TABLE 7.1  Classification of Sprains and Strains**

| DEGREE | SPRAIN | STRAIN |
|--------|--------|--------|
| First | Ligament stretches without tearing. Joint is stable and functional. | Overstretched muscle |
| Second | Ligament stretches and tears. Slight joint instability and limited functionality | Partial tear of the muscle |
| Third | Ligament stretches and tears leading to trauma to the tendon. The joint is unstable and functionality is severely lost. | Complete tear of the muscle |

- Protrusion at the trauma site (third degree)
- Unstable joint (third degree)

### 7.14.2   Medical Tests

- X-ray shows no fracture.

### 7.14.3   Treatment

- Administer
    - NSAIDs to decrease inflammation and aid in pain relief
        - Indomethacin, ibuprofen, naproxen
    - Analgesics to decrease pain
        - Anacin, Tylenol (acetaminophen)

### 7.14.4   Intervention

- Apply ice 20 minutes on and 20 minutes off for the first 24 hours to reduce swelling.
- Apply heat 20 minutes on and 20 minutes off for the second 24 hours to enhance the inflammation process, thus repairing tissue.
- Elevate trauma site.
- Indicate rest.
- Immobilize site (second and third degree).
- Prescribe follow-up with specialist (i.e., surgeon) and rehabilitation (three degree).
- Instruct the patient
    - Keep the site free from any binding such as jewelry that can inhibit circulation when the site is swollen.
    - Gradually reuse the muscle, but stop if there is pain.

## Solved Problems

7.1   What are the five Ps of a musculoskeletal injury?

- Pain
- Paralysis
- Paresthesia
- Pulse
- Pallor

**7.2** What is adduction and abduction?

- **Adduction:** moving the limb closer to the body (adding to the body)
- **Abduction:** moving the limb away from the body (subtracting from the body)

**7.3** What auscultation would you perform during a musculoskeletal assessment?

Listen for abnormal sounds during the range-of-motion inspection:

- Clicking
- Crunching
- Grating

**7.4** How do you assess the range of motion in TMJ?

For temporomandibular joint (TMJ)

- Place first two fingers on patient's ear.
- Ask patient to open and close his mouth.
- Place fingers into the depression over the joint.
- Ask patient to open and close his mouth.
- The patient should easily open and close his mouth without pain or discomfort.

**7.5** What is the first step before assessing the range of motion of the neck?

Rule out cervical spine injury through imaging study.

**7.6** How do you assess the range of motion of the neck?

Ask the patient to

- Touch right ear to right shoulder.
- Touch left ear to left shoulder.
- Touch chin to chest (45 degrees is normal).
- Move head back and look at the ceiling (55 degrees is normal).
- Turn head to each side.
- Move head in a circle (70 degrees is normal).

**7.7** How do you assess the patient's shoulders?

Shoulders should be symmetric and not deformed. Feel the:

- Bony landmarks with your fingers
- Shoulder muscles with your hand (muscles should be firm and symmetrical)
- Elbow and ulna

Ask the patient to:

- Extend his arms straight at his side (neutral position).
- Lift his arms straight to shoulder level.
- Bend his elbow at 90 degrees.
- Extend his arms out parallel to the floor, palms down and fingers extended.
- Extend his forearms up with fingers pointed to the ceiling. (Forearms should move 90 degrees.)
- Extend his forearms down with fingers pointing to the floor. (Forearms should move 90 degrees.)
- Extend his arms straight at his side (neutral position).
- Move arms forward and up over his head.
- Extend his arms straight at his side (neutral position).
- Move his arms as far back as possible. (Arms should bend 30 degrees.)
- Extend his arms straight at his side (neutral position).
- Move his arms away from his body (abduction). (Arms should move 180 degrees.)
- Extend his arms straight at his side (neutral position).
- Move his arms across the front of his body (adduction). (Arms should move 50 degrees.)
- Extend his arms straight at his side (neutral position).
- Flex his elbows. (Elbows should flex 90 degrees.)
- Place the side of his hand (thumbs facing up) on a flat surface.
- Rotate the palm of his hands down to the surface (pronation). (The elbow should rotate 90 degrees.)
- Rotate the palm of his hands upward from the surface (supination). (The elbow should rotate 90 degrees.)

**7.8**     What is a complete fracture?

Complete fracture is where the fracture is completely through the bone.

**7.9**     What is an open fracture?

Open fracture is when the fracture penetrates the skin.

**7.10**    What is compartment syndrome?

Compartment syndrome is when nerves, blood vessels, and muscles in a closed space caused by a facture are compressed, leading to tissue necrosis.

**7.11**    What is a delayed union?

Delayed union is a fracture that is not joined within six months.

**7.12**    What is a fat embolism?

Fat embolism is when yellow bone marrow releases fat into the bloodstream, resulting in emboli.

**7.13**   How do you grade muscle strength?

| Grade | Description |
|-------|-------------|
| 0 | No muscle contraction |
| 1 | Muscle contraction is felt, but joint does not move |
| 2 | Complete range of motion with assistance (passive range of motion) |
| 3 | Complete range of motion against gravity |
| 4 | Complete range of motion against gravity with moderate resistance |
| 5 | Complete range of motion against gravity with full resistance |

**7.14**   What are the signs of bleeding?

Increased pulse, increased respiration, and decreased blood pressure are the signs of bleeding.

**7.15**   Why should a patient perform range-of-motion exercise?

A patient should perform range-of-motion exercise to maintain muscle tone.

**7.16**   Why shouldn't a patient insert objects into a cast?

This can cause a breakdown of skin.

**7.17**   What is arthrocentesis?

Arthrocentesis is a procedure that collects a sample of synovial fluid from a joint for analysis by the lab. This is also referred to as tapping synovial fluid. The color and appearance of the synovial fluid might indicate the underlying cause of swelling:

- **Crystals:** arthritis, gout (foot)
- **Cloudy:** infection (white blood cells)
- **Red:** bleeding (red blood cells) related to trauma

**7.18**   When should a patient who uses an immobilizing device call his practitioner immediately?

The patient should contact the practitioner immediately if there are signs of

- Drainage
- Pain
- Swelling

**7.19**   What are the effects of a skeletal muscle relaxant?

Skeletal muscle relaxants are used to reduce muscle tone and to treat muscle spasms and hyperreflexia by either interfering with neurological transmission to the muscle or reducing the spasticity of the muscle.

**7.20**   What is a dislocation?

A dislocation is a traumatic injury causing two or more bones in an articulated joint to move out of anatomical alignment. The dislocation may result in injury to nerves, soft tissue, and circulation.

**7.21** What is a contusion?

A contusion is a hemorrhage beneath the skin as a result of blunt trauma to the site, leading to discoloration and discomfort at the site of the injury.

**7.22** Why do you outline a contusion with a marker?

A marker is used to outline a contusion to assess if bleeding has stopped. Discoloring increasing beyond the outline indicates that bleeding continues and may require intervention.

**7.23** What is a sprain?

A sprain is a traumatic injury resulting in stretching of ligaments (connect bone to bone) in a joint.

**7.24** Why should the patient remove jewelry from the site of a strain?

Inflammation at the site of the strain can cause swelling, and jewelry may bind the site, resulting in decreased circulation.

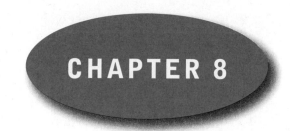

CHAPTER 8

# Genitourinary and Gynecologic Emergencies

## 8.1   Define

- Genitourinary and gynecologic emergencies are conditions that alter the urinary system or the reproductive system, resulting in the patient becoming unstable.

- Genitourinary and gynecologic physiology can be disrupted by an inflammation, infection, or trauma.

- A genitourinary or gynecologic emergency can be life threatening.

- A genitourinary or gynecologic emergency can result in pain, disfigurement, and disability.

- Focus on genitourinary and gynecologic symptoms after the patient's airway, breathing, circulation, cervical spine, and neurological system are stabilized.

- A genitourinary or gynecologic emergency requires immediate intervention.


### 8.1.1   Goal of Treating Genitourinary and Gynecologic Emergencies

- The goal of the emergency-department staff is to identify the genitourinary or gynecologic emergency and stabilize the patient. The underlying cause of the genitourinary or gynecologic emergency is treated in follow-up care unless the emergency department staff can address the underlying cause. For example, an antibiotic may be ordered for a patient diagnosed with a urinary tract infection who is then requested to follow up with a primary-care practitioner.

- Thoroughly assess the patient before beginning treatment. Administering medication may mask a sign or symptom that indicates a genitourinary or gynecologic emergency.

- Diagnose the acute problem.

- Stabilize the patient by relieving pain and treating the acute problem.

- Refer the patient to follow-up care.

**8.1.2   Genitourinary and Gynecologic Assessment**

- Assess the patient's urinary system first because this is the least sensitive system to discuss.
    - Kidneys
    - Ureters
    - Bladder
    - Urethra
- Assess the patient's reproductive system last because this is the most sensitive system to discuss.
    - Male:
        - Penis
        - Scrotum
        - Testicles
        - Epididymis
        - Vas deferens
        - Seminal vesicles
        - Prostate gland
    - Female:
        - Vagina
        - Uterus
        - Ovaries
        - Fallopian tubes
        - Vulva
        - Labia majora
        - Labia minora
        - Clitoris
        - Urethral meatus
        - Skene's glands
        - Bartholin's glands
- The genitourinary or gynecologic assessment interview
    - Ask open-ended questions.
        - Why did you come to the hospital today?
        - What makes you feel that something is wrong?
    - Look for clues for underlying cause of the genitourinary or gynecologic emergency.
        - What happened prior to your noticing this problem?
        - Have you recently undergone any medical procedure?
            - What medical procedure?
            - When was the medical procedure performed?

- ○ Follow-up questions help probe further into the presenting genitourinary or gynecologic problem.

  - When did this problem start?

  - How long have you had this problem?

  - Can you describe the problem?

  - How much does the problem bother you?

  - Where do you feel uncomfortable?

  - Is the problem spreading or does the problem remain in one place?

  - Does anything make the problem worse?

  - Does anything make the problem better?

  - Did you have this problem or a similar problem in the past?

    - □ Explain.

  - Have you been diagnosed with any medical condition (previous diagnosis and treatment)?

    - □ What medical condition?

      - ◆ Are you being treated for the medical condition?

      - ◆ What is the treatment?

      - ◆ Who is treating you?

  - What medications do you use?

    - □ Prescribed

    - □ Over-the-counter

    - □ Cultural

    - □ Herbal

- ○ Ask about the patient's urinary system.

  - Have there been any recent changes in your urination?

  - How frequently do you urinate?

  - Do you experience any burning during urination?

  - What color is your urine?

  - Does your urine emit an odor?

- ○ Ask about the patient's reproductive issues.

  - How many sexual partners have you had?

  - Do you engage in risk-taking behaviors?

  - What is your sexual preference?

  - Have you ever had or do you have an STD?

  - Do you know your HIV status?

  - Do you use birth control?

    - □ If so, what type?

  - Males:

    - □ Is there any discharge from your penis?

    - □ Do you experience any tenderness in your genitals?

- □ Did you notice any lumps or growths in your genitals?

- □ Do you experience any itching (pruritus) in your genitals?

- ■ Females:

  - □ Did you experience menopause?

    - ◆ When was your last menstrual period?

    - ◆ Do you experience vaginal dryness?

    - ◆ Do you experience vaginal itching?

    - ◆ Do you have hot flashes?

    - ◆ Do you experience flushing?

    - ◆ Do you have mood swings?

  - □ Do you have a menstrual cycle?

    - ◆ Describe your menstrual cycle.

    - ◆ Do you spot between menstruation cycles?

    - ◆ What is the length of your menstrual cycle?

    - ◆ When was your last menstrual period?

    - ◆ When was your first menstrual period?

    - ◆ Do you use tampons?

  - □ Is there any vaginal discharge?

  - □ Do you experience any unusual uterine bleeding?

  - □ Do you experience any vaginal itching (pruritus)?

  - □ Do you experience pain with intercourse?

  - □ When was your last intercourse?

  - □ When was your last Pap (Papanicolaou) test?

  - □ What was the result of your last Pap test?

  - □ Do you go for routine gynecological examinations?

    - ◆ When was your last gynecological examination?

- ○ Ask about the patient's family history.

  - ■ Does anyone in your family have diabetes or a history of diabetes?

  - ■ Does anyone in your family have hypertension or a history of hypertension?

  - ■ Does anyone in your family have cardiovascular disease or a history of cardiovascular disease?

  - ■ Does anyone in your family have kidney stones or a history of kidney stones?

- • Inspection

  - ○ Snow crystals on the skin (uremic frost) indicate increased retention of metabolic waste related to decreased renal function.

  - ○ Pale skin indicates decreased hemoglobin related to decreased renal function.

- The abdomen should

  - Be symmetrical when the patient lies on his or her back

  - Have no discolorations

  - Have no silvery streaks (striae). Silvery streaks indicate ascites related to nephrotic syndrome.

- Genitalia should

  - Have no discharge

  - Not appear inflamed

- Auscultation

  - Listen for abnormal sounds in the renal arteries.

    - Use the bell of the stethoscope.

    - Place the stethoscope at the midline of the abdomen.

    - Ask the patient to exhale.

    - Move the stethoscope left then right.

    - A turbulent sound (bruits) indicates a disruption in blood flow in the renal artery.

- Percussion

  - Percuss the kidneys.

    - Ask the patient to sit upright on the edge of the bed.

    - Place the ball of one hand on the patient's back over the kidney at the 12th rib.

    - Strike your hand with your other hand. You should hear a thud.

    - Repeat the percussion on the other kidney.

    - Tenderness may indicate a kidney infection.

  - Percuss the bladder.

    - Ask the patient to urinate immediately before the examination begins.

    - Ask the patient to lie on his back.

    - Place one hand on the abdomen.

    - Tap the middle finger with your other hand to hear tympany.

    - Start at the symphysis pubis and move up over the bladder.

    - A dull sound may indicate urine retention or a mass.

- Palpation

  - Palpate the kidneys.

  - Ask the patient to lie on his back.

  - Place one hand under the patient below the kidney.

  - Place the other hand above the patient by the kidney.

  - Ask the patient to inhale

  - Press your hands together.

  - Repeat this process on the other kidney.

  - You should not feel the kidney unless the kidney is enlarged.

### 8.1.2.1  Signs and Symptoms

Genitourinary and gynecologic assessments in an emergency situation require the nurse to recognize common signs and symptoms of underlying causes and then prepare for the anticipated treatment that the practitioner is likely to order.

Commonly seen signs and symptoms of urinary system problems:

- Not urinating (anuria)
- Excessive urinating (polyuria)
- Producing small amount of urine (oliguria)
- Painful urination (dysuria)
- Hesitancy to urinate
- Involuntary urination (incontinence)
- Getting up from sleep to urinate (nocturia)
- Odor from urine (bacterial infection)
- Cloudy urine (bacterial infection)
- Blood in urine (hematuria)
- Clear urine (overhydrated)
- Dark urine (dehydrated)

Commonly seen signs and symptoms of reproductive system problems:

- Males:
  - Itchiness (pruritus)
  - Penile discharge
  - Mass on genitals
  - Tenderness on genitals
- Females:
  - Vaginal discharge
  - Vaginal odor
  - Uterine bleeding
  - Vaginal itching (pruritus)
  - Cramps
  - Infrequent menstrual periods (oligomenorrhea)
  - Short menstrual periods (hypomenorrhea)
  - Painful menstrual periods (dysmenorrhea)
  - No menstrual periods (amenorrhea)
  - Frequent menstrual periods (polymenorrhea)
  - Spotting (metrorrhagia)
  - Long menstrual peirods (hypermenorrhea)

## 8.2 Genitourinary and Gynecologic Tests and Procedures

Genitourinary and gynecologic tests are designed to assess the effectiveness and the capability of the two systems to function. Emergency-department practitioners order genitourinary and gynecologic tests to collect objective data and to further assess and assist in stabilizing the patient. Once stabilized, the patient is transferred or referred to follow-up care designed to treat the underlying cause of the current episode, which may require additional genitourinary and gynecologic tests. Genitourinary and gynecologic procedures are performed to stabilize the patient.

The following are genitourinary and gynecologic tests and procedures commonly ordered by the emergency department's practitioners.

### 8.2.1 Genitourinary and Gynecologic CT Scan

A genitourinary and gynecologic CT scan provides a three-dimensional image of the genitourinary and gynecologic systems using x-rays that enable the practitioner to visualize normal and abnormal structures. A CT can be performed with or without a contrast agent. A contrast agent is iodine-based and enhances images of blood vessels and less-dense areas.

The practitioner typically orders a genitourinary and gynecologic CT scan to assess for:

- Inflammation
- Tumor
- Cysts
- Pseudocysts

**CT Scan Procedure**

- Assess if the patient is allergic to iodine or shellfish if the patient is undergoing a CT scan with contrast. Patients who are allergic to iodine or shellfish have a high likelihood of experiencing an allergic reaction to the contrast agent.

- Administer diphenhydramine (Benadryl) and prednisone (Deltasone) before the CT scan to reduce the risk of an allergic reaction to the contrast agent if a contrast agent is ordered.

- Administer the contrast agent through an IV. The patient may feel flushed and have a salty or metallic taste in his or her mouth.

- Explain to the patient that the contrast material typically discolors the urine for upward of 24 hours following the CT scan. The patient should increase fluid intake after the CT scan to flush the contrast agent from the patient's body, if a contrast agent is used for the CT scan.

- Assess if the patient is claustrophobic, as the patient will be placed in an enclosure during the test.

- Assess if the patient can remain still for 30 minutes during the CT scan, as the CT scanner encircles the patient for up to 30 minutes.

### 8.2.2 Genitourinary and Gynecologic MRI

A genitourinary and gynecologic magnetic resonance imaging (MRI) provides a three-dimensional view of the genitourinary and gynecologic systems using radio waves, a strong magnet, and a computer. An MRI is particularly used to assess fluid-filled soft tissue and to identify tumors from other structures within the genitourinary and gynecologic systems.

The practitioner typically orders a genitourinary and gynecologic MRI to assess for:

- Inflammation
- Tumor
- Cysts
- Pseudocysts

**Genitourinary and Gynecologic MRI Procedure**

- The patient may need to be NPO (nothing by mouth) for up to 12 hours before the test, depending on the site of the MRI.
- All metal must be removed from the patient.
- No metal must enter the room containing the MRI scanner. The MRI scanner's magnet is always activated.
- Assess if the patient is claustrophobic. If so, then ask the healthcare provider if an open MRI scanner should be used for the test, or if the patient should be sedated before the scan begins.
- The MRI scan takes about 30 minutes.
- The MRI scan is noninvasive. The patient will not feel any discomfort.

### 8.2.3  KUB Radiography

A KUB radiography provides an x-ray view of the kidneys, ureters, and bladder without using contrast. No special preparation is necessary. This test is typically performed at bedside using a portable x-ray machine.

The practitioner typically orders a KUB radiography to assess for:

- Lesions
- Calculi
- Position of kidneys

**KUB Radiography Procedure**

- The patient lies on his back.
- The x-ray machine is positioned.
- Images are recorded.

### 8.2.4  Genitourinary and Gynecologic Ultrasound

A genitourinary and gynecologic ultrasound provides a view of the kidneys, ureters, and bladder using high-frequency sound waves. No special preparation is necessary. This test can be performed at bedside or in an imaging room.

The practitioner typically orders a genitourinary and gynecologic ultrasound to assess:

- Underlying structure

**Genitourinary and Gynecologic Ultrasound Procedure**

- If the bladder is being examined, then the patient requires a full bladder during the test.

- The patient lies on his or her back or stomach depending on which structure is being examined.

- A conductive gel is placed on the site and on the ultrasound transducer.

- The ultrasound transducer is moved over the site.

## 8.2.5 Renal Scan

A renal scan provides a functional view of the kidneys. A radioactive tracer is injected into the patient's vein and is observed as the tracer flows through the kidneys. The renal scan is an alternative to the intravenous pyelogram (IVP) (see 8.2.6 Intravenous Pyelogram).

The practitioner typically orders a renal scan to assess for:

- Kidney function

- Blood flow through the kidneys

**Renal Scan Procedure**

- The patient drinks three glasses of water before the test.

- The patient lies on his or her back.

- A radioactive tracer is injected into the patient's vein.

- The renal scan camera is positioned.

- Function study is conducted.

  ○ An image is taken every 3 minutes for 30 minutes.

  ○ The patient may be administered a diuretic to increase kidney function during the test.

- Perfusion study is conducted.

  ○ A renogram is created showing movement of the tracer throughout the kidneys.

- Following the test, the patient drinks a lot of water to flush the tracer from his or her body.

- For two days following the renal scan, the patient must flush the toilet immediately after urinating and defecating. The radioactive tracer remains in urine and feces for two days.

## 8.2.6 Intravenous Pyelogram (IVP)

An intravenous pyelogram (IVP) provides an x-ray view of the kidneys, ureters, and bladder. A contrast material is injected into the patient's vein. Images are taken periodically for up to five minutes as the contrast material flows through the urinary system.

The practitioner typically orders an intravenous pyelogram to assess for:

- Obstructions

- Tumors

- Cysts

**Intravenous Pyelogram Procedure**

- The patient drinks at least three glasses of water before the test.

- The patient lies on his or her back.

- Contrast material is injected into the patient's vein.

- The x-ray machine is positioned.

- Several images are taken over a five-minute period.

## 8.2.7  Renal Angiograph

A renal angiograph provides a fluoroscopic view using x-rays of the arterial and venial blood flow in the kidneys. A contrast material is injected into the patient's artery. Images are taken continually as the contrast material flows through the kidneys.

The practitioner typically orders a renal angiograph to assess for:

- Blood clots

- Narrowing of blood vessels in the kidneys (renal stenosis)

- Aneurysm

- Pyelonephritis

- Kidney disorders

**Renal Angiograph Procedure**

- The patient lies on his or her back.

- The injection site near the groin is cleaned.

- Contrast material is injected into the patient's artery through a catheter.

- Fluoroscopic images are taken.

- Pressure is applied to the site for 15 minutes after the catheter is removed.

- The patient must keep the leg that was tested straight for six hours following the procedure.

- The healthcare provider monitors the patient's serum creatinine and BUN levels (see 8.2.8 Renal Blood Tests) following the test for signs of renal failure related to the contrast material.

## 8.2.8  Renal Blood Tests

Practitioners use blood studies to assist in diagnosing genitourinary disorders. A practitioner may order one or multiple of the following common blood studies:

- Blood urea nitrogen (BUN): BUN levels are compared with serum creatinine levels to assess if an increase in BUN level is caused by a renal disorder. Renal disorder is suspected if both BUN and serum creatinine levels are increased.

  - Increase may indicate:

    - Glomerulonephritis

    - Obstruction

    - Oliguria

- Serum creatinine: positively correlates with glomerular filtration rate (GFR)
  - Increase may indicate:
    - Renal disorder
- Serum osmolality
  - Increase may indicate renal disorder if urine osmolality decreases.
- Serum proteins
  - Decrease may indicate:
    - Nephrosis
    - Hephritis
- Creatinine clearance: positively correlates with glomerular filtration rate (GFR)
  - Decrease may indicate:
    - Pyelonephritis
    - Glomerulonephritis
    - Tubular necrosis
    - Nephrosclerosis
    - Decreased renal blood flow
    - Renal lesion
- Uric acid
  - Increase may indicate:
    - Decreased renal function
  - Decrease may indicate:
    - Tubular absorption disorder
- Urea clearance
  - Decrease may indicate:
    - Glomerulonephritis
    - Nephrosclerosis
    - Pyelonephritis
    - Renal blood flow disorder
    - Tubular necrosis
    - Dehydration
    - Renal lesion
    - Ureteral obstruction
- Complete blood count (CBC)
  - White blood cell count (WBC)
    - Increase may indicate:
      - Infection

- Red blood cell count (RBC)
    - Decrease may indicate:
        - Chronic renal insufficiency
- Hemoglobin (Hgb)
    - Decrease may indicate:
        - Chronic renal insufficiency
- Hematocrit (Hct)
    - Decrease may indicate:
        - Chronic renal insufficiency
- Electrolytes
    - Calcium
        - Decrease may indicate:
            - Renal failure
    - Phosphorus
        - Increase may indicate:
            - Renal failure
    - Chloride
        - Increase may indicate:
            - Renal failure
            - Tubular necrosis
            - Dehydration
        - Decrease may indicate:
            - Pyelonephritis
    - Potassium
        - Increase may indicate:
            - Acidosis
            - Renal insufficiency
            - Renal failure
        - Decrease may indicate:
            - Tubular disorder
    - Sodium
        - Decrease may indicate:
            - Renal failure

## 8.2.9 Urine Analysis

Practitioners use urine analysis to assist in diagnosing genitourinary disorders. A practitioner may order one or multiples of the following urine studies. Table 8.1 contains common urine studies.

**TABLE 8.1 Common Urine Studies**

| STUDY | ABNORMAL RESULTS | MAY INDICATE |
|---|---|---|
| pH | Alkaline >8.0 | Urinary tract infection |
| | | Chronic renal disease |
| | | Respiratory alkalosis |
| | | Metabolic alkalosis |
| | Acidic <4.5 | Acidosis |
| | | Tuberculosis |
| | | Phenylketonuria |
| Specific gravity | Decreased | Renal failure |
| | | Glomerulonephritis |
| | | Diabetes insipidus |
| | | Alkalosis |
| | | Pyelonephritis |
| | Increased | Nephrosis |
| | | Dehydration |
| Ketones | Found | Starvation |
| | | Diabetes mellitus |
| | | Vomiting |
| | | Diarrhea |
| Protein | Found | Renal disease |
| Odor/color | Fruity odor | Starvation |
| | | Dehydration |
| | | Diabetes mellitus |
| | Turbid | Renal infection |
| | Cloudy | Infection |
| | Dark | Dehydration |
| Epithelial cells | Many found | Tubular degeneration |
| Red blood cells | Many found | Urinary tract infection |
| | | Trauma |
| | | Renal hypertension |
| | | Inflammation |
| | | Obstruction |
| | | Hydronephrosis |
| | | Tuberculosis |
| | | Glomerulonephritis |
| | | Pyelonephritis |
| | | Bladder infection |
| Glucose | Found | Diabetes mellitus |
| Crystals | Calcium oxalate | Hypercalcemia |
| | Cystine crystals | Metabolic disorder |

*(Continued)*

**TABLE 8.1** **Common Urine Studies** (*Continued*)

| STUDY | ABNORMAL RESULTS | MAY INDICATE |
|---|---|---|
| White blood cells | Many found | Urinary tract infection |
| | | Pyelonephritis |
| | | Cystitis |
| Creatinine clearance | Decreased | Renal artery obstruction |
| | | Glomerulonephritis |
| | | Renal lesion |
| | | Dehydration |
| | | Nephrosclerosis |
| | | Heart failure |
| | | Tubular necrosis |
| Yeast cells | Found | Vaginitis |
| | | Prostatovesiculitis |
| | | Urethritis |
| | | Contaminated sample |
| Casts | Red blood cell casts | Renal infarction |
| | | Bacterial endocarditis |
| | | Malignant hypertension |
| | | Sickle-cell anemia |
| | | Collagen disorder |
| | | Glomerulonephritis |
| | White blood cell casts | Renal infection |
| | Many hyaline casts | Inflammation |
| | | Trauma |
| | | Renal parenchymal disorder |
| | Waxy casts | Chronic renal disease |
| | | Diabetes mellitus |
| | | Nephrotic syndrome |
| | Epithelial casts | Nephrosis |
| | | Chronic lead intoxication |
| | | Tubular disorder |
| | | Eclampsia |
| | Many casts | Renal disease |
| Parasites | Found | Contaminated sample |

## 8.2.10 Calculi Basketing

Calculi basketing is a procedure where a basketing device is inserted into the ureter using an ureteroscope or cystoscope to remove a ureteral calculus.

The practitioner typically orders a calculi basketing to:

- Remove a stone (calculi) that is too large to pass through the ureter

**Renal Angiograph Procedure**

- The patient lies on his back.

- Ureteroscope or cystoscope is inserted into the ureter.

- The basketing device is inserted into the urteroscope or cystoscope.

- The calculi is removed, as are the basketing device and urteroscope or cystoscope.

- An indwelling urinary catheter is inserted into the ureter.

- The patient is administered intravenous fluids for up to 48 hours.

- Fluid intake and output is measured.

- The indwelling urinary catheter is removed within 48 hours.

## 8.2.11   Extracorporeal Shock Wave Lilthotripsy (ESWL)

ESWL is a procedure where a high-energy shock wave is administered to the patient to break up calculi. The calculi then passes naturally through the ureter.

The practitioner typically orders ESWL to:

- Break up a stone (calculi) that is too large to pass through the ureter

**ESWL Procedure**

- The patient receives an anesthetic.

- The patient lies on his or her back.

- Shock waves are administered.

- An indwelling urinary catheter is inserted into the ureter.

- The patient is told to increase fluid intake to increase urine output.

- The patient is told to ambulate.

- The patient is told to urinate in container. Urine is then strained for calculi.

- The patient is told that there might be a small amount of blood in the urine for several days following the procedure.

- The patient should contact the practitioner immediately if there is persistent bleeding, persistent pain, fever, chills, nausea, vomiting, or an inability to urinate.

## 8.3   Genitourinary and Gynecologic Medication

Commonly used medications in genitourinary and gynecologic emergencies are nonsteroidal anti-inflammatory drugs, corticosteroids, analgesics, and antibiotics. These medications reduce pain and discomfort by reducing pressure on nerves caused by inflammation or blocking neurological transmission. Antibiotics assist the immune system in combatting bacterial infection.

### 8.3.1 Nonsteroidal Anti-Inflammatory Drugs (NSAIDs)

Nonsteroidal anti-inflammatory drugs are medications that reduce swelling, pain, and stiffness without exposing the patient to the adverse side effects that occur when using corticosteroid medications.

- Aspirin (ASA)
- Ibuprofen (Motrin, Advil, Nuprin)
- Naproxen (Naprosyn, Aleve)
- Oxaprozin (Daypro)
- Ketoprofen (Orudis)
- Diclofenac sodium (Voltaren)
- Ketorolac (Toradol)
- Velecoxib (Celebrex)

### 8.3.2 Corticosteroids

Corticosteroids are used to reduce inflammation and cerebral edema. Corticosteroids increase the risk of pancreatitis, heart failure, and thromboembolism.

- Dexamethasone (Dexasone, Decadron)
- Methylprednisolone (Solu-Medrol)

### 8.3.3 Analgesics

Analgesics are used to reduce pain.

- Oxycodone (OxyContin)
- Morphine (Duramorph)

### 8.3.4 Antibiotics

Antibiotics are used to treat bacterial infections such as gonorrhea, bacterial vaginosis, and urinary tract infection.

- Ceftriaxone for gonorrhea
- Tinidazole (Tindamax) for bacterial vaginosis
- Clindamycin (Cleocin) for bacterial vaginosis
- Metronidazole (Flagyl) for bacterial vaginosis
- Viprofloxacin (Cipro) for urinary tract infection
- Levofloxacin (Levaquin) for urinary tract infection
- Sulfamethoxazole-trimethoprim (Bactrim) for urinary tract infection

### 8.3.5 Antiparasitics

Antiparasitics are used to treat parasitic infections such as trichomoniasis.

- Metronidazole for trichomoniasis
- Tinidazole for trichomoniasis

### 8.3.6 Antifungals

Antifungal medications are used to treat fungus infections such as a vaginal yeast (candida) infection.

- Miconazole (Monistat) for vaginal yeast infection

## 8.4 Testicular Torsion

Testicular torsion is a disorder where the spermatic cord twists, resulting in strangulation of the testis that can lead to testicular infarction and disruption of blood flow to the testis. The disorder must be resolved within six hours of onset to maintain testicular functionality. Necrosis can occur after 12 hours.

There are two types of testicular torsion:

- Intravaginal torsion:
  - Within the tissue covering the testicles
  - Testis is free to rotate.
- Extravaginal torsion:
  - Outside the tissue covering the testicles
  - Spermatic cord twists above the testis.

### 8.4.1 Signs and Symptoms

- Scrotal swelling not relieved by elevation of the scrotum
- Severe pain in the scrotum
- Prehn's sign:
  - Elevate scrotum to symphysis pubis
    - Increased pain indicates positive Prehn's sign.
    - Decreased pain indicates negative Prehn's sign and is indicative of inflammation of testis (epididymitis), rather than testicular torsion.

### 8.4.2 Medical Tests

- Ultrasound shows testicular torsion.

### 8.4.3 Treatment

- Manual reduction by practitioner
- Surgical reduction
- Administer
  - Analgesic for symptom relief

### 8.4.4 Intervention

- Monitor vital signs.
- Prepare patient for surgery.
- Instruct the patient
  - Success rate for restoring testicular function is 75%.

## 8.5 Acute Glomerulonephritis

Acute glomerulonephritis is a kidney infection known as acute nephritic syndrome resulting from an ascending urinary infection or infection from elsewhere in the body.

### 8.5.1 Signs and Symptoms

- Oliguria
- Hematuria
- Peripheral edema
- Elevated blood pressure

### 8.5.2 Medical Tests

- BUN: elevated
- Albumin: decreased
- Glomerular filtration rate: decreased
- 24-hour urine: elevated protein
- Urinalysis: shows red blood cell casts
- Renal biopsy: identifies cause of infection

### 8.5.3 Treatment

- Administer
  - Diuretic
  - Plasmapheresis (if cause is an autoimmune disorder)

### 8.5.4   Intervention

- Monitor vital signs.

- Monitor intake and output.

- Weigh daily.

- Monitor extremities for edema.

- Instruct the patient to decrease fluid intake.

## 8.6   Kidney Trauma

Kidney trauma is damage to the kidney caused by either a blunt or penetrating injury. A blunt injury is commonly caused by a motor-vehicle accident, assault, fall, or sports injury. A penetrating injury is commonly caused by a blast, a knife wound, or gunshot.

Kidney trauma is classified by a five-grade scale as illustrated in Table 8.2.

### 8.6.1   Signs and Symptoms

- Sign of wound

- Flank bruising or hematoma

- Blue-red-purple or green-brown flank discoloration (Turner's sign)

- Flank tenderness or pain

- Blood in the urine (hematuria)

- Blood clots in urine

TABLE **8.2**  **Classification of Kidney Trauma**

| GRADE | DESCRIPTION |
|---|---|
| 1 | Superficial laceration of the renal cortex |
|  | Bruising (contusion) of the parenchyma |
| 2 | Hematoma of the kidney that does not expand |
|  | Laceration less than 1 cm of the parenchyma |
| 3 | Laceration 1 cm or more of the parenchyma |
|  | Collecting system intact |
| 4 | Thrombosis in a portion of the renal artery |
|  | Bleeding of renal artery and veins that is controllable |
|  | Laceration 1 cm or more of the collecting system |
|  | Leaking of fluid (extravasation) around and within the kidney |
| 5 | Fractured kidney |
|  | Tearing of the renal artery or vein |
|  | Thrombosis of the renal artery |

- Hypotension related to bleeding (grade 3, 4, or 5)
- Hypovolemic shock (grade 5)

### 8.6.2   Medical Tests

- KUB shows wound and kidney damage.
- IVP is used to grade trauma.
- Renal angiograph shows arterial damage.
- Blood test
  - CBC shows blood loss and clotting ability.
- Urinalysis shows presence of red blood cells.
- Ultrasound shows renal damage.
- CT scan with contrast shows renal damage.
- MRI shows renal damage.

### 8.6.3   Treatment

- Stabilize airway, breathing, cardiovascular functioning, and hemodynamics.
- Administer
  - Oxygen
  - Lactated Ringer's solution or normal saline
  - Antibiotic
  - Analgesic for symptom relief
- Surgical repair of kidney

### 8.6.4   Intervention

- Apply direct pressure on wound to control bleeding.
- Cover the wound.
- Insert two large-bore saline/heparin locks.
- Monitor vital signs every 15 minutes.
- Monitor for abdominal distention.
- Instruct the patient on the importance of rest.

## 8.7   Kidney Stones (Renal Calculi)

Kidney stones are also known as renal calculi and nephrolithiasis. Slow urine flow enables crystals to form from calcium, uric acid, cystine, or struvite in the kidneys or in the urinary tract. The crystals may block the ureter, causing hydronephrosis and swelling. There is a genetic predisposition to kidney stones.

### 8.7.1 Signs and Symptoms

- Unilateral extreme flank pain (renal colic) may radiate to lower abdomen, groin, scrotum, or labia.
- Hematuria
- Blood pressure elevated with pain
- Nausea
- Vomiting

### 8.7.2 Medical Tests

- Urinalysis shows leukocytosis.
- Ultrasound shows stones.
- X-ray of kidneys, ureters, and bladder (KUB) shows stones.
- CT scan shows stones.
- MRI shows stones.

### 8.7.3 Treatment

- Lithotripsy: shock waves break the stone into pieces so the stone can pass.
- Surgical removal of the stone
- Surgical insertion of stent
- Administer
    - Narcotics
    - Morphine
    - NSAIDs
    - Ketorolac

### 8.7.4 Intervention

- Monitor intake and output.
- Strain urine.
- Instruct the patient
    - Increase fluid intake.
    - Make dietary modification based on makeup of stone.

## 8.8 Sexual Assault

Sexual assault is nonconsensual, sexual contact that usually involves force or coercion. The objective is to treat the physical and emotional trauma of the sexual assault and to collect evidence based on the healthcare facility's protocol. Evidence may have to be collected by a certified sexual assault nurse examiner who is trained to collect and preserve evidence and follow the chain of evidence protocol. The chain of evidence (chain of custody) protocol requires detailed documentation of evidence commonly referred to as a paper trail, beginning with the person who collected the evidence, through presentation in court, and terminating when the evidence is destroyed after the case is closed.

### 8.8.1 Signs and Symptoms

- Patient is withdrawn.
- Outward signs of an assault (i.e., stains, torn clothing)
- Agitation, especially when close to staff
- Crying
- Flat affect
- Denial

### 8.8.2 Medical Tests

- X-ray: to rule out fractures
- Blood tests
  - Human chorionic gonadotropin (HCG) to rule out pregnancy
  - To rule out STDs

### 8.8.3 Treatment

- Care for patient's physical injuries.
- Administer medication to treat STDs, if present.
- Indicate follow-up treatment including psychological counseling, which should begin within 10 days of discharge from the emergency department.

### 8.8.4 Intervention

- Remain with the patient.
- Separate the patient from persons accompanying the patient to the emergency department until you are certain that the patient is comfortable with their presence.
- Assess if any person accompanying the patient to the emergency department is the possible attacker or possibly involved in the assault.
- Request that the patient not shower or change clothes until evidence is collected.
- Develop a therapeutic relationship with the patient.
- Ask the patient
  - To explain in detail how the patient was assaulted (i.e., date, time, areas of penetration, objects used)
  - What the patient did following the assault (e.g., urinate, shower)
  - To identify all sexual intercourse that occurred in the last 72 hours (consensual or nonconsensual)

- To explain any treatments and surgeries and when they occurred

- To sign a consent form for testing

- Provide psychological counseling immediately based on healthcare facility's protocol.

- Make sure that the patient has a safe place to stay following discharge from the emergency department. Social-service organizations are usually available to provide emergency housing.

- Instruct the patient

  - Evidence must be collected immediately and must follow strict procedures.

  - Authorities must be informed of the assault.

  - Counseling is highly recommended as soon as possible following discharge from the emergency department.

## 8.9 Pyelonephritis

This is an infection of the kidneys commonly from E. coli, klebsiella, enterobacter, proteus, pseudomonas, or *Staphylococcus saprophyticus* related to ascending urinary tract infection.

### 8.9.1 Signs and Symptoms

- Flank pain
- Fever
- Chills
- Urinary frequency
- Urinary urgency
- Costovertebral angle (CVA) tenderness
- Nausea
- Vomiting
- Diarrhea

### 8.9.2 Medical Tests

- Urinalysis shows red blood cells.
- Urine culture and sensitivity identifies organism and medication to treat the illness.
- CBC shows leukocytosis.

### 8.9.3 Treatment

- Administer
  - Antibiotics
    - Nitrofurantoin, ciprofloxacin, levofloxacin, ofloxacin, trimethoprim-sulfamethoxazole, ampicillin, amoxicillin

- ○ Antipyretics
- ○ Phenazopyridine

### 8.9.4   Intervention

- Monitor vital signs.
- Monitor intake and output.
- Increase fluid intake.
- Instruct the patient that Phenazopyridine will cause orange-colored urine.

## 8.10   Renal Failure

Renal failure is decreased renal function.

- **Acute:** sudden decrease in renal function
- **Prerenal:** caused by diminished renal perfusion
- **Hypovolemia:** caused by blood or fluid loss
- **Postrenal:** caused by urinary tract obstruction
- **Chronic:** progressive decrease in renal function due to irreversible renal disease

### 8.10.1   Signs and Symptoms

- Decreased urinary output
- Peripheral edema
- Abdominal bruit
- Weight loss
- Uremic pruritis

### 8.10.2   Medical Tests

- Renal ultrasound shows decrease in renal size.
- Blood tests
  - ○ BUN: elevated
  - ○ Creatinine: elevated
  - ○ Creatinine clearance: decreased
  - ○ Red blood cells: decreased
  - ○ Hemoglobin: decreased
  - ○ Urinalysis: shows proteinuria
  - ○ Glomerular filtration rate: decreased

### 8.10.3   Treatment

- Dialysis
- Stent placement or catheter to allow for drainage of urine
- Administer
  - Phosphate binders to reduce phosphate levels
  - Sodium polystyrene sulfonate to reduce potassium levels
  - Erythropoetin to treat anemia
  - Antibiotics for pyelonephritis

### 8.10.4   Intervention

- Monitor vital signs.
- Monitor intake and output.
- Monitor electrolyte levels.
- Monitor blood glucose levels.
- Do not use contrast-dye tests.
- Do not use nephrotoxic medication.
- Instruct the patient to restrict potassium, phosphate, sodium, and protein in diet.

## 8.11   Urinary Tract Infection

This is an infection of the urinary tract typically by a gram-negative bacteria such as E. coli found on the skin of the genital area or introduced by an invasive procedure.

### 8.11.1   Signs and Symptoms

- Dysuria
- Low back pain
- Feeling of fullness in suprapubic area
- Urinary frequency
- Urinary urgency

### 8.11.2   Medical Tests

- Urinalysis shows leukocytes, nitrites, red blood cells.
- Urine culture and sensitivity identifies microorganism and medication to treat microorganism.

### 8.11.3    Treatment

- Administer
  - Antibiotics
    - Nitrofurantoin, ciprofloxacin, levofloxacin, ofloxacin, trimethoprim-sulfamethoxazole, ampicillin, amoxicillin
  - Phenazopyridine

### 8.11.4    Intervention

- Increase fluid intake.
- Monitor intake and output.
- Monitor vital signs.
- Instruct the patient
  - Phenazopyridine will cause orange-colored urine.
  - Drink cranberry juice to acidify urine.

## 8.12    Ectopic Pregnancy

A fertilized egg implants outside the uterus, typically in the fallopian tube, increasing the risk that the fallopian tube will burst and result in hemorrhage should the fertilized egg continue to grow. There is a high risk of maternal death.

### 8.12.1    Signs and Symptoms

- Sharp, darting pain in the lower pelvic area
- Backache
- Vaginal bleeding
- Absence of menstruation (amenorrhea)

### 8.12.2    Medical Tests

- Urine pregnancy test: positive
- Blood test
  - Beta HCG: elevated, but lower than if pregnant
- Ultrasound: shows empty uterus

### 8.12.3    Treatment

- Surgical removal of the fertilized egg
- Surgical removal of partial or complete fallopian tube (salpingectomy)

### 8.12.4   Intervention

- Monitor vital signs.

- Monitor bowel sounds.

- Monitor abdominal distention.

- Monitor vaginal bleeding.

- Instruct the patient that there is an increased risk of future ectopic pregnancies.

## 8.13   Ovarian Cysts

Fluid-filled sacs, these cysts form on the ovary, and many are self-resolving. A follicle forms inside the ovary during ovulation and then ruptures, releasing the egg. A corpus luteum forms in the ruptured follicle and dissolves if there is no conception. Abnormal dissolving of the corpus luteum results in formation of a cyst. Types of ovarian cysts:

- **Endometrioma:** forms when uterus-lining tissue attaches to the ovaries

- **Dermoid:** cysts containing hair, skin, and other tissue

- **Polycystic ovarian disease:** a buildup of follicles resulting in enlarged ovaries with thick outer covering and leading to decreased or no ovulation. It may occur due to an imbalance of estrogen and progesterone.

- **Functional:** self-resolving within three menstrual cycles

- **Cystadenoma:** develops from the surface of the ovaries

An ovarian cyst can contain

- Fluid

- Semifluid

- Solid material

### 8.13.1   Signs and Symptoms

- Asymptomatic

- Menstruation changes

- Pelvic pain (unilateral, sharp)

### 8.13.2   Medical Tests

- Ultrasound shows cyst.

### 8.13.3 Treatment

- No treatment needed, self-resolving
- Administer
  - Nonsteroidal anti-inflammatory drugs (NSAIDs)
    - Ibuprofen (Motrin, Advil)
    - Naproxen (Naprosyn, Aleve)
  - Low-dose hormonal contraceptive
  - Clomiphene citrate (Clomid) to induce ovulation in polycystic disease
- Surgical removal of the cyst

### 8.13.4 Intervention

- Monitor vital signs.
- Monitor for signs and symptoms of hypovolemic shock.
- Instruct the patient
  - Most cysts are self-resolving.
  - Rest when pain is present.

## 8.14 Pelvic Inflammatory Disease

Pelvic inflammatory disease is the inflammation of the uterus, fallopian tubes, or other reproductive organs resulting from sexually transmitted disease and leading to ectopic pregnancy, abscess, chronic pelvic pain, or infertility.
Common causes of pelvic inflammatory disease are:

- Chlamydia trachomatis
- Neisseria gonorrhea
- Escherichia coli
- Bacteroides

### 8.14.1 Signs and Symptoms

- Vaginal discharge
- Fever
- Painful sexual intercourse (dyspareunia)
- Cervical motion tenderness

### 8.14.2 Medical Tests

- Chandelier sign positive
- Blood tests
  - Chlamydia test positive
  - Gonorrhea test positive

- VDRL test positive
- RPR test positive
- WBC elevated

### 8.14.3   Treatment

- Administer
  - Antibiotics
    - Ofloxacin and metronidazole; ceftriaxone and doxycycline; azithromycin and metronidazole; clindamycin and gentamycin

### 8.14.4   Intervention

- All sexual partners must be treated.
- Instruct the patient to take all prescribed antibiotics.

## 8.15   Preeclampsia and Eclampsia

- **Preeclampsia (toxemia):** high blood pressure, elevated urine protein, swollen hands and feet in second or third trimester of pregnancy
- **Eclampsia:** untreated preeclampsia leading to seizures, coma, and possible death during or after delivery of baby

### 8.15.1   Signs and Symptoms

- Preeclampsia:
  - Asymptomatic
  - Blood pressure >140/90
  - Headache
  - Weight gain (rapid)
  - Nausea and vomiting
  - Edema
  - Urine output decreased
- Eclampsia:
  - Seizure
  - Asymptomatic
  - Blood pressure >140/90
  - Headache
  - Weight gain (rapid)
  - Nausea and vomiting
  - Edema
  - Urine output decreased

### 8.15.2  Medical Tests

- Blood tests
  - Creatinine: elevated
  - Platelet count: decreased
  - RBC: decreased
  - Hgb: decreased
- Urine analysis:
  - Proteinuria >300 mg/24 hours
  - Creatinine elevated

### 8.15.3  Treatment

- Delivery of the baby
- Administer
  - Antihypertension medication
    - Hydralazine, labetolol, methyldopa, nifedipine
  - Antiseizure medication
    - Magnesium sulfate

### 8.15.4  Intervention

- Indicate bed rest.
- Monitor vital signs.
- Monitor intake and output.
- Instruct the patient to follow a low-salt diet.

## Solved Problems

**8.1**  What type of questions would the healthcare provider ask regarding the patient's reproductive issues?

- How many sexual partners have you had?
- Do you engage in risk-taking behaviors?
- What is your sexual preference?
- Have you ever had or do you currently have an STD?
- Do you know your HIV status?
- Do you use birth control?

**8.2**  What would snow crystals on the skin indicate?

Snow crystals on the skin (uremic frost) indicate increased retention of metabolic waste related to decreased renal function.

**8.3**   What is the significance of pale skin in a patient who may have a renal disorder?

Pale skin indicates decreased hemoglobin related to decreased renal function.

**8.4**   What is the purpose of listening to the patient's abdomen when doing a renal assessment?

The purpose is to listen for a turbulent sound (bruits) indicating a disruption in blood flow in the renal artery.

**8.5**   What should be heard when percussing the bladder?

Tympany should be heard.

**8.6**   What should the healthcare provider do before percussing the bladder?

The healthcare provider should ask the patient to empty his bladder.

**8.7**   Should the kidney be felt on palpation?

The kidney should not be felt unless the kidney is enlarged.

**8.8**   What is anuria?

The patient does not urinate.

**8.9**   What is oliguria?

The patient produces a small amount of urine.

**8.10**   What might cloudy urine indicate?

Bacterial infection may be indicated.

**8.11**   What might hematuria indicate?

A urinary tract infection may be indicated.

**8.12**   What might be indicated by dark urine?

Dehydration may be indicated.

**8.13**   What is metrorrhagia?

This is menstrual spotting.

**8.14**   What is a KUB?

KUB is an x-ray of the kidneys, ureters, and bladder without using contrast.

**8.15**   What is the purpose of the renal scan test?

The purpose is to assess kidney function and blood flow through the kidneys.

**8.16**   What is an IVP?

An intravenous pyelogram (IVP) provides an x-ray view of the kidneys, ureters, and bladder. A contrast material is injected into the patient's vein. Images are taken periodically for up to five minutes as the contrast material flows through the urinary system.

**8.17** Why is a renal angiograph ordered?

This is ordered to assess for:

- Blood clots

- Narrowing of blood vessels in the kidneys (renal stenosis)

- Aneurysm

- Pyelonephritis

- Kidney disorders

**8.18** What may decreased serum proteins indicate?

- Nephrosis

- Hephritis

**8.19** What may a decrease in uric acid indicate?

Tubular absorption disorder may be indicated.

**8.20** What is calculi basketing?

Calculi basketing is a procedure where a basketing device is inserted into the ureter using an ureteroscope or cystoscope to remove a ureteral calculus.

**8.21** What is testicular torsion?

Testicular torsion is a disorder where the spermatic cord twists, resulting in strangulation of the testis that can lead to testicular infarction and disruption of blood flow to the testis. The disorder must be resolved within six hours of onset to maintain testicular functionality. Necrosis can occur after 12 hours.

**8.22** What is renal failure?

Renal failure is decreased renal function.

- **Acute:** sudden decrease in renal function

- **Prerenal:** caused by diminished renal perfusion

- **Hypovolemia:** caused by blood or fluid loss

- **Postrenal:** caused by urinary tract obstruction

- **Chronic:** progressive decrease in renal function due to irreversible renal disease

**8.23** What is a urinary tract infection?

This is an infection of the urinary tract typically by a gram-negative bacteria such as E. coli found on the skin of the genital area or introduced by an invasive procedure.

**8.24** What is an ovarian cyst?

These are fluid-filled sacs that form on the ovary, many of which are self-resolving. A follicle forms inside the ovary during ovulation and then ruptures, releasing the egg. A corpus luteum forms in the ruptured follicle and dissolves if there is no conception. Abnormal dissolving of the corpus luteum results in formation of a cyst.

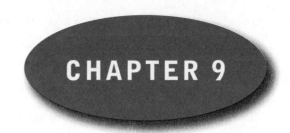

**CHAPTER 9**

# Maxillofacial and Ocular Emergencies

## 9.1 Define

- A maxillofacial or ocular emergency is a condition that alters eyes, ears, nose, mouth, or facial structure, resulting in the patient becoming unstable.

- Maxillofacial and ocular physiology can be disrupted by an inflammation, infection, or trauma.

- A maxillofacial and ocular emergency can be life threatening if the injury compromises the airway.

- A maxillofacial and ocular emergency can result in pain, discomfort, and disfigurement.

- Focus on maxillofacial and ocular injuries after the patient's airway, breathing, circulation, cervical spine, and neurological system are stabilized.

- A maxillofacial or ocular emergency requires immediate, quick assessment.

### 9.1.1 Goal of Treating Maxillofacial and Ocular Emergencies

- The goal of the emergency-department staff is to identify the maxillofacial or ocular emergency and stabilize the patient. The underlying cause of the maxillofacial or ocular emergency is treated in follow-up care unless the emergency-department staff can resolve the presenting problem. For example, a patient may have an object on the exterior of the eye, and the emergency-department staff may be able to remove the object and provide the patient with antibiotics and other medication. The patient is then requested to visit a primary-care practitioner for follow-up care.

- Thoroughly assess the patient before beginning treatment.

- Diagnose the acute problem.

- Stabilize the patient by relieving pain and treating the acute problem.

- Refer the patient to follow-up care.

### 9.1.2 Maxillofacial and Ocular Assessment

- The maxillofacial and ocular assessment interview
  - Ask open-ended questions.
    - Why did you come to the hospital today?
    - What makes you feel that something is wrong?

- Look for clues for underlying causes of the maxillofacial and ocular emergency.
  - What happened prior to your noticing this problem?
  - Have you recently undergone any medical procedure?
    - What medical procedure?
    - When was the medical procedure performed?
- Follow-up questions help probe further into the presenting maxillofacial and ocular problems.
  - When did this problem start?
  - How long have you had this problem?
  - Can you describe the problem?
  - How much does the problem bother you?
  - Where do you feel uncomfortable?
  - Is the problem spreading, or does the problem remain in one place?
  - Does anything make the problem worse?
  - Does anything make the problem better?
  - Did you have this problem or a similar problem in the past?
    - Explain.
  - Have you been diagnosed with any medical condition?
    - What medical condition?
      - Are you being treated for the medical condition?
        - What is your treatment?
        - Who is treating you?
  - What medications do you use?
    - Prescribed
    - Over-the-counter
    - Cultural
    - Herbal
- Ask about the patient's eyes.
  - Have there been any recent changes in your vision?
  - Do you wear corrective lenses (i.e., eyeglasses or contact lenses)?
    - Why do you wear corrective lenses?
  - Have you ever been diagnosed with an eye disorder (e.g., cataracts, glaucoma)?
  - Have you ever had an eye injury?
  - Have you ever had an eye infection?
  - Have you ever had eye surgery?
  - When was your last eye examination?
- Ask about the patient's ears.
  - Have there been any recent changes in your hearing?
  - Do you use any device to enhance your hearing (i.e., hearing aid)?

- Have you ever been diagnosed with an ear disorder?

- Have you ever had an ear injury?

- Have you ever had an ear infection?

- Have you ever had ear surgery?

- When was your last hearing examination?

  ○ Ask about the patient's nose and sinuses.

- Have there been any recent changes in your smelling or taste?

- Do you experience nose bleeds?

- Do you have any nasal discharge?

- Do you experience any postnasal drainage?

- Have you ever had a nose injury?

- Have you ever had a nasal infection?

- Have you ever had nasal surgery?

- Have you ever been diagnosed with a sinus disorder?

- Do you experience sinus headaches?

  ○ Ask about the patient's lifestyle.

- Are you exposed to dust, debris, or chemicals that may affect your eyes?

  □ Do you wear goggles when working?

  □ Are you exposed to loud sounds?

  ◆ Do you wear ear protection?

- Inspection

  ○ Ask the patient to look up while you pull down the lower eyelids.

  ○ Ask the patient to look up while you pull up the upper eyelids.

  ○ The eyes should be:

- Symmetrical

- Free from foreign bodies

  ○ The sclera should be:

- White

  □ Yellow indicates jaundice.

  □ Blue indicates that the sclera is thinning.

  □ Tan spots are common in African-American patients.

- Moist without excessive tearing

  ○ The eyelids should:

- Cover the top portion of the iris

- Open and close bilaterally completely

  □ Inability to close an eyelid may indicate facial palsy.

- Be free from
  - Lesions (e.g., stye)
  - Edema
  - Redness
  - Inflammation
  - Infection (e.g., conjunctivitis, commonly called pinkeye)
- Pupils should
  - Be checked for pupil assessment
    - PERRLA: Pupils Equal Round Reactive to Light and Accommodation
  - Be equal size and round
    - Unequal pupils may indicate:
      - Side effects of medication
      - Glaucoma
      - Neurologic disorder
      - Inflammation of the iris (iritis)
      - Aneurysm
      - Bleeding inside the skull
      - Increased intracranial pressure
      - Tumor
  - React to light
    - Shine a light into each eye.
      - Pupils react bilaterally when exposed to light.
        - Light shined into a seeing eye causes both pupils to react to the light.
        - Light shined into a blind eye results in no reaction by either pupil to the light.
      - Fixed pupils may indicate neurological disorder.
  - Accommodation test
    - Place your finger four inches from the patient's nose.
    - Ask the patient to look behind you.
    - Ask the patient to look at your finger.
    - Pupils constrict as the patient focuses on your finger.
- Corneal sensitivity test
  - Take a small piece of cotton.
  - Ask the patient to look straight ahead.
  - Lightly and carefully touch the cornea from the side with the tip of the cotton.
  - The patient should blink.
    - Failure to blink may indicate:
      - Cranial nerve V or cranial nerve VI disorder

- Ocular muscle
  - Corneal light reflex test
    - Ask the patient to look straight ahead.
    - Shine a light on the bridge of the patient's nose from a distance of 12 inches.
    - The light should reflect from the same position on each cornea.
    - Unequal reflection may indicate cross-eye (strabismus) resulting from decreased extraocular muscle coordination.
  - Cardinal positions of gaze test
    - Ask the patient to look straight ahead.
    - Hold a pen in your hand 18 inches from the patient's nose.
    - Ask the patient to hold his head straight and to follow your pen with his eyes.
    - Move the pen:
      - Center starting point in front of the patient's nose
      - Left up (superior)
      - Center starting point in front of the patient's nose
      - Left center (lateral)
      - Center starting point in front of the patient's nose
      - Left down (inferior)
      - Center starting point in front of the patient's nose
      - Right up (superior)
      - Center starting point in front of the patient's nose
      - Right center (lateral)
      - Center starting point in front of the patient's nose
      - Right down (inferior)
    - The patient's eyes should move in coordination.
  - Cover-uncover test
    - Perform this test only if there are abnormal findings from the corneal light reflex test and the cardinal positions of gaze test.
    - Ask the patient to stare at the far wall.
    - Ask the patient to cover one eye.
    - Observe movement of the uncovered eye.
    - Repeat this test with the other eye.
    - The uncovered eye should not move.
    - If the uncovered eye moves, then there might be a cranial nerve disorder resulting in abnormal functioning of the extraocular muscles.
- Peripheral vision test
  - Sit in front of the patient.
  - Ask the patient to look at your eyes.

- You look at the patient's eyes.

- Position your hand about two feet to the side of the patient's head at ear level.

- Make sure that you and the patient look at each other's eyes.

- Wiggle your fingers on the extended hand.

- Slowly bring your extended hand toward the patient's nose.

- Ask the patient when he first sees your wiggling fingers.

- Both of you should see the wiggling fingers at the same time.

- Repeat the test using your other hand.

- Gross hearing acuity test

  ○ Ask the patient to cover one ear.

  ○ Stand two feet in front of the covered ear.

  ○ Whisper "82."

  ○ Ask the patient to repeat the word.

  ○ Repeat the test using the opposite ear and whisper, "77."

  ○ The patient should be able to repeat the words.

- Inspect the patient's nose.

  ○ Describe the patient's nose:

    - Symmetry

    - Position

    - Size

    - Discoloration

    - Deformity

    - Nasal flaring (indication of respiratory distress)

  ○ Describe nasal discharge:

    - Consistency

    - Color

    - Amount

  ○ Nasal patency test

    - Acquire substances that have strong, different aromas, familiar to most patients. Make sure each is in the same kind of container with labels away from the patient.

    - Ask the patient to close one nostril.

    - Expose one substance to the open nostril.

    - Ask the patient to identify the aroma.

    - Repeat the test with the other nostril and a different aroma.

- Inspect the nasal cavity.

  ○ Use the otoscope to illuminate the nasal cavity.

  ○ Ask the patient to move his head back.

- Describe the nasal cavity:
  - Swelling
  - Redness
  - Nasal septum (perforation, deviation)
  - Mucosa (no lesion, moist, pink)
- Palpation
  - Palpate the nose.
    - Use your forefinger and thumb.
    - Lightly press against tissue around the nose.
    - Note:
      - Tenderness
      - Deformity
      - Swelling
  - Palpate the sinuses.
    - Use your fingertips.
    - Simultaneously press upward then laterally on both sides
    - Note:
      - Tenderness
      - Deformity
      - Swelling
  - Palpate the facial structures.
    - Use your fingertips.
    - Simultaneously press upward then laterally on both sides.
    - Both sides of the facial structure should be similar.
    - Note:
      - Tenderness
      - Deformity
      - Swelling

### 9.1.2.1  Signs and Symptoms

Maxillofacial and ocular assessment in an emergency situation requires the nurse to recognize common signs and symptoms of underlying causes and then prepare for the anticipated treatment that the practitioner is likely to order.

Commonly seen maxillofacial and ocular signs and symptoms are:

- Deformities (trauma, birth defect)
- Tenderness (inflammation, infection, trauma, lesion)
- Discoloration (inflammation, bleeding, cardiovascular disorder)

- Asymmetry (neurological disorder, trauma, birth defect)

- Nasal, eye, ear discharge (infection)

- Unequal pupils (neurological disorder)

- Unreactive pupils (neurological disorder, side effect of medication)

- Swelling (inflammation)

## 9.2 Maxillofacial and Ocular Tests

Maxillofacial and ocular tests are designed to assess the effectiveness and the capability of the maxillofacial and ocular systems to function. Emergency-department practitioners order maxillofacial and ocular tests to collect objective data to further assess and assist in stabilizing the patient. Once stabilized, the patient is transferred or referred to follow-up care designed to treat the underlying cause of the current episode, which may require additional maxillofacial and ocular tests. Maxillofacial and ocular procedures are performed to stabilize the patient.

The following are maxillofacial and ocular tests and procedures commonly ordered by the emergency department's practitioners.

### 9.2.1 Maxillofacial and Ocular CT Scan

A maxillofacial and ocular CT scan provides a three-dimensional image of the face and head using x-rays, enabling the practitioner to visualize normal and abnormal structures. A CT can be performed with or without a contrast agent. A contrast agent is iodine-based and enhances images of blood vessels and less-dense areas.

The practitioner typically orders a maxillofacial and ocular CT scan to assess for:

- Facial fractures
- Soft tissue injuries

**CT Scan Procedure**

- Assess if the patient is allergic to iodine or shellfish if the patient is undergoing a CT scan with contrast. Patients who are allergic to iodine or shellfish have a high likelihood of experiencing an allergic reaction to the contrast agent.

- Administer diphenhydramine (Benadryl) and prednisone (Deltasone) before the CT scan to reduce the risk of an allergic reaction to the contrast agent if a contrast agent is ordered.

- Administer the contrast agent through an IV. The patient may feel flushed and have a salty or metallic taste in his or her mouth.

- Explain to the patient that the contrast material typically discolors the urine for upward of 24 hours following the CT scan. The patient should increase fluid intake after the CT scan to flush the contrast agent from his or her body, if a contrast agent is used for the CT scan.

- Assess if the patient is claustrophobic. The patient will be placed in an enclosure during the test.

- Assess if the patient can remain still for 30 minutes during the CT scan, as the CT scanner encircles the patient for up to 30 minutes.

### 9.2.2 Fluorescein Staining

A fluorescein staining is a procedure used to stain ocular structures with a dye to make them easier to assess under a blue light. Once the stain is applied, a cobalt blue light is used to examine the structures. Variation in color may indicate an irregularity in the structure.

- **Bright green:** cornea abrasion
- **Orange-green:** irregular protective conjunctiva

The practitioner typically orders fluorescein staining to assess for:

- Cornea abrasion
- Trauma to the eye
- Infection
- Foreign bodies
- Dry eye

**Fluorescein Staining Procedure**

- Remove contact lenses if present.
- Wear gloves when handling the fluorescein strip.
- Moisten the fluorescein strip with normal saline.
- Pull down the patient's lower eyelid.
- Touch the moistened tip of the fluorescein strip to the outer surface of the eye (conjunctiva) near the lower eyelid (inner canthus).
- Ask the patient to blink his eyes.
- Look for colors on the eye using a cobalt blue light.
- Remove the fluorescein stain by flushing the eye with normal saline.
- Contact lenses can be reinserted an hour following the test.

### 9.2.3 Maxillofacial and Ocular Ultrasound

A maxillofacial and ocular ultrasound provides a view of the eye using high frequency sound waves. No special preparation is necessary. This test is can be performed at bedside or in an imaging room.
    The practitioner typically orders a maxillofacial and ocular ultrasound to assess for:

- Fundus
- Cataract
- Fractures
- Intraocular lens implant

**Maxillofacial and Ocular Ultrasound Procedure**

- A conductive gel is placed on the closed eyelid and on the ultrasound transducer.
- The ultrasound transducer is moved over the site.
- The patient is asked to move his eyes during the test.
- The conductive gel is removed from the eyelid after the test.

### 9.2.4 Fluorescein Angiograph

A fluorescein angiograph is a procedure used to assess blood vessels in the eye using sodium fluorescein contrast material that is injected into the patient's vein. A camera photographs the back of the inner eye (fundus), making blood vessels in the eye visible.

The practitioner typically orders fluorescein staining to assess for:

- Retinal circulation

- Trauma to the retinal vascular bed

- Microvascular structure functionality

**Fluorescein Angiograph Procedure**

- Determine if the patient is allergic to shellfish or contrast material.

- Determine if the patient has glaucoma or has used eye drops before the test.

- Administer miotic eye drops to dilate the pupils.

- Administer sodium fluorescein into the vein in the patient's arm. The patient may experience nausea and feel warm.

- Observe the patient for hypersensitivity to the sodium fluorescein:
  - Metallic taste in mouth
  - Dry mouth
  - Light-headedness
  - Vomiting
  - Fainting
  - Sneezing
  - Increased salivation

- A rapid sequence of photos is taken of the fundus.

- The patient may experience
  - Yellow skin and yellow urine for up to two days after the test
  - Blurred vision for up to 12 hours after the test

## 9.3 Maxillofacial and Ocular Medication

Commonly used medications in maxillofacial and ocular emergencies are ophthalmic drugs, nonsteroidal anti-inflammatory drugs, corticosteroids, analgesics, and antibiotics. These medications dilate or constrict the pupil, reduce pain and discomfort by reducing pressure on nerves caused by inflammation, and block neurological transmission. Antibiotics assist the immune system in combatting bacterial infection.

### 9.3.1 Nonsteroidal Anti-Inflammatory Drugs (NSAIDs)

Nonsteroidal anti-inflammatory drugs are medications that reduce swelling, pain, and stiffness without exposing the patient to the adverse side effects that occur when using corticosteroids.

- Aspirin (ASA)

- Ibuprofen (Motrin, Advil, Nuprin)

- Naproxen (Naprosyn, Aleve)

- Oxaprozin (Daypro)

- Ketoprofen (Orudis)

- Diclofenac sodium (Voltaren)

- Ketorolac (Toradol)

- Celecoxib (Celebrex)

### 9.3.2  Corticosteroids

Corticosteroids are used to reduce inflammation and cerebral edema. Corticosteroids increase the risk of pancreatitis, heart failure, and thromboembolism.

- Dexamethasone (Dexasone, Decadron)

- Methylprednisolone (Solu-Medrol)

### 9.3.3  Analgesics

Analgesics are used to reduce pain.

- Oxycodone (OxyContin)

- Morphine (Duramorph)

### 9.3.4  Antibiotics

Antibiotics are used to treat bacterial infections such as sinus infection and conjunctivitis.

- Bacitracin (Baciguent)

- Cefuroxime (Ceftin)

- Cephalexin (Keflex)

- Ceftibuten (Cedax)

- Erythromycin (Ilotycin)

- Gentamicin (Garamycin)

- Trimethoprim (Bactrim)

- Tobramycin (Tobrex)

### 9.3.5  Opthalmics

Opthalmics are used to change the size of the pupil, required for assessment and treatment. There are two categories of opthalmics.

- **Miotics:** constrict the pupil. Commonly prescribed miotics are:
  - Acetylcholine (Miochol)
  - Arbachol (Miostat)
  - Betaxolol (Betoptic)
- **Mydriatics:** dilate the pupil. Commonly prescribed mydriatics are:
  - Atropine (Atrisol)
  - Epinephrine (Epifrin)
  - Tropicamide (Mydriacyl Ophthalmic)

## 9.4  Epistaxis

Epistaxis is commonly known as a nosebleed. Mucous membranes in the nose contain blood vessels that rupture as a result of trauma, dry mucous membranes, hypertension, polyps, anticoagulant therapy, vitamin K deficiency, or infection. Bleeding can occur at the anterior or posterior of the nasal septum. Posterior bleeding is typically more serious than anterior bleeding. Typically epistaxis appears more serious than it is.

### 9.4.1  Signs and Symptoms

- Visible blood from the nostril(s)
  - Anterior bleeding: bright red
  - Posterior bleeding: red or dark red
- Bilateral bleeding may indicate trauma or blood disorder.

### 9.4.2  Medical Tests

- Blood tests
  - Complete blood count
  - PT/INR, PTT
- X-ray to rule out fracture

### 9.4.3  Treatment

- Remove blood clots using suctioning.
- Progressively apply:
  - Direct pressure for up to 10 minutes to stop bleeding
  - Ice compress to constrict blood vessels
  - Phenylephrine (Neo-Synephrine), lidocaine, or epinephrine topically to the site to constrict blood vessels
  - Nasal packing containing antibiotic ointment
  - Cauterization of the bleeding vessel, if bleeding has not stopped

### 9.4.4   Intervention

- Identify the location of the bleeding. Nasal bleeding may originate from other than the nose.

- Place the patient upright with head tilted downward.

- Monitor for signs of shock.

- Monitor vital signs.

- Instruct the patient

  - Breathe through his or her mouth.

  - Bleeding should resolve in less than 10 minutes.

  - Avoid nonsteroidal anti-inflammatory medications (NSAIDs), including aspirin.

  - Nasal packing can be removed in 48 hours by the practitioner, if packing is applied to the nostril.

  - Encourage patient to seek follow-up treatment for the underlying cause of the nosebleed.

  - Use a humidifier if nasal mucosa membranes are dry.


## 9.5   Chemical Eye Burn

A chemical burn occurs when an irritant, acidic, or alkaline material enters the eye, resulting in discomfort or damage to tissue on the eye. The extent of tissue damage depends on the nature of the material.

- Irritant:

  - pH 7

  - No injury to eye. The patient experiences discomfort.

  - Common irritant materials:

    - Household detergents

    - Pepper spray

- Acidic:

  - pH <7

  - Less severe damage to the eye because acidic material cannot penetrate the corneal epithelial layer of the eye and, with few exceptions, does not cause progressive damage

  - Common acidic materials:

    - Sulfuric acid (from battery explosion)

    - Hydrofluoric acid (in rust remover, cleaners, aluminum brighteners) causes progressive and severe damage.

    - Hydrochloric acid

    - Acetic acid

    - Chromic acid

    - Nitric acid

- Alkaline:

    ○ pH >7

    ○ Most severe damage to the eye because alkaline material can penetrate the eye within 15 minutes and injure internal structures of the eye

    ○ Common alkaline materials:

        ▪ Lime

        ▪ Lye

        ▪ Ammonia

        ▪ Cement

### 9.5.1   Signs and Symptoms

- Pain in the eye
- Redness
- Unable to keep eye open
- Feeling that something is in the eye
- Excessive tearing
- Blurred vision

### 9.5.2   Medical Tests

- Blood test

    ○ Serum calcium (hydrofluoric acid causes hypocalcemia)

### 9.5.3   Treatment

- Irrigate eye continuously for 30 minutes with normal saline.
- Administer

    ○ Corticosteroids

    ○ Cycloplegic medication to temporarily paralyze accommodation of the eye

    ○ Topical antibiotics

    ○ Opioid analgesia in severe burns

    ○ Beta-adrenergic blocker to lower intraocular pressure (if secondary glaucoma occurs)

### 9.5.4   Intervention

- Test the pH of the eye periodically during irrigation.

    ○ Normal: pH between 7.4 and 7.5

- Adjust the length of time irrigating the eye based on the pH test results.
- The practitioner will perform an ophthalmic examination once the pH level of the eye is within normal range.

- The patient may develop secondary glaucoma.

- Apply dressing and/or eye patch per practitioner's order.

- Instruct the patient

    ○ How to administer eye medication

    ○ How to avoid repeat exposure to the chemical (wear protective eye covering)

## 9.6   Facial Injury

A facial injury typically involves injury to soft tissue and alters the patient's physical appearance. Commonly seen facial injuries are:

- Abrasions

- Contusions

- Friction-related injuries

- Lacerations

### 9.6.1   Signs and Symptoms

- Bleeding

- Open wound

- Bruise

- Epidermal staining (friction-related injury)

- Unable to purse lips (facial nerve damage)

- Unable to close eye (facial nerve damage)

### 9.6.2   Medical Tests

- MRI of the head to rule out fracture

- CT scan of the head to rule out fracture

### 9.6.3   Treatment

- Control bleeding by placing pressure on wound.

- Suture lacerations immediately to reduce scarring.

- Perform debridement to remove necrosis.

- Request plastic surgeon consult immediately for severe injuries.

- Adminster rabies treatment if necessary for animal bite
- Administer
  - Corticosteroids
  - Antibiotics
  - Opioid analgesia in severe injuries
  - Tetanus

### 9.6.4   Intervention

- Irrigate wounds with normal saline.
- Scrub friction-related injuries with soap.
- Dress wound appropriately.
- Instruct the patient to visit the practitioner in seven days to remove any stitches.

## 9.7   Facial Fracture

A facial fracture is any broken bone in the face, commonly the result of a fall, motor-vehicle accident, sports injury, or assault. There are four categories of facial fractures.

- **Maxillary:** fracture of the upper jaw bone
- **Nasal:** fracture of the nose
- **Mandibular:** fracture to the lower jaw bone
- **Zygomatic arch:** fracture to the cheek bone

### 9.7.1   Signs and Symptoms

- Difficulty opening and closing jaw
- Swelling (edema)
- Pain at site of fracture
- Bloody nose (epistaxis)
- Running nose (rhinorrhea)
- Vision problems
- Grating, crackling, or popping sounds (crepitus)
- Bruise (ecchymosis)
- Asymmetric facial structure

### 9.7.2   Medical Tests

- MRI of the head to rule out fracture
- CT scan of the head to rule out fracture

### 9.7.3 Treatment

- Control bleeding by placing pressure on wound.

- Reduce the fracture surgically.

- Request plastic surgeon to consult immediately for severe injuries.

- Administer

  - Corticosteroids

  - Antibiotics

  - Opioid analgesia in severe injuries

  - Tetanus

### 9.7.4 Intervention

- Stabilize airway, breathing, and circulation.

- Monitor for intracranial pressure.

- Monitor vital signs.

- Immobilize cervical spine with cervical collar until the cervical spine is assessed by the practitioner as stable.

- Apply ice pack to site to reduce swelling.

- Instruct the patient

  - On the treatment and follow-up care once the practitioner has discussed the severity of the injury with the patient

  - Plastic surgeon will minimize scarring.

## 9.8 Detached Retina

The retina is the lining of the inner surface of the eye that is sensitive to light. A detached retina occurs when the outer portion of the inner surface separates, resulting in a subretinal space that fills with subretinal fluid. Common causes are degeneration of tissue, diabetes mellitus, inflammation, trauma, adverse effect of cataract surgery, and nearsightedness (myopia). The entire retina may become detached, leading to vision loss and blindness.

### 9.8.1 Signs and Symptoms

- Light flashes

- Painless loss of vision

- Watery vision

- Reduced field of vision commonly reported as curtain-blocking vision

- Eye floaters
- Feeling of heavy eyes

### 9.8.2   Medical Tests

- Ocular ultrasound
- Ophthalmoscopic examination

### 9.8.3   Treatment

- Surgery to reattach the retina
  - Vitrectomy
  - Pneumatic retinopexy
  - Scleral buckle surgery
- Cryotherapy
- Laser therapy

### 9.8.4   Intervention

- Indicate bed rest.
- Prescribe eye patches for both eyes.
- Position the head so that the site is lower than the eye, if the center of the retina (macula) is affected. Return to the normal upright position following surgery.
- Indicate no activities that increase intraocular pressure (IOP).
- Instruct the patient
  - Restrict eye movement until after surgery.
  - Do not bend over.
  - Avoid
    - Straining
    - Coughing
    - Vomiting
    - Sneezing
    - Driving
  - Use stool softeners.
  - For several days after surgery:
    - There will be blurred vision.
    - Do not drive.
    - Do not lift.
    - Follow practitioner's instructions.

## 9.9   Corneal Abrasion

A corneal abrasion is a scratch on the transparent tissue that covers the iris and pupil. Common causes of corneal abrasions are:

- Foreign object trapped under the eyelid

- Fingernail scratch

- Contact lenses worn for a long period of time

- Eye infection

### 9.9.1   Signs and Symptoms

- Increased tearing

- Redness

- Patient reports, "Something is in my eye."

- Pain

- Decreased vision

- Blurred vision

### 9.9.2   Medical Tests

- Fluorescein staining and assessing with cobalt blue light

### 9.9.3   Treatment

- Irrigate eye with normal saline solution if foreign object is visible.
- Practitioner removes foreign body.
- Administer
  - Topical anesthetic before and after the foreign object is removed
  - Antibiotic
  - Tetanus
  - NSAID eyedrops to reduce inflammation
  - Pain medication

### 9.9.4   Intervention

- Assess visual acuity before and after the foreign body is removed.
- Apply eye patch, if ordered.

- Instruct the patient
  - Apply antibiotic eyedrops properly.
  - Remove the eye patch after 12 hours.
  - Avoid activities that require depth perception until the eye patch is removed.
  - Corneal abrasion will heal within two days.

## 9.10 Corneal Ulceration

A corneal ulceration is an infection of the transparent tissue that covers the iris and pupil that disrupts the tissue, resulting in perforation and scarring that can impair vision and lead to blindness.
  Common causes of corneal ulceration are:

- Toxins
- Allergies
- Bacterial infections
- Viral infections
- Fungal infections
- Protozoan infections
- Trauma

### 9.10.1  Signs and Symptoms

- Pain when blinking
- Light sensitivity
- Increased tearing
- Discharge from the eye
- Blurred vision

### 9.10.2  Medical Tests

- Fluorescein staining and assessing with cobalt blue light
- Culture and sensitivity study

### 9.10.3  Treatment

- Administer
  - Antimicrobial medication to treat underlying infection
  - Topical anesthetic
  - Artificial tears
  - Topical antifungal agent

### 9.10.4 Intervention

- Assess visual acuity before and after treatment.
- Do not apply an eye patch. An eye patch can create an environment that fosters microbe growth.
- Apply a perforated shield.
- Keep room dark.
- Instruct the patient
  - Apply eye drops properly.
  - Report seeing halos or decreased vision.
  - Wear dark glasses, if sensitive to light.
  - Corneal abrasions generally heal within two days.

## 9.11  Foreign Body in Ear

The ear canal is obstructed by a foreign body that can decrease hearing and lead to infection. The most common cause is cerumen (earwax) that is impacted as a result of using cotton swabs to clear the cerumen from the ear canal.
   Other causes are:

- Insects
- Toys (children)
- Beads (children)

### 9.11.1  Signs and Symptoms

- Buzzing in ear
- Decreased hearing
- Ear drainage
- Foul smell from the ear
- Pain
- Dizziness

### 9.11.2  Medical Tests

- Hearing test
- Visual inspection with the otoscope

### 9.11.3 Treatment

- Physical removal of the foreign body
- Administer
  - Cerumenolytics to soften cerumen
  - Mineral-oil ear drops to kill live insect before removal

### 9.11.4 Intervention

- Irrigate the ear.
  - Use hydrogen peroxide and warm water in a ratio of 1:1
  - Don't irrigate the ear if:
    - There is an ear infection.
    - There is a ruptured tympanic membrane.
    - The foreign body absorbs water.
    - The patient is under six years of age.
- Explain to the patient
  - Do not use cotton swabs in the ear canal to remove cerumen.
  - Irrigate ears regularly with over-the-counter solutions to avoid buildup of cerumen.

## Solved Problems

9.1     How should the eyes appear on inspection?

They should appear symmetrical and free from foreign bodies.

9.2     What might blue sclera indicate?

Thinning of the sclera due to aging may be indicated.

9.3     What might be indicated if a patient's eyelid is unable to completely cover the eye?

Inability to close an eyelid may indicate facial palsy.

9.4     What would you suspect if the inside of the patient's eyelid is reddened?

Conjunctivitis, commonly called pinkeye, may be suspected.

9.5     What might unequal pupils indicate?

- Side effect of medication
- Glaucoma
- Neurologic disorder
- Inflammation of the iris (iritis)

**9.6**   How do you test accommodation?

- Place your finger 4 inches from the patient's nose.

- Ask the patient to look behind you.

- Ask the patient to look at your finger.

- Pupils constrict as the patient focuses on your finger.

**9.7**   What might be indicated if the patient does not blink during the corneal sensitivity test?

Cranial nerve V or cranial nerve VI disorder may be indicated.

**9.8**   What might be the cause of nasal flaring?

Respiratory distress may be the cause.

**9.9**   What might cause nasal, eye, or ear discharge?

Infection may be the cause.

**9.10**   What is the likely cause of swelling in the ear?

Inflammation is the likely cause.

**9.11**   What is fluorescein staining?

Fluorescein staining is a procedure used to stain ocular structures to make them easier to assess. Once the stain is applied, a cobalt blue light is used to examine the structures. Variation in color may indicate an irregularity in the structure.

**9.12**   What is a fluorescein angiograph?

A fluorescein angiograph is a procedure used to assess blood vessels in the eye using sodium fluorescein contrast material that is injected into the patient's vein. A camera photographs the back of the inner eye (fundus), making blood vessels in the eye visible.

**9.13**   How do you know if the patient is having a hypersensitivity reaction to sodium fluorescein?

- Metallic taste in the mouth

- Dry mouth

- Light-headedness

- Vomiting

- Fainting

- Sneezing

- Increased salivation

**9.14**   What would you say if the patient who has undergone fluorescein angiograph yesterday called and said her skin is yellow?

This is an expected side effect and will subside within a few days.

**9.15** What is the reaction of miotics?

The reaction is to constrict the pupil.

**9.16** Why are mydriatics prescribed?

Mydriatics dilate the pupil and are prescribed for eye examinations and for use in some procedures.

**9.17** What are the common causes of epistaxis?

Trauma, dry mucous membrane, hypertension, polyps, anticoagulant therapy, vitamin K deficiency, and infection are the common causes of epistaxis.

**9.18** What would you say to a family member of a patient who has an epistaxis?

Epistaxis appears more serious than it is.

**9.19** A patient reports that the practitioner said he had a chemical burn in his eye from an irritant. The patient wants to know if he is going to go blind. How would you respond?

An irritant causes discomfort to the patient but no injury to the eye because an irritant is chemically neutral. An irritant does not cause loss of sight.

**9.20** What is the response when a patient says something was sprayed into his eyes?

Irrigate the eye continuously for 30 minutes with normal saline. Test the pH of the eye periodically during irrigation.

**9.21** What would be suspected if a patient reported light flashes and the feeling that curtains are blocking his vision?

Detached retina would be suspected.

**9.22** Why would the practitioner order a stool softener for a patient who was treated for a detached retina?

The practitioner may order a stool softener to prevent straining during a bowel movement that may cause increased intraocular pressure (IOP).

**9.23** What can cause a corneal abrasion?

- A foreign object that is trapped under the eyelid
- Fingernail scratch
- Contact lenses worn for a long period of time

**9.24** Why is an eye patch not applied to a patient diagnosed with a corneal ulceration?

A corneal ulceration can be caused by a microorganism. The eye patch creates a warm, moist environment within which the microorganism can grow.

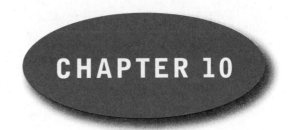

# Environmental Emergencies

## 10.1  Define

- An environmental emergency is a condition caused by factors such as temperature and exposure to materials that can cause burns and other injuries that alter any part of the body and result in the patient becoming unstable.

- The patient's physiology can be disrupted by an inflammation, infection, or trauma.

- An environmental emergency can be life threatening if the injury compromises the airway.

- An environmental emergency can result in pain, discomfort, and disfigurement.

- Focus on the site of the environmental emergency after the patient's airway, breathing, circulation, and cervical spine are stabilized.

- An environmental emergency requires immediate and quick assessment.

### 10.1.1  Goal of Treating Environmental Emergencies

- The goal of the emergency-department staff is to identify the environmental emergency and stabilize the patient.

- Thoroughly assess the patient before beginning treatment.

- Diagnose the acute problem.

- Stabilize the patient by relieving pain and treating the acute problem.

- Refer the patient to follow-up care.

### 10.1.2  Environmental Assessment

- The environmental assessment interview
  - Ask open-ended questions.
    - Why did you come to the hospital today?
    - What makes you feel that something is wrong?
  - Look for clues for underlying causes of the environmental emergency.
    - What happened prior to your noticing this problem?

- Have you recently undergone any medical procedure?
  - What medical procedure?
  - When was the medical procedure performed?
- Follow-up questions help probe further into the presenting environmental problem.
  - When did this problem start?
  - How long have you had this problem?
  - Can you describe the problem?
  - How much does the problem bother you?
  - Where do you feel uncomfortable?
  - Is the problem spreading, or does the problem remain in one place?
  - Does anything make the problem worse?
  - Does anything make the problem better?
  - Did you have this problem or a similar problem in the past?
    - Explain.
  - Have you been diagnosed with any medical condition?
    - What medical condition?
      - Are you being treated for the medical condition?
        - What is your treatment?
        - Who is treating you?
  - What medications do you use?
    - Prescribed
    - Over-the-counter
    - Cultural
    - Herbal
- Perform a physical assessment as described in Chapter 1 (1.9 Quick Assessments).
  - Inspection
    - Ask the patient to show you the site of the injury or confirm the site if the injury is visible.
    - Remove the patient's clothes and inspect the patient beginning with the head. Look for other sites of injury besides those presented by the patient.
  - Auscultation
    - In a fire, a patient's lungs may be burned without obvious signs and symptoms, resulting in pulmonary inflammation that can place the patient in respiratory distress. Pulmonary inflammation can occur at any time.
  - Percussion
  - Palpation

## 10.1.2.1 Signs and Symptoms

Environmental assessment in an emergency situation requires the nurse to recognize common signs and symptoms of underlying causes and then prepare for the anticipated treatment that the practitioner is likely to order.

Commonly seen environmental signs and symptoms are:

- Disruption of skin (burns)

- Abnormal lung sounds (rhonchi, stridor, crackles)

- Discoloration of skin (reddened, cyanotic)

- Pain (burn)

- Burning sensation

- Lack of pain in presence of severe burn (nerves are damaged)

- Change in voice (inflammation)

- Unusual breath odor (chemical ingestion)

- High or low temperature

- Loss of consciousness

## 10.2    Environmental Tests and Procedures

Environmental tests are designed to assess adverse environmental conditions on multisystems. Emergency-department practitioners order tests to collect objective data to further assess and assist in stabilizing the patient. Once stabilized, the patient is transferred or referred to follow-up care designed to treat the underlying cause of the current episode.

The following are commonly ordered environmental tests and procedures by the emergency department's practitioners.

### 10.2.1    Bronchoscopy

Bronchoscopy is a procedure that enables the healthcare provider to view the patient's larynx, trachea, and bronchi through the use of a bronchoscope. The bronchoscope is a flexible tube that uses fiber optics to display images of the respiratory structure. The healthcare provider uses the bronchoscope to remove airway obstructions, including mucus, tumors, and foreign bodies. The bronchoscope is also used to obtain specimens for further testing.

**Bronchoscopy Procedure**

- Administer atropine to decrease secretions.

- Administer midazolam (Versed) or other sedative and antianxiety medications to help relax the patient.

- Administer a topical anesthetic to the nasopharynx, vocal cords, and trachea to suppress the gagging reflex.

- Administer oxygen.

- Monitor vital signs.

- Insert the bronchoscope through the mouth or nose.

- Suction as necessary.

- Remove the obstruction or sample.

- After the bronchoscope is removed, raise the head of the bed 30 degrees or place the patient on his side.

- The patient must refrain from taking anything by mouth until the gag response returns.

- Test for the return of the gag response.

- Monitor the patient's vital signs until the gag response returns.

## 10.2.2 Arterial Blood Gas (ABG)

The arterial blood gas is a blood test where an arterial blood sample is taken from the patient and assessed for oxygen ($Pao_2$), carbon dioxide ($Paco_2$), bicarbonate ($HCO_3-$), saturation oxygen ($Sao_2$), and pH levels in the blood.
Normal ranges are:

| | |
|---|---|
| $Pao_2$ | 80 to 100 mm Hg |
| $Paco_2$ | 35 to 45 mm Hg |
| $HCO_3-$ | 22 to 26 mEq/L |
| $Sao_2$ | 95% to 100% of hemoglobin |
| pH | 7.35 to 7.45 |

The pH value measures the concentration of hydrogen ions in arterial blood. A value greater than 7.45 indicates alkalosis and a value lower than 7.35 indicate acidosis. The patient's blood must be within normal limits to be considered stabilized. Abnormal values indicate that the patient's body is trying to reestablish the acid-base (alkalosis) balance by having the metabolic system work together with the respiratory system to compensate for the acid-base imbalance.

The imbalance can be caused by a problem with the respiratory system. This is referred to as respiratory acidosis or respiratory alkalosis. The imbalance can also be caused by a problem with the metabolic system. This is referred to as metabolic acidosis or metabolic alkalosis. The results of the arterial blood gas can help identify the underlying cause as shown in Table 10.1.

It is important that any supplemental oxygen administered to the patient shortly before or when the sample is taken is noted on the sample documentation. This enables the lab to adjust the results accordingly.

Since the sample is taken from an artery, it is necessary to apply pressure to the puncture site for 5 minutes and apply a pressure dressing for 30 minutes once the bleeding stops. The site then needs to be monitored regularly to ensure there is no residual bleeding.

## 10.2.3 Blood Chemistry

Blood chemistry is a laboratory test of venous blood that examines levels of enzymes, electrolytes, and various elements in the blood to develop a profile of the patient's health. This test is usually performed routinely for emergency-department patients because results provide the healthcare provider with objective information about how well the patient's systems are functioning.
Blood chemistry results typically include:

- Electrolyte balance (sodium, potassium, bicarbonate, magnesium, calcium, phosphorus)

- Kidney function (BUN, creatinine)

- Liver function (AST/ALT)

- Diabetes (serum glucose)

- Cholesterol level (cholesterol, LDL, HDL, triglycerides)

Enzymes are normally inside the cell. As cells rupture during normal events, enzymes leave the cell and enter the bloodstream. The laboratory determines the normal level of a particular enzyme in the blood. A level greater than the normal level indicates more than the normal number of cells were injured, indicating something unusual is happening with the patient.

**TABLE 10.1  Acid-Base Values**

| | pH | Paco$_2$ | HCO$_3$– | SIGNS | CAUSES |
|---|---|---|---|---|---|
| Respiratory acidosis (too much carbon dioxide retained) | <7.35 | >45 mm Hg | >26 mEq/L (metabolic system compensating) | Flushed face Sweating Restlessness Tachycardia Headache | Hypoventilation Asphyxia Decreased central nervous system function Acute/chronic lung disease Sedatives Trauma Neuromuscular disease |
| Respiratory alkalosis (too little carbon dioxide retained) | >7.45 | <35 mm Hg | <22 mEq/L | Anxiety Rapid, deep breathing Light-headedness | Hyperventilation Gram-negative bacteria infection Increased respiratory function related to medication Anxiety Liver failure Sepsis |
| Metabolic acidosis (too little bicarbonate retained) | <7.35 | <35 mm Hg (respiratory system compensating) | <22 mEq/L (metabolic system compensating) | Drowsiness Vomiting Nausea Rapid, deep breathing Fruity breath Headache | Diarrhea Hyperkalemia Renal disease Hepatic disease Medication Intoxication Shock Endocrine disorder |
| Metabolic alkalosis (too much bicarbonate retained) | >7.45 | >45 mm Hg (respiratory system compensating) | >26 mEq/L | Ringing in the ear Confusion Slow, shallow breathing Irritability | Vomiting Gastric suctioning Steroid administration Diuretic therapy Decreased potassium levels (hypokalemia) |

Enzyme levels might increase gradually and then return to normal level This might occur with a myocardial infarction when blood supply to a port of cardiac tissue is interrupted, leading to the death of some cardiac tissue. Several hours may pass before the enzyme levels are abnormal and then decrease hours later when no more cardiac tissue is injured.

It is important to look for obvious reasons why enzyme levels or other values are abnormal before assuming that the patient is unstable related to the test results. For example, a patient who exercised before coming to the emergency department will have elevated muscle cell enzymes because exercising injures muscles. Likewise, a patient who ate a normal breakfast before visiting the emergency department will have a high blood-glucose level.

## 10.2.4  Hematologic Studies

Hematologic studies profile the patient's blood and include:

- RBC count

- WBC count indicating inflammation

- Erythrocyte sedimentation rate (ESR)

- Bleeding (prothrombin time, INR, partial thromboplastin time, platelet count)

- Hemoblogin and hematocrit (Hgb, Hct)

## 10.2.5  Gastric Lavage

Gastric lavage is a procedure used to flush the stomach of ingested material using a lavage tube that is inserted into the patient's mouth, nose, esophagus, and stomach. Gastric lavage is typically used following some poisoning, resulting in decreased gag reflex, as directed by poison control. Gastric lavage is only effective within a half hour following ingestion of the toxic material. Gastric lavage is contraindicated when an antidote for ingested corrosive substance, hydrocarbon, or poison is available. Likewise, gastric lavage is contraindicated when a patient has an unprotected or a compromised airway or if the patient is at risk for G.I. perforation or hemorrhage. Placement of the gastric lavage tube must be confirmed by insertion of air into the tube while auscultating the stomach or by pH test.

Oral activated charcoal can be used as an alternative for binding poisons, resulting in no absorption by the G.I. tract. Activated charcoal (see 10.3.6 Activated Charcoal) is administered following gastric lavage and if more than a half hour has passed since the patient ingested the toxin.

Don't use gastric lavage if you suspect that the following material was ingested because the material may compromise the integrity of the gastric lavage tube, resulting in the material injuring the esophagus:

- Ammonia

- Mineral acids

- Petroleum products

- Alkalis

- Corrosive material

The material may remain corrosive once removed from the patient and therefore must be disposed of appropriately based on hospital policy.

## 10.2.6  Dialysis

Dialysis is a mechanical/chemical process that is used to assist the kidneys in removing toxins from the blood when an antidote is unavailable and gastric lavage and activated charcoal are ineffective or not appropriate. In dialysis, the patient's vascular system is attached to the dialysis device that filters the blood, replacing the function of the kidneys.

During dialysis:

- Monitor vital signs constantly or at least every 15 minutes per practitioner's order.

- Perform a INR/PT/PTT blood test periodically to assess for clotting.

## 10.3   Environmental Medication

Commonly used medications in environmental emergencies are nonsteroidal anti-inflammatory drugs, corticosteroids, analgesics, and antibiotics. These medications reduce pain and discomfort by reducing pressure on nerves caused by inflammation and block neurological transmission. Antibiotics assist the immune system in combatting bacterial infection.

### 10.3.1   Nonsteroidal Anti-Inflammatory Drugs (NSAIDs)

Nonsteroidal anti-inflammatory drugs are medications that reduce swelling, pain, and stiffness without exposing the patient to the adverse side effects that occur when using corticosteroids.

- Aspirin (ASA)

- Ibuprofen (Motrin, Advil, Nuprin)

- Naproxen (Naprosyn, Aleve)

- Oxaprozin (Daypro)

- Ketoprofen (Orudis)

- Diclofenac sodium (Voltaren)

- Ketorolac (Toradol)

- Celecoxib (Celebrex)

### 10.3.2   Corticosteroids

Corticosteroids are used to reduce inflammation and cerebral edema. Corticosteroids increase the risk of pancreatitis, heart failure, and thromboembolism.

- Dexamethasone (Dexasone, Decadron)

- Methylprednisolone (Solu-Medrol)

Side effects of corticosteroids include:

- Increased appetite

- Increased bruising

- Hypertension

- Osteoporosis

- Fluid retention (lower extremities)

- Blurred vision

- Decreased resistance to infection

- Increased impact of diabetes

### 10.3.3    Analgesics

Analgesics are used to reduce pain.

- Oxycodone (OxyContin)
- Morphine (Duramorph)

### 10.3.4    Antibiotics

Antibiotics are used to treat bacterial infections.

- Bacitracin (Baciguent)
- Cefuroxime (Ceftin)
- Cephalexin (Keflex)
- Ceftibuten (Cedax)
- Erythromycin (Ilotycin)
- Gentamicin (Garamycin)
- Trimethoprim (Bactrim)
- Tobramycin (Tobrex)

### 10.3.5    Activated Charcoal

Activated charcoal is used to treat ingestion of toxic chemicals or drugs by absorbing the toxin in the gastro-intestinal tract. The patient ingests the fine, black powder—activated charcoal—which absorbs up to 60% of the toxin using the process called adsorption. Adsorption is where the toxin attaches to the activated charcoal. Activated charcoal is not absorbed by the body and therefore passes through the gastrointestinal tract and is eliminated through a bowel movement. Activated charcoal is administered in conjunction with sorbitol (see 10.3.6 Sorbitol).

Activated charcoal is administered:

- **Patient awake and alert:** patient drinks a black liquid.
- **Patient vomiting:** a nasogastric or orogastric tube is inserted.

Activated charcoal does not bind well with:

- Sodium
- Iron
- Lithium
- Iodine
- Boric acid
- Fluorine
- Lead
- Iron
- Alcohol
- Acetone

- Petroleum products
- Plant oils

Do not administer activated charcoal if:

- There is an intestinal obstruction.
- Corrosive (acid/alkali) toxin was ingested.
- An antidote was administered.

### 10.3.6   Sorbitol

Sorbitol is a sugar substitute that stimulates the bowels and is used in conjunction with activated charcoal to move the activated charcoal through the gastrointestinal tract quickly, reducing the risk of constipation, which is a side effect of activated charcoal. Monitor the patient for dehydration and chemical imbalance since frequent doses of sorbitol can cause diarrhea.
Don't administer sorbitol if

- The patient is less than one year old, since doing so can result in excessive fluid losses.
- The patient is fructose intolerant.

## 10.4   Hyperthermia

Hyperthermia is a condition where body temperature is greater than 99° F, resulting from the body's inability to dissipate heat sufficiently to maintain normal body temperature. Heat is generated by ambient temperature such as being exposed to very hot temperatures. Heat can also increase when the body's temperature-regulating mechanism has malfunctioned. The hypothalamus coordinates changes in the neurological and cardiovascular systems to regulate body temperature. Veins dilate with hot temperatures to help cool blood. Sweat glands excrete fluids to cool the skin. Veins contract in cold temperatures to help warm the blood. Disorders such as cardiovascular disorders and dehydration can lead to malfunction of the temperature-regulating system, leading to hyperthermia and the risk of hypovolemic shock.
There are three classifications of hyperthermia.

- **Mild:** severe heat cramps, excessive perspiration, weakness, nausea, and tachycardia. Temperature is 99° to 102° F.
- **Moderate:** heat exhaustion, excessive perspiration, excessive thirst, weakness, muscle cramps, nausea, vomiting, tachycardia, and fainting (syncope). Blood accumulates in the skin, decreasing the amount of circulating blood. Temperature ranges from 98.4° F to 105° F.
- **Critical:** this is caused by the body's inability to dissipate heat and cool the body. This is heatstroke. Internal organs are affected. Temperature must be reduced rapidly to avoid permanent damage. Temperature is greater than 104° F.

### 10.4.1   Signs and Symptoms

- Skin: moist, cool (mild)
- Skin: pale, moist (moderate)

- Skin: hot, dry, reddened (critical)
- Hypertension (mild)
- Hypotension (moderate)
- Agitation (mild)
- Confusion (moderate)
- Combativeness (critical)
- Nausea (mild)
- Vomiting (moderate)
- Tachycardia (mild, moderate, critical)
- Loss of consciousness (critical)
- Muscle spasms (mild)
- Syncope (moderate)
- Dizziness (moderate)
- Low-urine output, or oliguria (moderate)
- Fixed, dilated pupils (critical)
- Weakness (moderate)
- Seizures (critical)
- Tachypnea (critical)

### 10.4.2   Medical Tests

- Urinalysis
  - Protein increased
  - Concentrated urine
  - Myoglobin
  - Tubular casts
- Complete blood count
  - Hematocrit increased
  - White blood cells increased
  - BUN elevated

### 10.4.3   Treatment

- Remove the patient from the heat source.
- Remove patient's clothes.
- Replace electrolytes.
- Apply cooling blankets.
- Apply ice packs to arm pits (axilla), neck, and groin area for patients experiencing heat stroke.

- Avoid cooling too quickly as that might result in shivering and lead to decreased circulation and increased oxygen demand.

- Administer

  ○ Chlorpromazine (Thorazine) or diazepam (Valium) to reduce shivering

  ○ Oxygen

### 10.4.4   Intervention

- Monitor vital signs.

- Classify the degree of hyperthermia.

- Monitor renal functions.

- Monitor fluids and electrolytes.

- Monitor cardiac function using an ECG.

- Instruct the patient

  ○ How to avoid hyperthermia

  ○ How to recognize signs of hyperthermia

  ○ To avoid outdoor exercise in very hot weather

## 10.5   Hypothermia

Hypothermia is a condition where the body temperature is less than 95° F resulting from the body's inability to retain heat sufficiently and to maintain normal body temperature. Heat is lost by exposure to very cold temperature. Heat can also be lost when the body's temperature-regulating mechanism has malfunctioned. Veins contract in cold temperatures to help warm the blood. The body shivers to stay warm, resulting in decreased circulation and increased oxygen demand.

There are three classifications of hypothermia.

- **Mild:** patient is alert and oriented. Shivering, slurred speech, loss of coordination, and amnesia. Temperature ranges from 93.2° to 96.8° F.

- **Moderate:** cyanosis, rigidity, and unresponsiveness. Temperature ranges from 86° to 93.2° F.

- **Critical:** no pulse, absence of deep tendon reflexes, pupils dilated, ventricular fibrillation. Temperature is below 86° F.

**Cautions**

- Don't use tympanic thermometer to measure temperature.

- Surface warming alone is ineffective in critical hypothermia.

- Lidocaine is ineffective in ventricular dysrhythmias related to hypothermia.

- Don't perform chest compressions if the patient's chest is frozen.

- Don't defibrillate when patient's temperature is below 86° F.

## 10.5.1 Signs and Symptoms

- Slurred speech (mild)
- Shivering (mild)
- Cyanosis (moderate)
- Amnesia (mild)
- Atrial fibrillation (critical)
- Ventricular fibrillation (critical)
- Pupils dilated (critical)
- Absence of deep tendon reflex (critical)
- Rigidity (moderate)
- Unresponsive (critical)
- No pulse (critical)

## 10.5.2 Medical Tests

- Doppler: used to locate pulse
- Pletysmograph: used to assess the impact of frostbite
- Pertechnetate scan: shows perfusion and assesses damage to deep tissue

## 10.5.3 Treatment

- Remove patient's wet clothes and replace with dry clothes.
- Provide external warming with heated blankets and radiated heat lamps.
- Provide extracorporeal rewarming to rewarm core blood.
- Prescribe full-body immersion in warm water (Hubbard tank technique).
- Administer
  - Heated normal saline IV
  - Oxygen

## 10.5.4 Intervention

- Monitor vital signs.
- Monitor cardiac rhythms with an ECG.
- Measure core temperatures with rectal, esophageal, or bladder thermometer. Make sure that the thermometer can measure very low temperatures. Do not insert rectal thermometer into stool.
- Classify the degree of hypothermia.
- Be alert for sudden drop in blood pressure (warming shock).

- Carefully handle the patient in moderate to critical hypothermia to prevent cardiac degeneration.

- Instruct the patient

  ○ Avoid exposure to cold temperature.

  ○ Remove wet clothes immediately.

## 10.6  Burns

A burn is damage to the skin as a result of exposure to an external heat source such as fire, electricity, frostbite, or chemicals. Cells die directly from the trauma or as a results of decreased circulation to the affected area. Collagen in the skin is destroyed, leading to intravascular fluid moving into interstitial spaces. There is increased capillary permeability as the inflammation process mediates the burn site.

Burns are described by their depth:

- **Superficial burn (first degree):** affecting the surface of the epidermis. There is pain and redness, but no blister.

- **Superficial, partial thickness (first degree):** affecting the epidermis. The injury is painful. The skin remains a barrier between the environment and internal structures.

- **Deep, partial thickness (second degree):** affecting the epidermis and dermis. Blisters form. There is swelling (edema) and pain. Hair follicles remain functional. There is less pain because of neurological damage at the site. The skin no longer remains a barrier between the environment and internal structures.

- **Full thickness (third degree):** affecting the epidermis, dermis, subcutaneous tissues, and muscle. There is swelling, but little pain due to neurological damage at the site.

Measure the burn size using the Body Surface Area (BSA) charts, the Rule of Nines, and the Lund and Browder Classification to estimate the amount of fluids that need to be replaced. There are two BSA charts used to estimate the size of the burn, the adult BSA chart (Figure 10.1) and the infant BSA chart (Figure 10.2).

The Rule of Nines is used estimate the burn size of an adult. Each area of the body is assigned a percentage based on the number nine except for the groin area. This enables quick assessment of the size of the burn.

The Lund and Browder Classification is used to estimate the burn size for infants and children because of their different body shapes. Table 10.2 lists the burn percentage by age to determine the Lund and Browder Classification of the patient.

**TABLE 10.2  Lund and Browder Classification**

| AT BIRTH | 0 TO 1 YEAR | 1 TO 4 YEARS | 5 TO 9 YEARS | 10 TO 15 YEARS | ADULT |
|---|---|---|---|---|---|
| A: Half of head | | | | | |
| 10.5% | 8.5% | 6.5% | 5.5% | 4.5% | 4.3% |
| B. Half of one thigh | | | | | |
| 2.75% | 3.25% | 4.0% | 4.25% | 4.25% | 4.75% |
| C. Half of one leg | | | | | |
| 2.5% | 2.5% | 2.75% | 3% | 3.25% | 3.5% |

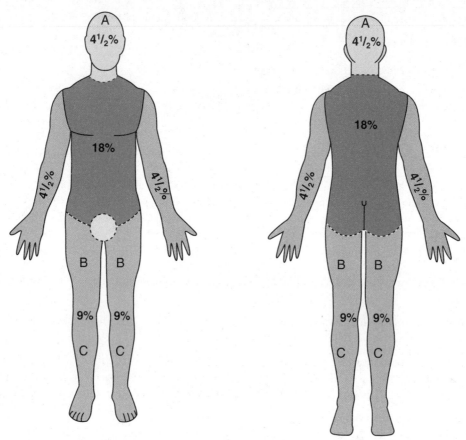

Figure 10.1 Apply the Rule of Nines to calculate the size of the burn for adults.

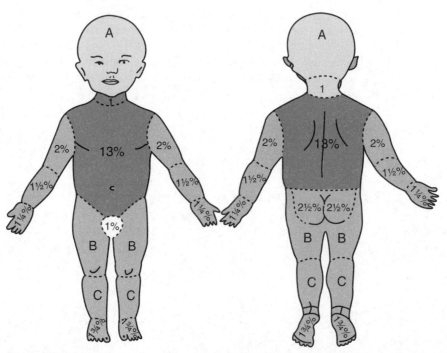

Figure 10.2 Apply the Lund and Browder Classification to calculate the size of the burn for infants and children.

Burns are classified as:

- Minor
  - Deep, partial thickness <15% in adults and <10% in infants and children
  - Full thickness <2%

- Moderate
  - Deep, partial thickness between 15% and 25% in adults and between 10% and 20% in infants and children
  - Full thickness between 2% and 10%

- Major
  - Deep, partial thickness >25% in adults and <20% in infants and children
  - Full thickness <10%
  - Electrical burn
  - High-risk patient related to co-diagnosis
  - Involvement of
    - Respiratory system
    - Fractures
    - Face
    - Hands
    - Genitalia
    - Feet

## 10.6.1   Signs and Symptoms

- Reddened skin (erythemia): superficial
- Swelling (edema): deep, partial thickness
- Nausea/vomiting: deep, partial thickness
- Shivers: superficial, partial thickness
- Blister: superficial, partial thickness
- Charred site: electrical
- Waxy, white color: deep, partial thickness
- Leathery appearance: full thickness
- Blood clot seen in blood vessels: full thickness
- Black, brown, white color: full thickness
- Caution: respiratory compromise can occur with little or no outward signs of burns if respiratory tissues are damaged. Signs of risk for respiratory compromise are:
  - Mucosal burns
  - Changes in voice
  - Wheezing
  - Singed nasal hairs
  - Dark sputum

- ○ Coughing
- ○ Darkened nose and mouth
- ○ Burns on the neck or chest

## 10.6.2   Medical Tests

- Urine tests
  - ○ Myoglobin: present, indicating renal involvement
- Blood tests
  - ○ Creatine kinase (CK): elevated, indicating muscle damage
  - ○ Myoglobin: elevated, indicating muscle damage
  - ○ Carboxyhemoglobin: elevated, indicating smoke inhalation
  - ○ BUN: elevated, related to increased protein breakdown and fluid loss
  - ○ Total protein: decreased, indicating protein breakdown
  - ○ Albumin: decreased, indicating fluid switch to interstitial space
  - ○ Hematocrit (Hct): increased, related to decrease in fluid
  - ○ White blood cells: increased, related to inflammation or infection
  - ○ Hemoglobin: decreased, related to the breakdown of red blood cells
  - ○ Sodium: decreased, related to fluid shift
  - ○ Potassium: increased, related to the destruction of cells and fluid shift

## 10.6.3   Treatment

- Irrigate chemical burns with saline solution.
- Insert nasogastric tube to suction and aspirate stomach contents.
- Insert indwelling urinary catheter to monitor urinary output.
- Fluid replacement
  - ○ Lactated Ringer's solution: use the Parkland formula to calculate the amount of lactated Ringer's solution to administer over the first 24-hour period.
    - Amount to infuse = 4 ml × weight in kilograms × BSA % of affected area
  - ○ Administer the total amount to infuse
    - 50% within first 8 hours of time of injury—not time of arrival
    - 50% over the next 16 hours
- Administer
  - ○ Humidified oxygen
  - ○ Nonsteroidal anti-inflammatory drugs
    - Ibuprofen
    - Naproxen
    - Ansaid
    - Anaprox

- Topical Antibiotic
    - Neosporin (superficial)
    - Bacitracin (superficial and ocular burns)
    - Silvadene (severe dermal burns)
- Analgesics
    - Morphine sulfate
    - Demerol
    - Vicodin
- Diuretics
    - Mannitol (restores urinary output)

### 10.6.4   Intervention

- Maintain cervical spine immobilization if spinal injury is suspected.
- Monitor airway, breathing, and circulation.
- Indicate nothing by mouth (NPO).
- Position patient in semi-Fowler's position.
- Intubate if airway is compromised.
- Remove patient's clothes. Clothes may contain the material that caused the burn.
- Cover burn site with sterile, dry bed sheets.
- Monitor signs of overreplacement of fluid.
    - Pulmonary edema
    - Cardiac failure
- Monitor signs of underreplacement of fluid
    - Hypovolemic shock
- Administer medication by IV and not IM, due to impaired absorptions of damaged muscle tissue.
- Monitor signs of compartment syndrome in full thickness burns. As tissue rehydrates from infusion of fluids, the inelasticity of burnt tissue can decrease circulation, resulting in decreased pulse in the affected area. The practitioner may perform an escharotomy, a surgical procedure to exposes fatty tissue below the site resulting in reduced constriction.
- Transfer patient to an appropriate burn center.
- Transfer to a hyperbaric chamber if appropriate.
- Instruct the patient
    - About ongoing treatment
    - About the prognosis

## 10.7   Poisoning

A poison is a material that produces a chemical reaction that disrupts bodily functions, resulting in nausea, vomiting, changes in heart rate, changes in breathing, confusion, or seizures. Symptoms reflect the type of poison and can occur immediately or hours, days, or months following exposure. The goal is to identify the poison and to prevent or reduce the absorption of the poison by administering an antidote or eliminating the poison from the body.

A poison enters the body

- Through ingestion
- Through the skin
- By inhalation
- By injection
- Through an animal bite

### 10.7.1  Signs and Symptoms

- Delayed symptoms
- Increased or decreased heart rate
- Increased or decreased respiration
- Dilated or constricted pupils
- Low level of consciousness or hyperactivity
- Sweating or excessive dryness

### 10.7.2  Medical Tests

- Toxicology screen: tests for common poisons
- Electrocardiogram (ECG): assesses for abnormal cardiac activity related to a poison
- Brain CT scan: assesses structural changes in the brain related to a poison

### 10.7.3  Treatment

- Intubate if the patient is unconscious.
- Call poison control (1-800-222-1222) and follow their advice.
- Administer gastric lavage, if not caustic material and material has not passed the stomach.
- Administer
  - Poison-specific antidote indicated by poison control
  - Activated charcoal, if caustic material and if material has passed the stomach
  - Whole bowel irrigant to flush the gastrointestinal tract to prevent absorption
    - Golytely
  - Sedative, if patient is agitated
    - Clonazepam (Klonopin)
    - Diazepam (Valium)
  - Antiseizure medication, if patient has a seizure
    - Lorazepam (Ativan)

## 10.7.4   Intervention

- Monitor airway, breathing, and circulation.

- Perform gastric lavage.

- Ask the patient, friends, or relatives for information that may lead you to identify the poison. Make sure everyone knows that telling the truth may save the patient's life. Some patients, friends, and relatives may conceal the truth to avoid undesirable consequences related to the poisoning.

- Determine medication that is accessible to the patient—either prescribed to the patient or to friends and family.

- Determine if the patient uses street drugs.

- Assess what poisonous materials may be around the patient's house or workplace.

- Ask if the patient was bitten or was outdoors any time prior to the signs and symptoms of the poisoning.

- Estimate the time that the poison was introduced into the patient's body.

- Assume that the material is caustic until proven otherwise.

- Assume that the patient has been poisoned even if no signs and symptoms are present, if the patient, friends, or family have reason to believe that a poisoning may have occurred. Signs and symptoms of poisoning can be delayed.

- Assess the patient's general medical condition. Signs and symptoms of poisoning may actually be signs and symptoms of an underlying medical condition rather than a poison.

- Instruct the patient
    - Treatment will minimize the impact of the poison on the patient's body.
    - How to avoid accidental poisoning
    - What to do if an accidental poisoning occurs again, and the importance of getting medical help immediately

## Solved Problems

**10.1**   Why is it important to know the time that the patient was burned?

The time the patient was burned is used to estimate the amount of fluid that must be replaced by the healthcare team.

**10.2**   What should you suspect if you smell an unusual odor from the patient's mouth?

The patient may have ingested a chemical that might be poison.

**10.3**   What is gastric lavage?

Gastric lavage is a procedure used to flush the stomach of ingested material using a lavage tube that is inserted into the patient's esophagus and stomach.

**10.4**   Why would a healthcare provider check whether a patient is undergoing dialysis?

To assess the patient's clotting ability and risk for bleeding.

**10.5** When shouldn't the healthcare provider use gastric lavage?

Don't use gastric lavage if the following materials may have been ingested because the material may compromise the integrity of the gastric lavage tube, resulting in the material injuring the esophagus:

- Ammonia
- Mineral acids
- Petroleum products
- Alkalis
- Corrosive material

**10.6** What is the purpose of activated charcoal used in treating poison?

Activated charcoal is used to treat ingestion of toxic chemicals or drugs by absorbing the toxin in the gastrointestinal tract.

**10.7** When shouldn't activated charcoal be used?

Do not administer activated charcoal if:

- There is an intestinal obstruction.
- Corrosive (acid/alkali) toxin was ingested.
- An antidote was administered.

**10.8** Why would sorbitol be administered to treat poison?

Sorbitol is a sugar substitute that stimulates the bowels and is used in conjunction with activated charcoal to move the activated charcoal through the gastrointestinal tract quickly, thereby reducing the risk of constipation, which is a side effect of activated charcoal.

**10.9** When shouldn't sorbitol be administered?

Don't administer sorbitol if:

- The patient is less than one year old, since doing so can result in excessive fluid losses.
- The patient is fructose intolerant.

**10.10** What is hyperthermia?

Hyperthermia is a condition where body temperature is greater than 99° F, resulting from the body's inability to dissipate heat sufficiently to maintain normal body temperature.

**10.11** What are the classifications of hyperthermia?

There are three classifications of hyperthermia.

- **Mild:** heat cramps, excessive perspiration, temperature is 99° to 102° F.
- **Moderate:** heat exhaustion, blood accumulates in the skin decreasing the amount of circulating blood, temperature is 104° to 106° F.
- **Critical:** heatstroke, internal organs are affected, temperature is greater than 106° F.

**10.12**   What are the signs and symptoms of hyperthermia?

- Skin: moist, cool (mild)

- Skin: pale, moist (moderate)

- Skin: hot, dry, reddened (critical)

- Hypertension (mild)

- Hypotension (moderate)

- Agitation (mild)

- Confusion (moderate)

- Combativeness (critical)

- Nausea (mild)

- Vomiting (moderate)

- Tachycardia (mild, moderate, critical)

- Loss of consciousness (critical)

- Muscle spasms (mild)

- Syncope (moderate)

- Dizziness (moderate)

- Low urine output, or oliguria (moderate)

- Fixed, dilated pupils (critical)

- Weakness (moderate)

- Seizures (critical)

- Tachypnea (critical)

**10.13**   Why is it important not to cool the patient too quickly if the patient has hyperthermia?

Avoid cooling too quickly as it might result in shivering that leads to decreased circulation and increased oxygen demand.

**10.14**   What is hypothermia?

Hypothermia is a condition where body temperature is less than 95° F, resulting from the body's inability to retain heat sufficiently to maintain normal body temperature.

**10.15**   What are the classifications of hypothermia?

There are three classifications of hypothermia.

- **Mild:** shivering, slurred speech, loss of coordination, and amnesia. Temperature ranges from 93.2° to 96.8° F.

- **Moderate:** cyanosis, rigidity, and unresponsive. Temperature ranges from 86° to 93.2° degrees F.

- **Critical:** heatstroke, no pulse, absence of deep tendon reflexes, pupils dilated, ventricular fibrillation. Temperature is below 86° F.

**10.16**   Why is a pletymograph used to assess a patient with hypothermia?

It is used to assess the impact of frostbite.

**10.17**   What is the purpose of using the Hubbard tank technique in hypothermia?

The Hubbard tank contains warm water. The patient who has hypothermia is fully immersed in the Hubbard tank to warm the patient.

**10.18**   What is warming shock?

This is a sudden drop in blood pressure if the patient who has hypothermia is warmed too quickly.

**10.19**   Why does intravascular fluid move into interstitial spaces in a burn?

Collagen in the skin is destroyed, leading to intravascular fluid moving into interstitial spaces.

**10.20**   How is the depth of burns described?

- **Superficial burn (first degree):** affecting the surface of the epidermis. There is pain and redness, but no blister.

- **Superficial, partial thickness (first degree):** affecting the epidermis. The injury is painful. The skin remains a barrier between the environment and internal structures.

- **Deep, partial thickness (second degree):** affecting the epidermis and dermis. Blisters form. There is swelling (edema) and pain. Hair follicles remain functional. There is less pain because of neurological damage at the site. The skin no longer remains a barrier between the environment and internal structures.

- **Full thickness (third degree):** affecting the epidermis, dermis, subcutaneous tissues, and muscle. There is swelling, but little pain due to the neurological damage at the site.

**10.21**   What is the purpose of using the Lund and Browder Classification?

The Lund and Browder Classification is used to estimate the burn size for infants and children because of their different body shapes.

**10.22**   What is the purpose of using the Rule of Nines?

The Rule of Nines is used to estimate the burn size of an adult.

**10.23**   How would you classify a burn when the skin appears a leathery black, brown, and white color?

This would be classified as a full thickness burn.

**10.24**   What would the healthcare provider suspect if a patient arrives from a fire to be "checked out" and his nasal hairs are singed?

Respiratory compromise with delayed presentation of signs and symptoms would be suspected.

**10.25**   How does the practitioner estimate the amount of fluid to replace in a patient who has suffered burns?

Use the Parkland formula to calculate the amount of lactated Ringer's solution to administer over the first 24 hour period.

- Amount to infuse = 4 ml × weight in kilograms × BSA % of affected area

- Administer the total amount to infuse:

    ○ 50% within first 8 hours of time of injury—not time of arrival

    ○ 50% over the next 16 hours

# Index